Biological Oxidants: Generation and Injurious Consequences

Cellular and Molecular Mechanisms of Inflammation

VOLUME 1
Receptors of Inflammatory Cells: Structure–Function Relationships

VOLUME 2
Vascular Adhesion Molecules

VOLUME 3
Signal Transduction in Inflammatory Cells Part A

VOLUME 4
Biological Oxidants: Generation and Injurious Consequences

Biological Oxidants: Generation and Injurious Consequences

Edited by

Charles G. Cochrane
Department of Immunology
Research Institute of Scripps Clinic
La Jolla, California

Michael A. Gimbrone, Jr.
Department of Pathology
Brigham and Women's Hospital
Harvard Medical School
Boston, Massachusetts

Academic Press, Inc.
Harcourt Brace Jovanovich, Publishers
San Diego New York Boston London Sydney Tokyo Toronto

This book is printed on acid-free paper. ♾

Academic Press, Inc.
1250 Sixth Avenue, San Diego, California 92101-4311

United Kingdom Edition published by
Academic Press Limited
24–28 Oval Road, London NW1 7DX

International Standard Serial Number: 1052-5882

International Standard Book Number: 0-12-150404-2

PRINTED IN THE UNITED STATES OF AMERICA
92 93 94 95 96 97 BB 9 8 7 6 5 4 3 2 1

Table of Contents

Preface

One of the major effector systems participating in a variety of human diseases appears to be that involving the generation of oxidant free radicals. In numerous forms of inflammation, the development of genetic mutations and malignant transformations, the generation of atherosclerotic plaques in arterial walls, and the process of aging all have in common the presence and participation of oxidant free radicals.

The past few years have witnessed a surge of information on the molecular events involved in the process of oxidant generation and its consequences in cells and tissues. In particular, knowledge of the molecules of the intracellular and plasma membrane generating system in leukocytes and other cells, the intracellular events involved in oxidant-induced cellular injury, mutational events and malignant transformation, and novel intracellular mechanisms of oxidant formation itself have taken a giant leap.

We have therefore thought it of value to bring together some of these important developments with selections from some of the most active and highly respected laboratories contributing to the new knowledge. In this volume, the reader will be exposed to the latest information from which a clear perception can be obtained of the fundamental bases of the several pathological processes mentioned above.

The information presented in this volume also contains the seeds of potential novel therapeutics that may be applied to oxidant systems. An understanding of the intracellular pathways responsible for the generation of oxidants, the formation of abnormal bases in the DNA, and the pathways leading to cell injury will be rewarding, if not essential, in the future development of specific therapies.

Under any circumstances, we are certain that the information in this volume will be of great interest to the reader.

Charles G. Cochrane
Michael A. Gimbrone, Jr.

CHAPTER 1

Composition and Function of the NADPH Oxidase of Phagocytic Cells with Particular Reference to Redox Components Located within the Plasma Membrane

Anthony W. Segal* and Jonathan H. A. Nugent†

Department of Medicine* and Biology†
University College London
London WC1E 6JJ, England

I. Introduction

Electron transport chains provide the biochemical basis for photosynthesis and respiration, and drug metabolism by the mixed-function oxidases. Oxidoreductases in the plasma membrane appear to be important for a wide range of cellular functions including the control of cell division,

Cellular and Molecular Mechanisms of Inflammation, Volume 4

transmembrane signaling, regulation of intracellular pH, reduction of extracellular oxidants, and many others, in both plant and animal cells (1).

The NADPH oxidase present in "professional" phagocytic cells, neutrophils, monocytes, macrophages, and eosinophils, which generates superoxide and hydrogen peroxide in the endocytic vacuole, is the best characterized of the plasma membrane oxidoreductases. The "extra respiration of phagocytosis" produced by this NADPH oxidase was first observed in 1933 (2). The unusual nature of the process was only revealed in 1959 when it was discovered that it was not inhibited by classic mitochondrial poisons like cyanide and azide (3), indicating that it was not simply a reflection of the enhanced energy requirements of phagocytosis. The obvious importance of the oxidase for the efficient killing of ingested microbes is best demonstrated by the consequences of its absence in the syndrome of chronic granulomatous disease (CGD), which is characterized by a profound, often fatal, predisposition to infection associated with widespread granuloma formation (4).

The mechanism by which the products of the oxidase optimize killing have yet to be fully elucidated. They might have a direct microbicidal effect or produce substrate for myeloperoxidase-mediated halogenation. However, they also elevate the phagosomal pH by pumping electrons, unaccompanied by protons, across the vacuolar membrane, an alkalinization that is important for optimal digestion by neutral proteinases and other enzymes (5).

An extensive series of investigations have been undertaken in an attempt to define the nature of this oxidase and the molecular basis of CGD. This chapter complements recent reviews on the subject (6–9) and will outline our current understanding of the structure and function of this oxidase. Emphasis will be placed on those components that are located within the plasma membrane and in particular on our recent discovery of a flavocytochrome *b* as the central electron-transporting molecule of this system.

II. Early Attempts to Identify the Oxidase System in Cells, Organelles, and Extracts

The earliest experiments attempted to purify the oxidase from whole-cell homogenates and crude subcellular fractions. These were incubated with a variety of potential substrates in an attempt to demonstrate oxidase or diaphorase activity (10). The dramatic increase in the activity of the hexose monophosphate shunt in association with the respiratory burst (11) indicated one of its products, NADPH (12), as the most physiological of these substrates. A variety of activities were detected, but the interpretation of these experiments was complicated by the lack of specificity of the oxidation of many of these substrates and the autocatalytic nature of many of the resulting reactions. A number of "enzymes" were discovered and described as defective in CGD (10).

The next advance in this approach came with the solubilization of an active oxidase from activated cells (13). Despite this achievement, complete purification of the source of the detectible activity was prevented by the instability of the system, particularly its sensitivity to salts, which prevented separations on most chromatographic media (14).

III. Identification of Cytochrome b_{-245} and Recognition of the Oxidase as an Electron Transport

In 1978 a cytochrome *b* was identified in human neutrophils (15), having been previously seen in animal cells (16). This discovery seemed significant as this was the sort of molecule that might be expected to accomplish the one-electron reduction of oxygen to form superoxide, and it pointed the way to the identification of the "NADPH oxidase" as an electron transport chain rather than a single enzyme. With few exceptions the cytochrome has been found by spectral analysis to be missing from cells of subjects having CGD with the commoner inheritance through a lesion on the X chromosome and normal in those with an autosomal recessive pattern (17–19).

In man this cytochrome was found in the "professional" phagocytic cells, neutrophils, monocytes, macrophages, and eosinophils, but not in a variety of other cell types (20). Its identity in these different cells was established by the determination of its midpoint redox potential ($Em_{7.0}$, see below). It is present in myeloid HL60 cells, a human promyelocytic cell line that can be induced to differentiate into cells resembling neutrophils, and in the U937 (21) monocyte/macrophage cell line. Uninduced cells are grossly deficient in all known specialized components of the oxidase, which accumulate on differentiation in association with the development of NADPH oxidase activity (22). In HL60 cells, the induction of differentiation with dimethyl sulfoxide was associated with the development of oxidase activity and a parallel increase in the concentration of this cytochrome (22).

In phagocytic cells the cytochrome is found in the plasma membrane and becomes incorporated into the wall of the phagocytic vacuole as it is formed by an invagination of this membrane (23). In neutrophils an additional pool of the cytochrome is detected in the membrane of the specific granules which also transfers to the membrane of the phagocytic vacuole (24).

IV. Biochemical Properties

Spectroscopy in alkaline pyridine reveals the spectrum of a protoheme pyridine hemochrome characteristic of a *b*-type cytochrome (25) which is present in neutrophils and monocytes at a concentration of approximately 100 pmol/mg protein (17).

The function of a redox molecule is dependent on its midpoint redox potential (26), which governs its bioenergetic structure in the heirarchy of components of an electron transport chain. At −245 mV (27) this cytochrome has the lowest midpoint potential of any mammalian cytochrome *b,* which provides it with the capability of directly reducing oxygen to superoxide (28). This measurement gives a considerable degree of discrimination between otherwise apparently similar molecules, and it is for this reason that we refer to it as cytochrome b_{-245}. It is also called cytochrome *b*-558, the 558 referring to the wavelength of its α band of light absorption.

Another unusual property of this cytochrome, not seen in other mammalian cytochromes *b* but shared with bacterial cytochromes *o* (29), is that it binds CO (27,30). The recombination time after flash dissociation of the complex is approximately 6 msec, which indicates that it probably binds oxygen. The oxidation of the reduced cytochrome is very rapid, with a half-time of 4.7 msec (30). The cytochrome b_{-245} represents the terminal component of the electron transport chain. Recent studies in which cytochrome b_{-245} was shown to be capable of reduction by cytochrome *P*-450 reductase, and that this resulted in the generation of superoxide (31), confirmed this.

NADPH reduces the cytochrome in preparations of the solubilized oxidase, but only at a very slow rate. This slow rate of reduction had been thought by some (32) to preclude its participation as a component of the oxidase. The kinetics of reduction of a molecule in an electron transport chain under anaerobic conditions, however, might bear no relationship to its normal physiological function in the presence of an electron acceptor which can help to pull electrons through the system. When the steady-state kinetics of reduction of the cytochrome were determined in the presence of oxygen, they correlated almost exactly with the observed rate of O_2^- generation (33).

V. Purification and Identification of Cytochrome b_{-245}

The purification of this molecule and identification of its apoprotein polypeptide proved difficult. The four initial purification schemes described isolated polypeptides of different molecular sizes, varying between 11 and 127 kDa (34–37). The main causes of these difficulties in the identification of the molecule were proteolysis, the neutrophil being richly endowed with a wide range of potent proteolytic enzymes, and anomalous behavior of the apoprotein(s) on sodium dodecyl sulfate–polyacrylamide gel electrophoresis (SDS-PAGE) (38).

Two reliable methods now exist for the purification of cytochrome b_{-245}, both of which resulted in the purification of not one but two proteins. Therefore cytochrome *b* is a heterodimer composed of α and β subunits with apparent molecular masses on SDS-PAGE of 23 and 76–92 kDa, respectively. The association of these two molecules has been established by their copurification with the heme of the cytochrome, their association on gel-filtration chromatography, sucrose density, and pH gradients, and cross-linking studies. Both proteins are missing from cells of patients with X-linked CGD (39–41), indicating that both subunits are required for mutual stability. A number of these heterodimers might be associated to form a macromolecular complex.

The larger β subunit migrates on SDS-PAGE as a broad band, an electrophoretic property characteristic of glycoproteins, with an apparent molecular mass of about 60–90 kDa. It was therefore not surprising when this molecule was shown to be heavily glycosylated (38) with about 21% carbohydrate, predominantly of the N-linked high-lactosamine complex-type oligosaccharide moieties.

VI. Molecular Biology of Genes Coding for Cytochrome b_{-245} and Their Abnormality in Chronic Granulomatous Disease

A number of different patterns of inheritance are found in CGD, indicating different genetic mechanisms and molecular lesions (18,19,42). The genetic lesion in patients with X-linked CGD was identified through the elegant application of "reverse genetics" (43). The gene was shown to code for the β subunit of the cytochrome by obtaining N-terminal amino acid sequence from this protein. This sequence was found to correspond to the DNA sequence in a region of the X-linked CGD gene originally designated as noncoding as a result of a nucleotide sequencing error (44), adding 101 amino acids to the transation product with a predicted size of 65 kDa. This observation, together with binding studies with an antibody made to the fusion protein product of their gene (45), unequivocally identified the primary lesion in X-linked CGD patients in the gene coding for the β chain of cytochrome b_{-245}.

The gene coding for the α subunit is located on chromosome 16 (46,47), and rare patients with CGD with an autosomal recessive inheritance result from lesions in this gene. Unlike the gene for the β subunit, the transcription of which is largely confined to the myeloid cell lineage, that for the α subunit is apparently transcribed in a number of cell types other than phagocytic cells (48). If this is correct, and the protein is translated, it will be interesting to determine its function in cells that do not demonstrate overt oxidase activity.

VII. Flavocytochrome Component of the Oxidase

Although the involvement of a flavoprotein in this oxidase was postulated by Cagan and Karnovsky as long ago as 1964 (49), identification of the NADPH-binding flavoprotein that transports electrons from the substrate to the cytochrome b eluded identification until recently.

Apart from the almost universal observation that the nucleotide-binding protein in electron transport chains is a flavoprotein, there is little doubt that a FAD-containing flavoprotein is an essential component of this NADPH oxidase. FAD enhances (50) and the analog 5-deaza-FAD inhibits activity of the solubilized oxidase (51). Diphenylene iodonium (DPI), a potent inhibitor of electron transport that is thought to act at the site of the flavoprotein, is a potent inhibitor of this oxidase (52). Most convincingly, an FAD semiquinone free radical was demonstrated by electron paramagnetic resonance (EPR) after the addition of NADPH to membranes from activated but not unstimulated neutrophils (53). Analysis of the flavin content of these membranes revealed that it was almost exclusively FAD, and that this FAD was released by denaturation with little covalently bound flavin. In addition, the amounts of FAD in the membranes of neutrophils from patients with CGD lacking cytochrome b_{-245} have been found to be variable but generally diminished when compared with normal cells or those with an autosomal recessive pattern of inheritance (18,19,54,55). Some partially purified preparations of the solubilized oxidase were found to contain both FAD and heme (56), which are reduced on the addition of NADPH (57); others contained FAD alone (14),58) or no cofactor (59).

Neutrophils contain both NADH cytochrome-b_5 reductase (60) and *P*-450 reductase (61) which is capable of reducing cytochrome b_{-245} (31), but neither has been shown to have any direct association with the NADPH oxidase. A 45-kDa DPI-binding protein has been purified that appeared to most closely match the properties expected of this reductase (62).

We decided to address the problem of the identity of the flavoprotein afresh and have discovered that cytochrome b_{-245} is a flavocytochrome containing both the heme and FAD redox centers (62a).

A. The FAD-Containing Flavoprotein Is Located in the Membranes

Our initial aim was to determine the location of the FAD component of the NADPH oxidase within the cell. The active oxidase is present in neutrophil membranes, and FAD was measured in this compartment to establish whether it was present there in resting cells, or recruited in part or in whole from the cytosol on activation. FAD was determined by the highly sensitive and specific assay that depends on its ability to reconstitute the activity of inactive apo-D-amino-acid oxidase rather than by the conventional fluorescence techniques (54).

The activated membranes demonstrated a marked increase in the capacity to generate superoxide, indicating the presence of an active NADPH oxidase system. The concentration of FAD in the membranes of resting cells was very similar to that in activated cells. The slight increase in specific activity of the FAD on activation was mirrored by a similar increase in that of the heme spectrum, so that the ratio of FAD to heme remained fairly constant. The slight increase in specific activity of both FAD and heme could result from phorbol myristate acetate (PMA)-induced degranulation of the specific granules (24), resulting in the incorporation of their membranes, possibly with a higher specific activity of redox molecules, into the membrane pool.

The cytochrome *b* is membrane bound, and the maintenance of a constant ratio of FAD to heme on activation indicates that the FAD, like the cytochrome, is present in the membranes from the outset, and that no additional FAD is recruited from the cytosol. These results support similar experiments with membranes purified from activated bovine cells, indicating a primary location of the flavoprotein in the membranes (53), and studies involving the cell-free system in which it was shown that cytosolic components functioned well although almost free of flavins (63).

The concentrations of FAD in membranes from patients with X-linked CGD were then measured. We (54), and others (18,19,55), had previously observed a reduction in the FAD content of membranes of neutrophils from these patients to about half of the normal levels. Some of these studies had produced inconsistent results (18,19), possibly because the measurements were made by fluorescence on relatively small amounts of material. We observed markedly reduced levels of FAD, to less than 30% of normal, in six patients with X-linked CGD. Normal concentrations of FAD were detected in membranes from the four patients with autosomal recessive CGD whose cells were deficient in the cytosolic factor p47-*phox*.

To determine the role of the small amount of FAD in X-linked CGD membranes, FAD was measured in membranes from uninduced HL60 cells. Concentrations of FAD in undifferentiated HL60 cells, with very low levels of oxidase activity, and of cytochrome *b* were similar to those observed in X-linked CGD. This suggests that the low concentrations of FAD found in the membranes of uninduced HL60 cells, and X-linked CGD cells, are probably unrelated to the NADPH oxidase.

Subtracting this presumed unrelated FAD from the total membrane FAD provided a concentration of presumed oxidase-specific FAD that can be related to the heme concentration in the specific cytochrome *b*. This comparison yielded a ratio of FAD to heme of roughly 1:2 in membranes from unstimulated and stimulated normal neutrophils and those from patients with autosomal recessive CGD. A similar ratio of FAD to heme was obtained by Bellavite and colleagues (56) in peak fractions of a partially purified solubilized oxidase. This ratio is important because it provides a mechanism by which the two electrons donated by NADPH and carried by FAD could be separately donated to oxygen to form superoxide, each being transported by one of the two hemes.

B. Electron Paramagnetic Resonance of the Flavocytochrome

Previous attempts to identify EPR signals from cytochrome b_{-245} have proved inconclusive, mainly due to attempts to assign signals obtained from impure cytochrome preparations. Kakinuma and co-workers (53) characterized a $g = 2.004$ signal in neutrophil membranes as a neutral flavosemiquinone radical and suggested that its relaxation properties indicated a nearby transition metal center. They subsequently suggested (64) that a high-spin heme signal present in partially purified preparations was from this cytochrome *b*. This indicated a possible five-coordinate iron with oxygen able to bind as the sixth ligand.

Recent studies have cast doubt on some of these findings. Hurst *et al.* (65), in a study using EPR and Raman spectrometry, failed to detect an EPR signal from the partially purified cytochrome. This suggested that interactions between, for example, two nearby hemes might decrease or eliminate the expected signal. The Raman study of the heme environment indicated a low-spin six-coordinate heme with axial imidazole or imidazolate ligands. The stability of the ferric state showed strong donation from the axial ligands which in turn indicated a degree of covalency. It was suggested that the high-spin signal previously described (64) was due to a damaged protein or to contamination.

Ueno *et al.* (66) have investigated the EPR properties of whole neutrophils at 4.2 K and, setting aside signals due to myeloperoxidase, ascribed signals with g values of 2.85, 2.17, and 1.67 to this cytochrome *b*. On this rather uncertain basis they speculated that this cytochrome is a low-spin six-coordinate heme with bisimidazole ligation, possibly involving both subunits.

We have investigated the EPR properties of purified cytochrome b_{-245} in concentrated samples and have now detected a weak low-spin EPR signal. The low-spin cytochrome heme has a g_z peak at $g = 3.31$. Additional signals were seen near $g = 2$ and $g = 1.5$, but no signals were observed near $g = 6$ from high-spin heme. The $g = 1.5$ signal is probably the g_x or g_y resonance of the heme. The g_y resonance, however, might be located near $g = 2$ where there is an overlap of signals from Cu^{2+} and an organic radical, possibly the flavoseminiquinone. The g value of the g_z peak is high for a simple bishistidine-liganded cytochrome, indicating a deviation from parallel orientation of axial histidine ligands (67,68) or perhaps an axial ligand which is not histidine.

The cytochrome spectrum is a weak feature for the concentration of heme, which suggests an interaction with a nearby spin, supporting the circular dichroism (CD) spectrum (69) that was interpreted as indicating an interaction of two heme centers in the protein. Our results are consistent with those of Hurst *et al.* (65), as the signal was perhaps below their level of detection. The spectrum is unlike any previously attributed to this cytochrome in impure preparations, suggesting that previous assignments were due to impurities or to damaged complexes.

C. The Flavocytochrome Shows Sequence Homology with the Flavin Nucleotide Family of Reductases

The absence of both the hemocytochrome *b* and FAD in X-linked CGD suggested that these two redox centers were likely to be located on the α and β subunits of the cytochrome *b*, which are both absent in this condition. Recent studies have demonstrated strong homologies in flavin and NADPH binding domains in the reductase family of proteins (70–72). This is a rapidly growing family of closely related molecules, the most recent addition to which is nitric oxide synthase (72). They are organized in a modular structure, with distinct regions that bind FMN, FAD, and NADPH (71). We therefore examined the sequences of the cytochrome subunits for homology with these reductases, paying particular attention to the nucleotide binding domains.

Initial searches on general homology and against libraries of common nucleotide binding sites (73) and general motifs [PROSITE (74)] were unrewarding. However, a search specifically with the conserved glycine-rich region in the proposed NADPH binding site of the flavin nucleotide reductase (FNR) flavoenzyme family (71) was more productive, showing close homology between the β subunit of cytochrome b_{-245} and other members of this family (Fig. 1) (74a). All the NADPH-binding proteins exhibited homology with Gly-Xaa-Gly-Xaa-Gly-Xaa-Xaa-Pro-Phe, whereas the sequences from the two NADH-binding proteins, nitrate and cytochrome-b_5 reductases, started with Gly-Gly.

In addition, there was some evidence for the presence of the other conserved sequence in the adenine binding region of the NAD(P)H binding site, Cys-Gly, in the cytochrome b_{-245} molecule. There was also weak homology in the region of the FAD-isoalloxazine in the appropriate region of the protein, approximately 90 amino acids upstream of the NADPH–ribose binding site. The structural differences in this region might explain the relative instability of FAD binding as compared with other members of this family.

The most related sequence is that of yeast ferric reductase (74a). In addition to homology in the above-mentioned regions, it shares some sequence homology with cytochrome b_{-245} throughout the proposed NAD/P and FAD domains. The conserved positively charged region shown in Fig. 1 may bind a negatively charged group such as a phosphate group of a cofactor.

```
   A. FAD-               B.  NAD/P-                        C. NAD/P-
    isoalloxazine             ribose                          adenine

   712               784                                880
1.   R A Y T P S S     A M I A G - - - G T G I T P V      L A A C G P
    66               150                                245
2.   R P Y T P I S     G M I A G - - - G T G I T P M      V L M C G P

   462               528                                649
3.   H P F T V L S     R N L V G V A A G L G V A A I      F Y S C G P

   337               403                         *      533
4.   H P F T L T S     V M L V G - - A G I G V T P F      V F L C G P
     #   # #     #       # # # #       #   # # #   #    # # # # #

   386               453                                549
5.   R L Y S I A S     V I M I G - - P G T G I A P F      I Y V C G D
    93               166                                269
6.   R L Y S I A S     I I M L G - - T G T G I A P F      V Y M C G L
   454               526                                627
7.   R Y Y S I A S     V I M V G - - P G T G I A P F      I Y V C G D
  1173              1242                               1345
8.   R Y Y S I S S     C I L V G - - P G T G I A P F      I Y V C G D


       D.  Pyrophosphate?

       431
    3.   K K P K F F K Y Q V G
       312
    4.   K K - K G F K M E V G
         # #   #   # # # # # #
```

NADH reductases

1. NADH	Nitrate reductase	Tomato
2. NADH	Cytochrome b5 reductase	Human
3. ?	Ferric reductase	Saccharomyces cerevisiae

NADPH reductases

4. NADPH	**Cytochrome b_{-245} β chain**	**Human**
5. NADPH	Sulphite reductase	Escherichia coli
6. NADPH	Ferredoxin reductase	Tomato
7. NADPH	Cytochrome P450 reductase	Rat
8. NADPH	Nitric oxide synthase	Rat

FIGURE 1

Sequence alignment of the cytochrome b_{-245} β chain and related reductases. The regions shown are the proposed FAD and NADPH binding sites. The site of the proline/histidine mutation in the patient with X-linked CGD (65) is indicated (*). The sites were identified from the crystal structure of NADPH ferredoxin reductase (70). # indicates amino acid identity or conservation of function. The most closely related protein, yeast ferric reductase (74a), shows additional homology, including a positively charged region which we propose may bind the pyrophosphate group of a cofactor.

A single patient with CGD (75) has been described in whom the pattern of inheritance was clearly X-linked and yet the cytochrome b_{-245} was clearly present. The cytochrome in this patient had normal light and Raman spectra and midpoint redox potential, indicating little if any abnormality of the heme environment (65). FAD concentrations in the membranes were normal. A point mutation has been identified in the β chain gene, however, resulting in the substitution of histidine for proline at amino acid 414 (415 including N-terminal methionine) (75). It is significant that this substitution is located in the glycine-rich region of the predicted NADPH binding pocket (indicated Fig. 1), a change that would be expected to severely impair its affinity for this nucleotide.

One X-linked patient has been identified in whom normal amounts of membrane heme are associated with deficient FAD (55). It seems probable that this mutation would involve the FAD binding site.

Secondary structure prediction using the amino acid sequences of both the α (48) and β (43,44) subunits indicate that both subunits have transmembrane helical spans. There are up to six helical hydrophobic regions in the β subunit, suggesting up to six possible membrane spans, and probably two membrane-spanning helices in the α subunit. The initial 240 amino acids of the 569 in the β subunit form a hydrophobic domain and contain five of the six possible membrane spans. From approximately residue 240 the character of the protein changes to a predominantly hydrophilic sequence containing the NADPH consensus binding site and possibly the site of FAD binding.

We propose therefore that the cytochrome b_{-245} β chain has a modular structure containing the NADPH and FAD binding sites. The hydrophobic domain not found in other members of the reductase family may form at least part of the heme binding site.

D. NADPH Affinity Labeling of Membranes and Cytosol

Having identified the probable NADPH binding site, we attempted to strengthen this evidence by demonstrating direct binding of the nucleotide to the β subunit of the cytochrome. Dialdehydes of reduced pyridine nucleotides have been used as inhibitors of, and affinity ligands to, the binding sites of dehydrogenases (76).

A number of attempts have been made to identify the pyridine nucleotide binding site by the use of NADPH dialdehyde followed by reduction by tritiated sodium borohydride. Although a large number of proteins in the cytosol and membranes were labeled with this method, the predominant membrane proteins, thought by Minakami and co-workers to represent the oxidase nucleotide binding site, had a size of 66 kDa on SDS-PAGE (77). Babior, Curnutte, and colleagues believe the NADPH binding site to be in a cytosolic protein that translocates to the membrane. This was first identified as a 66-kDa protein (78) but more recently as 32 kDa (79). In view of the previous uncertainties we decided to use the photoaffinity ligand AZIDO-NADPH (80). In cytosol, this agent almost exclusively labeled two bands of about 65 and 67 kDa.

In membranes, a number of bands were seen to label. One of these was located in the region of the large subunit of the cytochrome and was completely competed off by 1 m*M* NADP. Identification was hampered by the diffuse band of migration of this heavily glycosylated protein (38). This protein was also found to be labeled when the cytochrome was purified after labeling of the membranes, and this labeling was reduced by 100 μM cold NADP.

Radiolabeling of the β subunit of the cytochrome was defective in the X-linked CGD patient with the proline to histidine mutation at the putative NADPH binding site. These results suggest that NADPH binds to the cytochrome.

E. Reflavination of Cytochrome *b*

Solubilization of membranes with Triton X-100 and N-101, octyl glucoside, or dodecyl maltoside released most of the membrane cytochrome *b* and FAD. However, the FAD was not associated with protein, being almost entirely included in Sephadex G-10 desalting columns. This calls into question those studies conducted on "flavoproteins" solubilized by detergents from neutrophil membranes (81,82). It seems probable that under these conditions the properties observed were those of the free FAD.

Attempts to stabilize the protein-bound FAD by cross-linking with ethyl dimethylaminopropyl carbodiimide (EDC), which has been shown to stabilize the solubilized oxidase (83), were unsuccessful. Pick and co-workers had shown that the cytochrome *b*, which was free of FAD, could alone replace whole membranes in the cell-free system, but only if it was relipidated before use (84). We therefore attempted to reflavinate this molecule after purification, by incubation with FAD and detergent-solubilized lipid followed by removal of the detergent by dialysis. The cytochrome *b* was then separated from free FAD on sucrose gradients. We were able to obtain the association of FAD with the cytochrome in a flavin to haem ratio of $(0.10 \pm 0.08):1$ ($n = 8$), indicating reflavination of 20% of the cytochrome given the observed 0.5:1 ratio in membranes. The FAD did not associate with the cytochrome in the absence of lipid, nor with lipid in the absence of the cytochrome.

F. Location of the Heme on the Flavocytochrome

The FAD and NADPH binding sites are located on the β subunit, as discussed above. However, none of the other members of the FNR family so far identified contain heme. Therefore the heme is likely to be located on either the α subunit and/or the hydrophobic domain of the β subunit.

Yamaguchi *et al.* claim to have partially dissociated the subunits in octyl glucoside and separated the small subunit together with the heme, and to have obtained a midpoint potential of -210 mV for this molecule (69). However, the amino acid composition of their preparation was very different from that of the α subunit. Equilibrium centrifugation in the presence of octyl glucoside appeared to separate the subunits, and caused the heme to associate with the small one (85). In addition, radiation inactivation analysis indicated a size of about 21 kDa for the heme binding domain (85). Purification studies from different cell types (86) indicated a close correlation between the heme and amount of α, but not β, subunit.

Thus the evidence favored the location of the heme on the α subunit. However, Raman spectroscopy indicated that the heme was probably liganded to two histidines (65). The α subunit has two histidines, but one of these is the site of a polymorphism that does not affect heme binding (46). The other, histidine-93, is in an area of homology (V-L-H-L) shared with the heme-binding subunit of cytochrome-*c* oxidase (48). This suggests that the heme is on the α subunit with an unusual ligand, is bound between two α subunits, or that it has one ligand on the α and the other on the β subunit.

The α subunit has two predicted transmembrane helices. With this structure, the invariant histidine lies in close proximity to a cysteine residue that could form the other heme ligand, toward the external surface of a transmembrane helix in an ideal position to produce and release superoxide from this membrane surface.

VIII. Terminology

The constituent molecules of this NADPH oxidase have been accorded a variety of labels. The suffix *phox* (identifying them as components of the *ph*agocyte *ox*idase) has been attached to these proteins. The two subunits of the cytochrome *b* have been referred to as the α and β subunits or p22-*phox* and gp91-*phox*, respectively. Now that the redox components of the oxidase have been shown to reside on the two subunits of a flavocytochrome, we would appear to have two choices, either to refer to the α subunit as the cytochrome β component and the β subunit as the flavoreductase, or refer to the complex as a flavocytochrome. We favor the latter as it accentuates the interrelationship and structural interdependence of the two proteins, and suggest that the complex be called flavocytochrome-b_{-245}

IX. Cytosolic Factors

A. p47-*phox* and p67-*phox*

Cells from most patients with CGD with an autosomal recessive inheritance contain normal amounts of an apparently normal flavocytochrome-*b* (17), but they are unable to pass electrons onto the heme (87). This indicates an abnormality of the activation process or the absence or malfunction of a proximal electron-transferring molecule, or molecules. These patients lack one of two cytosolic proteins. Most commonly they are deficient in p47-*phox*. This protein is heavily phosphorylated on activation of the oxidase (88,89), and a small proportion of the total translocates to the membrane where it appears to associate with the β subunit of the cytochrome *b*. It is defective in approximately 90% of autosomal recessive CGD because of a GT deletion at the site of a GTGT tandem repeat located at the first splice junction of the gene (90). This genetic lesion is carried with a frequency of about 1 in 2000 in the general population. Rarely, a deficiency of another cytosolic protein, p67-*phox*, results in autosomal recessive CGD.

The function of both these cytosolic factors is unknown. They both contain two SH3 (*src* homology 3) domains which might be important for interactions between proteins. It has also been suggested that they are associated with the cytoskeleton (91). We are less certain of the veracity of this cytoskeletal attachment hypothesis, as it was based solely on the failure of the proteins to be solubilized by Triton. Although this is a standard technique in erythrocytes, it may not be equally applicable to more complex cells that contain nuclei and intracytoplasmic organelles like granules to which the proteins could adsorb.

B. A Small GTP-Binding Protein, p21*rac*1

The cell-free system is a model in which oxidase activity can be initiated in a mixture of membranes and cytosol from resting cells by the addition of anionic amphiphiles such as arachidonic acid (92,93) or sodium dodecyl sulfate (94). For activation, both membranes and cytosol are required, and these components can be fractionated to reveal their functional constituents. The membrane contributes the flavocytochrome-*phox* (15,84). The cytoplasm contains p47-*phox*, p67-*phox*, and a third component, called sigma 1 (95), that is separated from the other cytosolic components by fractionation with 37% ammonium sulfate.

Sigma 1 contains two proteins with apparent molecular masses of 22 and 26 kDa under denaturing conditions that associate as a heterodimer. We have identified these two proteins as p21*rac*1 and GDP dissociation inhibition factor (GDI), respectively (96). This observation is consistent with a considerable body of evidence in support of the involvement of a G protein in the cell-free system (97–100).

It has been reported that the small GTP-binding protein p21rap copurifies with the flavocytochrome-*phox* (101). Whether this small G protein also plays a role in the oxidase remains to be established. We have found that it progressively dissociates from the flavocytochrome during the purification of the molecule.

Exactly how p21*rac*1 contributes to activation of the oxidase system is not clear, it might be involved in catalyzing the formation of an active oxidase complex at the membrane (102), perhaps in combination with cytoskeletal elements.

X. Model of the Oxidase Electron Transport System

Our model of the NADPH oxidase (Fig. 2) places the complete redox system in the flavocytochrome-b_{-245}. This probably has two small α subunits, each with one heme, mounted on a single β subunit containing the FAD and NADPH binding site. The interaction of the redox cofactors and topology and conformation of the protein transport of electrons from one site to the other side of the membrane.

An interesting feature of the oxidase is that it is maintained in a completely dormant state until stimulated by surface receptors, whereon it is activated, after a brief lag period, to produce relatively large quantities of superoxide, before being inactivated. It is very likely that the

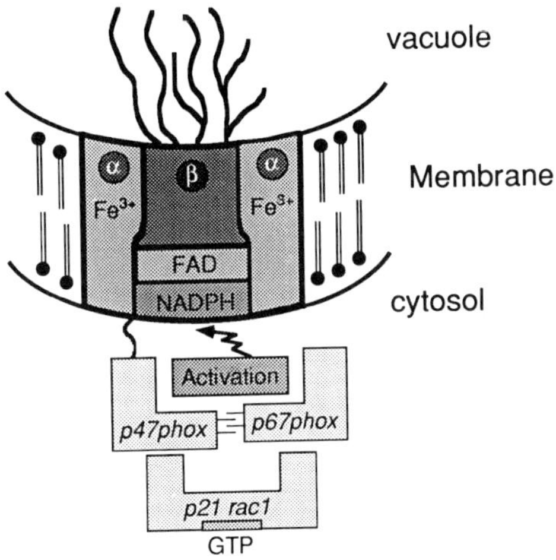

FIGURE 2

Schematic representation of NADPH oxidase. The flavocytochrome b_{-245} in the wall of the phagocytic vacuole is composed of a large, glycosylated β subunit that binds FAD and NADPH, and smaller α subunits that probably bind heme. The heme and FAD appear to be present in a ratio of 2:1, suggesting that the α and β subunits might associate in similar proportions. Activation of electron transport requires the presence of the cytosolic proteins p47-*phox*, p67-*phox*, and p21*rac*1. The precise activation mechanism remains to be determined.

cytosolic factors, p47-*phox*, p67-*phox*, and p21*rac*1, are intimately involved in the regulation of this activity. It remains to be discovered what role these proteins play in these processes, whether other proteins are involved, and how they exert their effect on the flavocytochrome-b_{-245}.

Acknowledgments

We would like to thank the Wellcome Trust for support.

References

1. P. M. McLoughlin, I. L. Sun, and F. L. Crane, *Biochim. Biophys. Acta* **802,** 71–76 (1984).
2. C. W. Baldridge and R. W. Gerard, *Am. J. Physiol.* **103,** 235–236 (1933).

3. A. J. Sbarra and M. L. Karnovsky, *J. Biol. Chem.* **234,** 1355–1362 (1959).
4. P. G. Quie, J. G. White, B. Holmes, and R. A. Good, *J. Clin. Invest.* **46,** 668–679 (1967).
5. A. W. Segal, M. Geisow, R. Garcia, A. Harper, and R. Miller, *Nature (London)* **290,** 406–409 (1981).
6. A. W. Segal, *J. Clin. Invest.* **83,** 1785–1793 (1989).
7. A. R. Cross and O. T. G. Jones, *Biochim. Biophys. Acta* **1057,** 281–298 (1991).
8. F. Rossi, *Biochim. Biophys. Acta* **853,** 65–89 (1986).
9. F. Morel, J. Doussiere, and P. V. Vignais, *Eur. J. Biochem.* **201,** 523–546 (1991).
10. S. J. Klebanoff, *Annu. Rev. Med.* **22,** 39–62 (1971).
11. R. Sternholm and R. C. Manak, *J. Reticuloendothel. Soc.* **8,** 550–560 (1970).
12. F. Rossi, *Biochim. Biophys. Acta* **853,** 65–89 (1986).
13. P. Bellavite, *Free Radical Biol. Med.* 225–261 (1988).
14. M. Markert, G. A. Glass, and B. M. Babior, *Proc. Natl. Acad. Sci. U.S.A.* **82,** 3144–3148 (1985).
15. A. W. Segal and O. T. G. Jones, *Nature (London)* **276,** 515–517 (1978).
16. H. Hattori, *Nagoya J. Med. Sci.* **23,** 362–378 (1961).
17. A. W. Segal, A. R. Cross, R. C. Garcia, N. Borregaard, N. H. Valerius, J. F. Soothill, and O. T. Jones, *N. Engl. J. Med.* **308,** 245–251 (1983).
18. M. C. Bohler, R. A. Seger, R. Mouy, E. Vilmer, A. Fischer, and C. Griscelli, *J. Clin. Immunol.* **6,** 136–145 (1986).
19. Y. Ohno, E. S. Buescher, R. Roberts, J. A. Metcalf, and J. I. Gallin, *Blood* **67,** 1132–1138 (1986).
20. A. W. Segal, R. Garcia, H. Goldstone, A. R. Cross, and O. T. Jones, *Biochem. J.* **196,** 363–367 (1981).
21. R. C. Garcia, A. R. Cross, and A. W. Segal, *Biochem. J.* **239,** 647–651 (1986).
22. P. J. Roberts, A. R. Cross, O. T. Jones, and A. W. Segal, *J. Cell Biol.* **95,** 720–726 (1982).
23. A. W. Segal and O. T. Jones, *Biochem. Biophys. Res. Commun.* **92,** 710–715 (1980).
24. R. C. Garcia and A. W. Segal, *Biochem. J.* **219,** 233–242 (1984).
25. A. W. Segal and O. T. Jones, *Biochem. J.* **182,** 181–188 (1979).
26. W. M. Clark, "Oxidation–Reduction Potentials of Organic Systems." Williams & Wilkins, Baltimore, Maryland, 1960.
27. A. R. Cross, O. T. Jones, A. M. Harper, and A. W. Segal, *Biochem. J.* **194,** 599–606 (1981).
28. P. M. Wood, *Trends Biochem. Sci.* **12,** 250–251 (1987).
29. R. K. Poole, *Biochim. Biophys. Acta* **726,** 205–243 (1983).
30. A. R. Cross, F. K. Higson, O. T. Jones, A. M. Harper, and A. W. Segal, *Biochem. J.* **204,** 479–485 (1982).
31. Y. Isogai, Y. Shiro, A. Nasuda-Kouyama, and T. Iizuka, *J. Biol. Chem.* **266,** 13481–13484 (1991).
32. B. M. Babior, *Trends Biochem. Sci.* **12,** 241–243 (1987).
33. A. R. Cross, J. F. Parkinson, and O. T. Jones, *Biochem. J.* **226,** 881–884 (1985).
34. A. M. Harper, M. J. Dunne, and A. W. Segal, *Biochem. J.* **219,** 519–527 (1984).
35. S. O. Pember, B. L. Heyl, J. M. Kinkade, Jr., and J. D. Lambeth, *J. Biol. Chem.* **259,** 10590–10595 (1984).
36. R. Lutter, M. L. J. van Schaik, R. van Zwieten, R. Ever, D. Roos, and M. N. Hamers, *J. Biol. Chem.* **260,** 2237–2244 (1985).
37. M. C. Serra, P. Bellavite, A. Davoli, J. V. Bannister, and F. Rossi, *Biochim. Biophys. Acta* **788,** 138–146 (1984).
38. A. M. Harper, M. F. Chaplin, and A. W. Segal, *Biochem. J.* **227,** 783–788 (1985).
39. A. W. Segal, *Nature (London)* **326,** 88–91 (1987).

40. C. A. Parkos, R. A. Allen, C. G. Cochrane, and A. J. Jesaitis, *J. Clin. Invest.* **80,** 732–742 (1987).
41. C. A. Parkos, R. A. Allen, C. G. Cochrane, and A. J. Jesaitis, *Biochim. Biophys. Acta* **932,** 71–83 (1988).
42. R. S. Weening, L. Corbeel, M. de Boer, R. Lutter, R. van Zwieten, and D. Roos, *J. Clin. Invest.* **75,** 915–920 (1985).
43. B. Royer-Pokora, L. M. Kunkel, A. P. Monaco, S. C. Goff, P. E. Newburger, R. L. Baehner, F. S. Cole, J. T. Curnutte, and S. H. Orkin, *Nature (London)* **322,** 32–38 (1986).
44. C. Teahan, P. Rowe, P. Parker, N. Totty, and A. W. Segal, *Nature (London)* **327,** 720–721 (1987).
45. M. C. Dinauer, S. H. Orkin, R. Brown, A. J. Jesaitis, and C. A. Parkos, *Nature (London)* **327,** 717–720 (1987).
46. M. C. Dinauer, E. A. Pierce, G. A. P. Bruns, J. T. Curnutte, and S. H. Orkin, *J. Clin. Invest.* **86,** 1729–1737 (1990).
47. H. N. Bu-Ghanim, C. M. Casimir, S. Povey, and A. W. Segal, *Genomics* **8,** 568–570 (1990).
48. C. A. Parkos, M. C. Dinauer, L. E. Walker, R. A. Allen, A. J. Jesaitis, and S. H. Orkin, *Proc. Natl. Acad. Sci. U.S.A.* **85,** 3319–3323 (1988).
49. R. H. Cagan and M. L. Karnovsky, *Nature (London)* **204,** 255–257 (1964).
50. B. M. Babior and R. S. Kipnes, *Blood* **50,** 517–524 (1977).
51. D. R. Light, C. Walsh, A. M. O'Callaghan, E. J. Goetzl, and A. I. Tauber, *Biochemistry* **20,** 1468–1476 (1981).
52. A. R. Cross, *Biochem. Pharmacol.* **36,** 489–493 (1987).
53. K. Kakinuma, M. Kaneda, T. Chiba, and T. Ohnishi, *J. Biol. Chem.* **261,** 9426–9432 (1986).
54. A. R. Cross, O. T. Jones, R. Garcia, and A. W. Segal, *Biochem. J.* **208,** 759–763 (1982).
55. T. G. Gabig and B. A. Lefker, *J. Clin. Invest.* **73,** 701–705 (1984).
56. P. Bellavite, A. R. Cross, M. C. Serra, A. Davoli, O. T. Jones, and F. Rossi, *Biochim. Biophys. Acta* **746,** 40–47 (1983).
57. A. R. Cross, J. F. Parkinson, and O. T. Jones, *Biochem. J.* **223,** 337–344 (1984).
58. K. Kakinuma, Y. Fukuhara, and M. Kaneda, *J. Biol. Chem.* **262,** 12316–12322 (1987).
59. J. Doussiere and P. V. Vignais, *Biochemistry* **24,** 7231–7239 (1985).
60. J. A. Badwey, A. I. Tauber, and M. L. Karnovsky, *Blood* **62,** 152–157 (1983).
61. H. Kojima, K. Takahashi, F. Sakane, and J. Koyama, *J. Biochem. (Tokyo)* **102,** 1083–1088 (1987).
62. C. M. Yea, A. R. Cross, and O. T. G. Jones, *Biochem. J.* **265,** 95–100 (1990).
62a. A. W. Segal, I. West, F. Wientjes, J. H. A. Nugent, A. J. Chavan, B. Haley, R. C. Garcia, H. Rosen, and G. Scrace, *Biochem J.* **284,** 781–788 (1992).
63. T. Chiba, M. Kaneda, H. Fujii, R. A. Clark, and W. M. Nauseef, *Biochem. Biiophys. Res. Commun.* **173,** 376–381 (1990).
64. A. Hata Tanaka, T. Chiba, and K. Kakinuma, *FEBS Lett.* **214,** 279–284 (1987).
65. J. K. Hurst, T. M. Loehr, J. T. Curnutte, and H. Rosen, *J. Biol. Chem.* **266,** 1627–1634 (1991).
66. I. Ueno, S. Fujii, H. Ohya-Nishiguchi, T. Iizuka, and S. Kanegasaki, *FEBS Lett.* **281,** 130–132 (1991).
67. G. T. Babcock, W. R. Widger, W. A. Cramer, W. A. Oertling, and J. G. Metz, *Biochemistry* **24,** 3638–3645 (1985).
68. M. K. Safo, G. P. Gupta, F. A. Walker, and W. R. Scheidt, *J. Am. Chem. Soc.* **113,** 5497–5510 (1991).
69. T. Yamaguchi, T. Hayakawa, M. Kaneda, K. Kakinuma, and A. Yoshikawa, *J. Biol. Chem.* **264,** 112–118 (1989).

70. P. A. Karplus, M. J. Daniels, and J. R. Herriott, *Science* **251,** 60–66 (1991).
71. T. D. Porter, *Trends Biochem. Sci.* **16,** 154–158 (1991).
72. D. S. Bredt, P. M. Hwang, C. E. Glatt, C. Lowenstein, R. R. Reed, and S. H. Snyder, *Nature (London)* **351,** 714–718 (1991).
73. P. Bork and C. Grunwald, *Eur. J. Biochem.* **191,** 347–358 (1990).
74. M. J. E. Sternberg, *Nature (London)* **349,** 111 (1991).
74a. A. Dancis, D. G. Roman, G. J. Anderson, A. G. Hinnebusch, and R. D. Klausner, *Proc. Natl. Acad. Sci. U.S.A.* **89,** 3869–3873 (1992).
75. M. C. Dinauer, J. T. Curnutte, H. Rosen, and S. H. Orkin. *J. Clin. Invest.* **84,** 2012–2016 (1989).
76. R. F. Coleman, *Annu. Rev. Biochem.* **52,** 67–91 (1983).
77. T. Umei, K. Takeshige, and S. Minakami, *J. Biol. Chem.* **261,** 5229–5232 (1986).
78. R. M. Smith, J. T. Curnutte, and B. M. Babior, *J. Biol. Chem.* **264,** 1958–1962 (1989).
79. T. Umei, B. M. Babior, J. T. Curnutte, and R. M. Smith, *J. Biol. Chem.* **266,** 6019–6022 (1991).
80. H. Kim and B. E. Haley, *J. Biol. Chem.* **265,** 3636–3641 (1990).
81. T. G. Gabig and B. A. Lefker, *Biochem. Biophys. Res. Commun.* **118,** 430–436 (1984).
82. T. R. Green and K. L. Pratt, *J. Biol. Chem.* **263,** 5617–5623 (1988).
83. M. Tamura, T. Tamura, D. N. Burnham, D. J. Uhlinger, and J. D. Lambeth, *Arch. Biochem. Biophys.* **275,** 23–32 (1989).
84. S. Knoller, S. Shpungin, and E. Pick, *J. Biol. Chem.* **266,** 2795–2804 (1991).
85. J. H. A. Nugent, W. Gratzer, and A. W. Segal, *Biochem. J.* **264,** 921–924 (1989).
86. C. Capeillere-Blandin, A. Masson, and B. Decsamps-Latscha, *Biochim. Biophys. Acta* **1094,** 55–65 (1991).
87. A. W. Segal and O. T. G. Jones, *FEBS Lett.* **110,** 111–114 (1980).
88. A. W. Segal, P. G. Heyworth, S. Cockcroft, and M. M. Barrowman, *Nature (London)* **316,** 547–549 (1985).
89. D. Rotrosen and T. L. Leto, *J. Biol. Chem.* **265,** 19910–19915 (1990).
90. C. M. Casimir, H. N. Bu-Ghanim, A. R. F. Rodaway, D. L. Bentley, P. Rowe, and A. W. Segal, *Proc. Natl. Acad. Sci. U.S.A.* **88,** 2753–2757 (1991).
91. R. C. Woodman, J. M. Ruedi, A. J. Jesaitis, N. Okamura, M. T. Quinn, R. M. Smith, J. T. Curnutte, and B. M. Babior, *J. Clin. Invest.* **87,** 1345–1351 (1991).
92. Y. Bromberg and E. Pick, *Cell. Immunol.* **88,** 213–221 (1984).
93. R. A. Heyneman and R. E. Vercauteren, *J. Leukocyte Biol.* **36,** 751–759 (1984).
94. Y. Bromberg and E. Pick, *J. Biol. Chem.* **260,** 13539–13545 (1985).
95. E. Pick, T. Kroizman, and A. Abo, *J. Immunol.* **143,** 4180–4187 (1989).
96. A. Abo, E. Pick, A. Hall, N. Totty, C. G. Teahan, and A. W. Segal, *Nature (London)* **353,** 668–670 (1991).
97. R. Seifert, W. Rosenthal, and G. Schultz, *FEBS Lett.* **205,** 161–165 (1986).
98. T. G. Gabig, D. English, L. P. Akard, and M. J. Schell, *J. Biol. Chem.* **262,** 1685–1690 (1987).
99. E. Ligeti, J. Doussiere, and P. V. Vignais, *Biochemistry* **27,** 193–200 (1988).
100. I. Aharoni and E. Pick, *J. Leukocyte Biol.* **48,** 107–115 (1990).
101. M. T. Quinn, C. A. Parkos, L. Walker, S. H. Orkin, M. C. Dinauer, and A. J. Jesaitis, *Nature (London)* **342,** 198–200 (1989).
102. M. Isomura, A. Kikuchi, N. Ohga, and Y. Takai, *Oncogene* **6,** 119–124 (1991).

CHAPTER 2

Early Injury of Cells by External Oxidants and the Consequences of DNA Damage

Ingrid U. Schraufstatter and Janis H. Jackson

Department of Immunology
The Scripps Research Institute
La Jolla, California 92037

I. Introduction

Oxidants, generated by stimulated leukocytes, induce a variety of distinct biochemical changes in target cells. Hydrogen peroxide diffuses into target cells where site-directed hydroxyl radical formation, which is transition metal-dependent, injures specific targets. DNA is particularly sensitive to ·OH-induced damage: both DNA strand breakage and base hydroxylations can be detected. Formation of DNA strand breaks activates poly(ADP-ribose) polymerase, a DNA-binding protein which forms polymers of ADP-ribose bound to various nuclear proteins using NAD as its substrate. NAD turnover under these circumstances increases so dramatically that it affects ATP synthesis. First, a low NAD/NADH ratio functionally inhibits glyceraldehyde-3-phosphate dehydrogenase (GAPDH) of the glycolytic pathway. In addition, GAPDH becomes di-

Cellular and Molecular Mechanisms of Inflammation, Volume 4

rectly inactivated due to sulfhydryl oxidation, leading to further inhibition of glycolysis. Second, NAD resynthesis leads to depletion of phosphoribosyl pyrophosphate, a cofactor for the synthesis of all four nucleotides. In addition, with higher concentrations of H_2O_2 mitochondrial ATP synthesis becomes inactivated.

If the concentration of H_2O_2 is high enough, these pathways will lead to cell death, and, therefore, H_2O_2-induced alterations will not be passed on to future cell generations. If, however, cells are exposed to sublethal concentrations of H_2O_2, the ensuing injury could cause permanent and transmissible cellular alterations which could be biologically detrimental. For instance, if ·OH-induced DNA damage fails to be repaired or is improperly repaired, this DNA damage could lead to genetic alterations such as mutations, deletions, and rearrangements. Moreover, if these genetic alterations occur in critical genes that are involved in cell growth and differentiation, they could lead to disregulated cell growth and differentiation and ultimately contribute to the malignant transformation of cells. We will discuss the current evidence that leukocyte-derived ·OH-induced DNA damage contributes to carcinogenesis.

Hypochlorous acid formed by myeloperoxidase in the presence of H_2O_2 and Cl^- is a potent bactericidal agent, which may oxidize any electron donor at the site of its production. When cells are exposed to HOCl in protein-free medium, various plasma membrane proteins (glucose transporter, amino acid transporters, etc.) are inactivated, and the cell loses its ionic balance, swells, and lyses.

Oxidants Produced by Stimulated Neutrophils

The local concentrations of oxidants formed by polymorphonuclear leukocytes (PMNs) can be extremely high: 2×10^6 PMNs stimulated with 10^{-8} *M* fMet-Leu-Phe produce 10 nmol O_2^- within 1 min in a volume of 1–2 μl. In the absence of O_2^--degrading pathways, this would be a local concentration of 5–10 m*M*. Superoxide itself is not indiscriminately reactive, although it selectively damages a limited number of targets (e.g., catalase). Its protonated form, $HO_2\cdot$(pK_a 4.8), can, however, directly attack polyunsaturated fatty acids, similar to ·OH. Superoxide quickly dismutates to H_2O_2. For extracellular O_2^-, this reaction can occur nonenzymatically and is presumably supported by the acidic pH in the proximity of stimulated PMNs. In the presence of transition metal ions, the extremely reactive ·OH radical can be formed in a Fenton-type reaction:

$$Fe^{2+} + H_2O_2 \rightarrow Fe^{3+} + \cdot OH + OH^-$$

Fe^{3+}can be rereduced by O_2^- or other reducing agents (e.g., ascorbate, glutathione):

$$Fe^{3+} + O_2^- \rightarrow Fe^{2+} + O_2$$

Since H_2O_2 easily diffuses through cell membranes, ·OH formation may occur extra- or intracellularly, depending on the availability of transition metals. Because of its high reactivity, ·OH will always cause site-directed damage at the site of its formation.

Myeloperoxidase, abundantly present in PMNs and released during the respiratory burst, converts H_2O_2 to HOCl, a very reactive oxidant which can further react to form more long-lived chloramines. This chapter will focus on cellular damage caused by H_2O_2 and its product ·OH as well as on HOCl.

II. Biochemical Pathways Affected by Oxidants

A. Oxidant Effects on Cellular Energy Systems

Early observations from our laboratory indicated that ATP levels were depleted in $P388D_1$ and cultured endothelial cells after being exposed to a bolus of H_2O_2. Reduction was observed within 2–3 min, and levels below 10% of control values could be observed within 10 min at high oxidant concentrations (Fig. 1) (1).

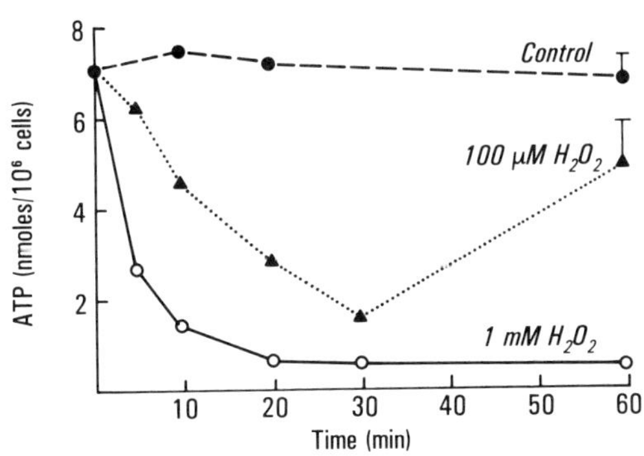

FIGURE 1

Time course of ATP depletion in $P388D_1$ cells exposed to a bolus of 100 μM or 1 mM H_2O_2.

The loss of ATP could result from either accelerated consumption or diminished formation. To examine the rate of consumption in P388D_1 cells exposed to oxidants, the rate of loss of ATP was followed in cells exposed to H_2O_2 in which both glycolytic and mitochondrial synthesis were blocked (2-deoxyglucose plus atractyloside). A calculated loss of 2.3 nmol ATP/min/10^6 cells compared favorably with the rate in cells not exposed to H_2O_2 and to the rate of synthesis in control cells of 2.1 nmol/min/10^6 cells (2). Thus, an increase in catabolism was an unlikely explanation of the drop in ATP levels in these cells.

B. Effect of Oxidants on the Glycolytic Synthesis of ATP

By contrast, both glycolytic and mitochondrial syntheses were profoundly affected by exposure to H_2O_2 (2). In P388D_1 cells, the glycolytic pathway was inhibited at the level of glyceraldehyde-3-phosphate dehydrogenase. Of the eleven enzymes of the glycolytic pathway analyzed, only GAPDH showed a significant decrease in V_{max}. The K_m of any enzyme was affected by less than 10%. The V_{max} of GAPDH in cells exposed to 0.5 m*M* H_2O_2 fell from 78.1 ± 8.7 to 0.8 ± 0.1 nmol/min/10^6 cells, and nearly total inhibition of activity was determined at 1 m*M* H_2O_2. This was accompanied by an elevation of the products of the glycolytic pathway immediately preceding the GAPDH step, namely, glyceraldehyde 3-phosphate and dihydroxyacetone phosphate. The combined levels were increased approximately 6-fold in the 10 min after exposure to H_2O_2. Lactate production decreased in proportion.

The inhibitory effect on the GAPDH step resulted from three independent factors: a direct attack of H_2O_2 on GAPDH, a decrease in the ratio of NAD and NADH, and a small shift in pH in the cell responding to H_2O_2. As to the first, not only was a decrease in V_{max} of GAPDH measured in oxidant-exposed P388D_1 cells (with an IC_{50} of ~100 μM H_2O_2), but isolated rabbit muscle GAPDH also was inactivated by H_2O_2 with an IC_{50} of 10 μM H_2O_2. Further studies have indicated that loss of activity of GAPDH is associated with loss of two SH groups and formation of an S—S bond. The SH groups involved were found to be cysteines 149 and 153 which from crystallographic studies are known to be spatially opposed in one turn of an α helix. Disulfide formation between these cysteines inhibits activity (P. A. Hyslop, unpublished observations), possibly by preventing binding of NAD.

The second major influence on GAPDH activity was found to be a fall in the ratio of NAD to NADH (2), NAD being the cofactor for GAPDH. In H_2O_2-injured cells NAD levels fall relative to NADH in cells that

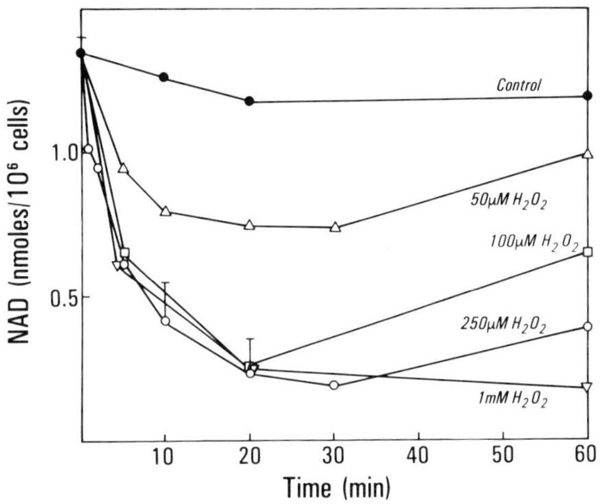

FIGURE 2

Diminution in levels of nicotinamide adenine dinucleotide (NAD) in P388D_1 cells exposed to various initial concentrations of H_2O_2.

contain poly(ADP-ribose) polymerase (Fig. 2) (3,4). When this enzyme becomes activated it consumes NAD (5); the two products of NAD during hydrolysis by the poly(ADP-ribose) polymerase are nicotinamide (NA) and ADP-ribose polymers which are bound to various nuclear proteins. NA formation in P388D_1 cells paralleled stoichiometrically the loss of NAD. ADP-ribosylation of nuclear proteins, primarily histones, occurred simultaneously.

The effects of the direct inactivation of GAPDH by H_2O_2, diminishing levels of cofactor NAD relative to NADH and slight but significant lowering of pH, in combination appear to produce the inhibition of the glycolytic pathway at this step. The concentration of H_2O_2 that would induce inhibition of glycolytic ATP formation varies, however, in different cell types. Whereas the IC_{50} for lactate production was 110 and 150 μM in P388D_1 cells and GM1380 fibroblasts, respectively, it was greater than 1 mM in bovine aortic endothelial cells. GAPDH is not normally the rate-limiting step of the glycolytic pathway, and variable regulation of the glycolytic flux in different cell types may explain this observation.

A relationship between the activation of poly(ADP-ribose) polymerase and the fall in NAD levels was observed employing inhibitors of the polymerase (Fig. 3). 3-Aminobenzamide, nicotinamide, and theophylline each inhibited poly(ADP-ribose) polymerase as measured by protein

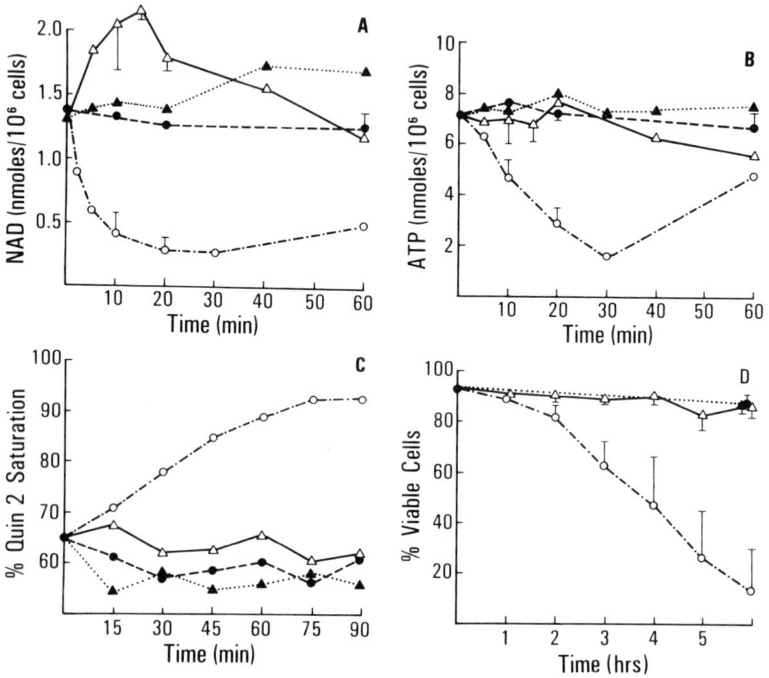

FIGURE 3

The capacity of 2.5 m*M* 3-aminobenzamide to inhibit biochemical alterations in 2×10^6 target P388D$_1$ cells induced by H_2O_2. (A) NAD levels: ●, untreated; ○, exposed to 250 μ*M* H_2O_2; △, treated with 2.5 m*M* 3-aminobenzamide; ▲, treated with 2.5 m*M* 3-aminobenzamide followed by 250 μ*M* H_2O_2. (B) ATP levels. Symbols same as in (A). (C) Intracellular Ca^{2+} levels as indicated by quin-2 fluorescence in the presence of 2.5 m*M* H_2O_2. Symbols same as in (A). (D) Viability in the presence of 2.5 m*M* H_2O_2. Symbols same as in (A).

ribosylation and prevented the loss of NAD (6) in P388D$_1$ cells. More surprisingly these cells were also protected from ATP depletion. With concentrations of H_2O_2 greater than 250 μ*M*, 3-aminobenzamide only partially protected from ATP loss, as would be expected from the direct effect of H_2O_2 on glycolytic and mitochondrial ATP synthesis, but still prevented an increase in intracellular free Ca^{2+} as well as cell lysis.

It should be noted that treatment of cells with 3-aminobenzamide did not affect the half-life of H_2O_2 (which was 7.5 min) and did not affect certain polymerase-independent effects of H_2O_2 such as the loss of total cellular Ca^{2+} from cells exposed to H_2O_2 (6). Thus, in P388D$_1$ cells, NAD cofactor appeared to be a critical modulating factor in oxidant damage.

C. Effect of Oxidants on Oxidative Phosphorylation

The second ATP-generating system, namely, oxidative phosphorylation by the mitochondria, was also affected by exposure to H_2O_2. Of interest, at H_2O_2 concentrations of 100–300 μM, an increase in net mitochondrial synthesis of ATP occurred. Nevertheless, over the same concentration range of H_2O_2 and above, the activity of ATP synthetase (ADP phosphorylation) consistently beclined (2).

Thus both glycolytic and oxidative phosphorylation pathways of ATP formation are affected by exposure of cells to oxidants. The balance of effect on one versus the other pathway will likely vary with cell type and oxidant concentration. Those cells heavily dependent on mitochondrial oxidative phosphorylation will not be as subject to ATP loss caused by inhibition of GAPDH as those more dependent on glycolysis. The reverse would be true for cells more dependent on glycolysis.

D. Effect of Oxidants on Nucleotide Synthesis

Inhibition of glycolytic and mitochondrial ATP synthesis seemed to fully explain the H_2O_2-induced depletion of ATP in P388D_1 cells. There were, however, cell types in which the drop in ATP needed additional explanation. For example, in WI38VA13 fibroblasts 150 μM H_2O_2 depleted ATP by 50% but had no effect on lactate formation as an indirect measure of glycolytic activity; mitochondrial respiration, which accounted for only 19% of cellular ATP synthesis in these transformed cells, gave no explanation either. It was furthermore observed that susceptibility to H_2O_2-induced NAD depletion in seven different cell types correlated well with the susceptibility to ATP depletion (Fig. 4).

Thus a third pathway of inhibition of ATP synthesis had to be operative. Careful kinetic analysis of NAD, ATP, and phosphoribosyl pyrophosphate (PRPP) synthesis and turnover in P388D_1 cells (Fig. 5) indicated that activation of poly(ADP-ribose) polymerase initiated such a high degree of NAD turnover (NAD synthesis between 5 and 10 min was increased 5-fold in P388D_1 cells exposed to 150 μM H_2O_2) in spite of severe depletion of NAD that PRPP became insufficient to support *de novo* and salvage pathway nucleotide synthesis (Ref. 7; I.U. Schraufstatter, unpublished results). This pathway of ATP depletion also explains the depletion of the other nucleotides which had been observed in our initial experiments (1). This mechanism was missed originally when decreased ATP synthesis rates were extrapolated from initial rates of ATP depletion, since it is of no importance during the first 5 min.

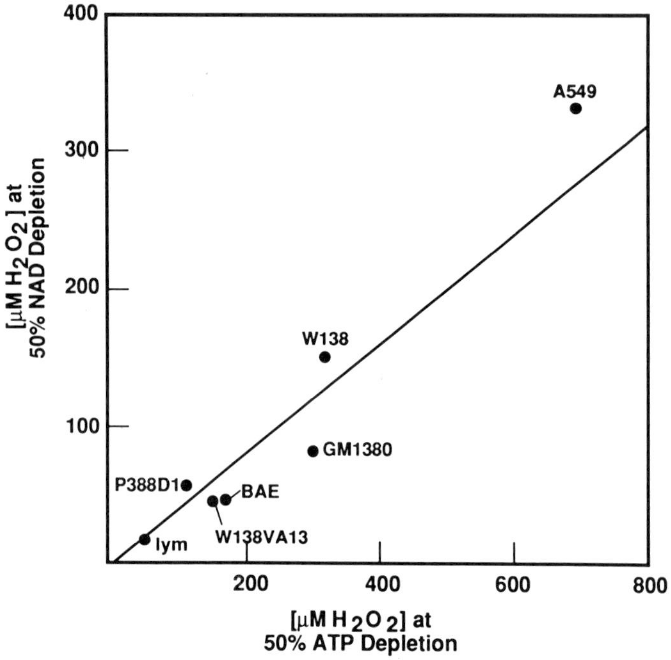

FIGURE 4

Correlation between ATP and NAD depletion in seven different cell types, extrapolated from dose–response curves determined 30 min after exposure to various doses of H_2O_2. The cell types used were human peripheral lymphocytes (lym), $P388D_1$ murine leukemia cells, GM1380 and W138 human lung fibroblasts and their SV40-transformed counterpart W138VA13, bovine aortic endothelial cells (BAE), and human lung carcinoma A549 cells.

Activation of poly(ADP-ribose) polymerase causes increased NAD turnover and depletion. The hatched area of Fig. 6 indicates metabolites with greatly increased turnover. Increased NAD synthesis leads to depletion of PRPP which is necessary for *de novo* and salvage nucleotide synthesis, and thus decreases ATP synthesis. At the same time GAPDH becomes inactivated either directly through sulfhydryl oxidation or following depletion of its cofactor NAD. This pathway can further deplete ATP synthesis through glycolysis, concomitantly leading to a transient increase of ADP (1). ADP, also formed by degradation of poly(ADP-ribose), inhibits PRPP synthetase, which forms PRPP from ribose 5-phosphate and may thus further enhance depletion of PRPP, although this pathway has not been investigated.

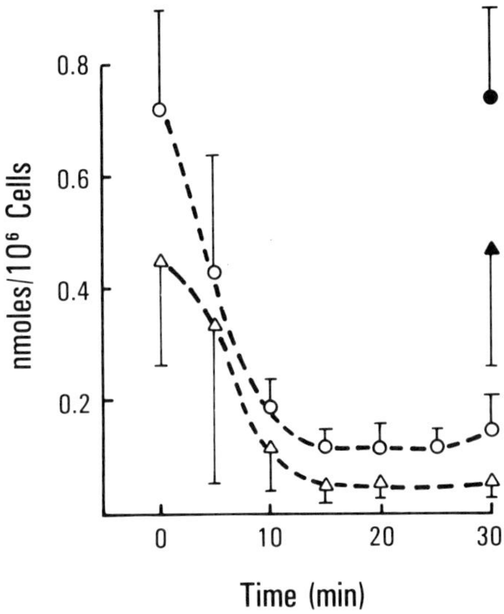

FIGURE 5

Effect of 150 μM H_2O_2 on NAD (○) and PRPP levels (△) in P388D$_1$ cells. Closed symbols show protection from 150 μM H_2O_2-induced NAD (●) and PRPP (▲) depletion in the presence of 3-aminobenzamide.

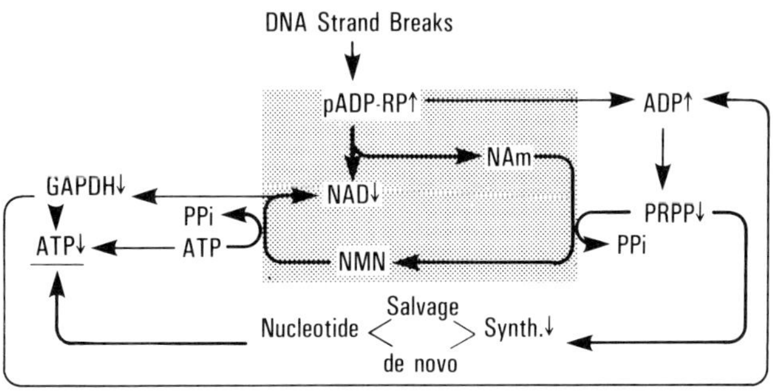

FIGURE 6

Network of metabolic pathways activated by H_2O_2-induced DNA strand breaks that lead to ATP depletion.

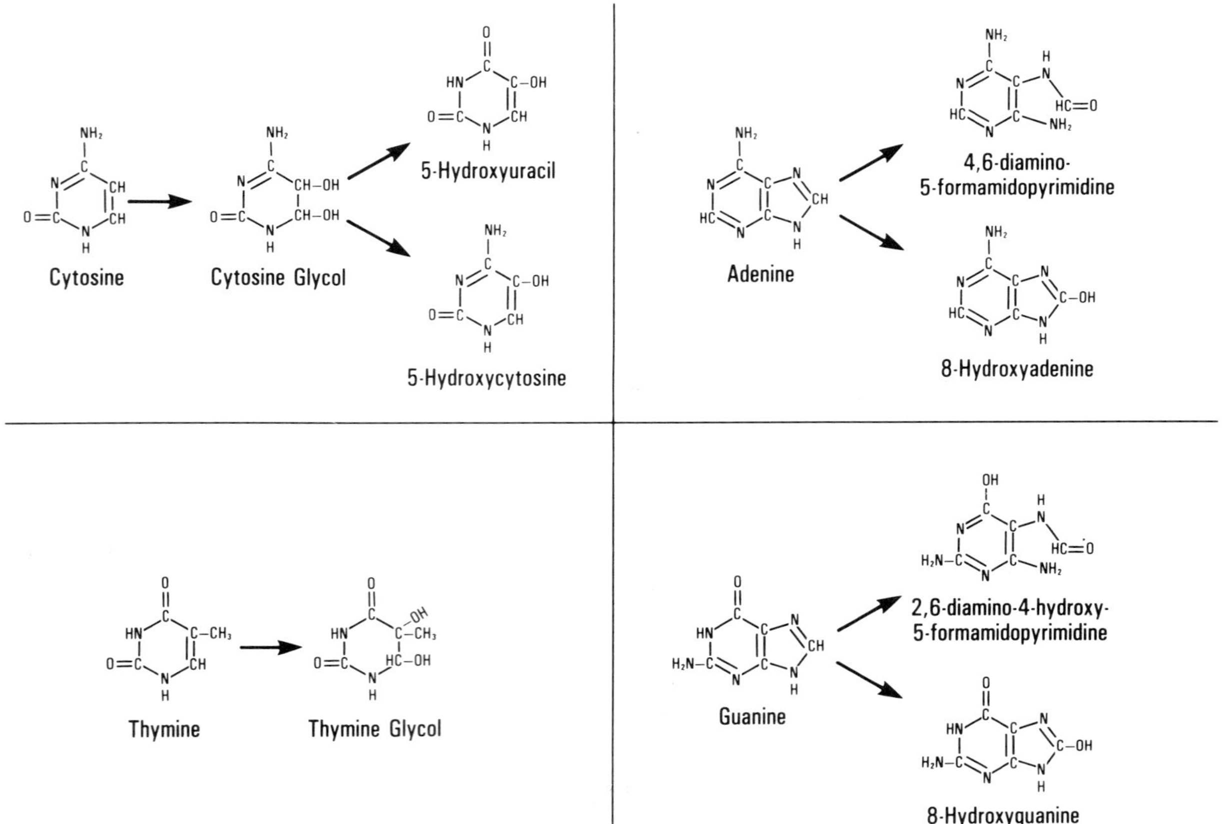

FIGURE 7

Chemical structures of modified bases identified in DNA treated with PMA-stimulated leukocytes.

E. Oxidant Damage of Cellular DNA

Since poly(ADP-ribose) polymerase is activated under conditions of DNA strand breakage (8,9), we reasoned that DNA damage might have occurred in cells exposed to oxidants. This has proved to be the case. Concentrations of H_2O_2 of 20–120 μM, well within the range produced by stimulated PMNs, caused formation of DNA strand breaks in various target cells (10–12). These strand breaks were observed within seconds after the addition of oxidant, and they could be prevented by the addition of catalase or cell-permeable iron-chelators (phenanthroline, deferrithiocine, and prolonged incubation with deferoxamine). H_2O_2-induced DNA strand breaks in isolated DNA were iron-dependent and inhibitable by ·OH scavengers (13). Moreover, the amount of strand breaks formed in isolated DNA mixtures exposed to H_2O_2 and Fe^{2+} was shown to correlate directly with the level of ·OH detected in these mixtures by electron paramagnetic resonance spectroscopy (14).

In addition to DNA strand breaks, H_2O_2 exposure also causes a number of different DNA base modifications. Specifically, by utilizing gas chromatography–mass spectroscopy with selected ion monitoring (GC-MS/SIM), it was shown that approximately 7 out of every 1000 DNA bases became modified when isolated DNA was exposed to physiological concentrations of stimulated neutrophils and Fe^{2+} (15). The specific base modifications detected included (in order of decreasing yield) 8-hydroxyguanine,* 8-hydroxyadenine,* cytosine glycol, 2,6-diamino-4-hydroxy-5-formamidopyrimidine, thymine glycol, and 4,6-diamino-5-formamidopyrimidine. The modified DNA bases are depicted in Fig. 7. The chemical structures of these modified bases are consistent with what would be expected from ·OH attack. Moreover, the facts that iron ions were required and that ·OH scavengers, superoxide dismutase (SOD), catalase, or iron chelators prevented the formation of these modified DNA bases (15) provide strong evidence that each of these base modifications occurred as a direct result of ·OH attack on the DNA. Some of these neutrophil-induced DNA base modifications have also been detected by high-performance liquid chromatography (HPLC) with electrochemical detection (16,17). In addition, similar base hydroxylations have been demonstrated to occur in intact cells exposed to H_2O_2 (12) or oxygen (18), and in isolated DNA exposed to chemically generated H_2O_2 and Fe^{2+} (19). Therefore, it appears that ·OH, or a transition metal–H_2O_2 complex

* These compounds are more correctly referred to as 7,8-dihydro-8-oxoguanine and 7,8-dihydro-8-oxoadenine. However, strictly speaking, this nomenclature is also not completely chemically correct.

with the reactivity of $\cdot OH$, was ultimately responsible for damage in isolated DNA and presumably also in whole cells.

Susceptibility to H_2O_2-induced DNA strand breaks in different cell types was inversely correlated with H_2O_2 degrading capacity, which at this concentration of H_2O_2 is primarily a function of catalase content.

Low doses of H_2O_2 (20–200 μM) cause DNA strand breaks and transient NAD and ATP depletion, but do not result in cell death. These strand breaks are repaired within 2–4 hr, and, although cell replication is delayed, it will occur eventually. Hence, there is the risk of misrepair of DNA and of H_2O_2-induced somatic mutations.

Higher doses of H_2O_2 result in cell lysis. Mechanisms of cell lysis may include severe energy depletion and the loss of ionic homeostasis (20,21). Programmed cell death (apoptosis) (22) causing similar histological changes, for example, cell blebbing, as those observed during H_2O_2-induced cell lysis (21,23) is associated with activation of a Ca^{2+}-dependent endonuclease (24) which leads to degradation of DNA into nucleosomal fragments. These fragments are detected by separating isolated DNA on agarose gels. While such fragment formation was observed 4 hr but not earlier after the addition of 250 μM H_2O_2 to bovine aortic endothelial cells or lymphocytes, no such endonuclease-induced DNA cleavage was observed in $P388D_1$ cells or W138VA13 cells exposed to up to 1 mM H_2O_2. This pathway thus does not appear obligatory for cell death, although it will certainly kill the cells in which it occurs.

F. Role of Oxidant-Induced DNA Damage in Carcinogenesis

As mentioned above, target cells exposed to H_2O_2 undergo DNA damage and a variety of other biochemical events. When the concentration of H_2O_2 to which cells are exposed is sufficiently high, these biochemical events are irreversible and ultimately culminate in cell lysis. This cell lysis may, therefore, represent a protective suicidal mechanism, because it prevents severely damaged cells from replicating and transmitting their potentially deleterious alterations to future cell generations. When, however, the concentration of H_2O_2 to which cells are exposed is low (i.e., 20–200 μM), the aforementioned cascade of biochemical changes is reversible, and the cells are able to repair their DNA damage and remain viable.

Although cellular DNA repair mechanisms are extremely efficient and reliable (25,26), there remains a slight, but inescapable, risk that a small proportion of H_2O_2-induced DNA damage will either escape repair or be improperly repaired. While most of these errors in repair are likely to be silent and of no biological consequence, errors in the repair of critical cellular genes, such as those involved in cell growth and/or differentiation, could cause genetic alterations which could lead to disregulated cell growth and differentiation. Moreover, since these genetic alterations could be passed on to future cell generations, errors in the repair of H_2O_2-induced DNA damage could ultimately contribute to the malignant transformation of cells.

A number of observations support the premise that leukocyte-derived H_2O_2-induced DNA damage contributes to carcinogenesis. For instance, it has long been recognized that epithelial tissues which are chronically infiltrated with inflammatory leukocytes have an increased incidence of developing malignant tumors (27). Specifically, it has been estimated that anywhere from 10 to 60% of patients with ulcerative colitis, a disease characterized by chronic infiltration of the colon with leukocytes, will eventually develop colon cancer (28,29). Similarly, chronic inflammation of the skin (29–31), urinary bladder (32,33), gallbladder (34), stomach (35), esophogus (31,36,37), and bone (31) is associated with an increased incidence of malignancy in these organs. In addition, it has been shown that inflammatory leukocytes can transform cultured mouse fibroblast cells into malignant cells that form tumors when injected into nude mice, and this transformation can be inhibited by agents which decrease ·OH concentrations (Refs. 38–40; J. H. Jackson, unpublished results).

As mentioned previously, one potential mechanism by which leukocytes might contribute to carcinogenesis is DNA damage. However, despite the large body of evidence demonstrating that leukocyte-derived ·OH causes DNA strand breaks, DNA base modifications, sister chromatid exchanges, and mutations (3,6,15–17,41–45), it remains unknown to what (if any) degree ·OH-induced DNA damage contributes to the ability of leukocytes to malignantly transform cells. One difficulty, which has impaired our ability to directly implicate leukocyte-derived ·OH-induced DNA damage in carcinogenesis, is the fact that leukocyte-derived ·OH can cause a variety of other cellular effects in addition to DNA damage, such as nonspecific stimulation of cell proliferation (due to cytotoxicity), activation of procarcinogens into carcinogens, and conversion of endogenous compounds to genotoxic intermediates (27). Since each of these effects could contribute to carcinogenesis, it has been difficult to ascertain whether leukocyte-induced cell transformation occurs as a result of direct ·OH-induced DNA damage or as a result of indirect or epigenetic mechanisms. We will, however, present the evidence available to date which supports the notion that ·OH-induced DNA damage contributes to carcinogenesis.

First, utilizing GC-MS/SIM, Malins and Haimanot (46) recently demonstrated that human breast cancer tissues had an 8- to 17-fold higher level of 8-hydroxyguanine, 8-hydroxyadenine, and 2,6-diamino-4-hydroxy-5-formamidopyrimidine, in comparison to surrounding noncancerous breast tissues. (The levels of 4,6-diamino-5-formamidopyrimidine were very low in both cancerous and noncancerous tissues, and the levels of cytosine glycol and thymine glycol in cancerous or noncancerous breast tissues were not measured.) Interestingly, the pattern of DNA base modification in these cancer tissues was identical to the pattern we had detected in isolated DNA exposed to leukocyte-derived ·OH (15) (i.e., the levels of 8-hydroxyguanine and 8-hydroxyadenine were highest, while the levels of 4,6-diamino-5-formamidopyrimidine were very low).

The origin of the ·OH that induced the DNA base damage in the breast cancer tissues is uncertain, but it is possible that H_2O_2, generated by cytochrome *P*-450-mediated oxidation of estrogen, could be responsible. Indeed, a recent study (47) showed that cytochrome *P*-450-mediated oxidation of estrogen generates H_2O_2, and treatment of hamsters with estrogen has been shown to cause increased kidney tissue levels of 8-hydroxyguanine as well as kidney carcinomas. In addition, a recent study (48) also demonstrated that several ·OH-induced DNA base modifications could be detected by GC-MS/SIM in cancerous liver tissues of English sole fish exposed to creosote hydrocarbons, but were not detected in surrounding noncancerous tissues. [Creosote hydrocarbons are believed to uncouple the liver cytochrome *P*-450 system and lead to increased levels of H_2O_2 production (49).]

The finding that the levels of ·OH-modified DNA bases were increased in cancerous tissues but were not increased in closely surrounding noncancerous tissues is an intriguing but unexpected finding. If one assumes that a cell which becomes malignant and immediately contiguous cells which do not become malignant are exposed to equal levels of ·OH, one would expect malignant and surrounding nonmalignant cells to have equal levels of ·OH-modified DNA bases. Accordingly, one would hypothesize that the reason one ·OH-exposed cell (but not similarly exposed neighboring cells) became malignant was that this cell acquired a procarcinogenic genetic alteration as a result of a rare error in the replication or repair of an ·OH-modified DNA base.

However, the finding that ·OH-modified DNA bases are increased in cancerous but not normal surrounding breast tissues suggests that this hypothesis may be too simplistic. It is possible, for instance, that the cell which became malignant underwent some preceding genetic or epigenetic event which made it much more susceptible to ·OH-induced DNA damage (i.e., it had reduced antioxidant defense mechanisms) and/or increased its level of intracellular ·OH production (i.e., it had increased levels of intracellular H_2O_2 production, increased levels of intracellular iron, etc.). In this regard, a recent study by Szatrowski and Nathan (50) demonstrated that one of the salient features of tumor cells is their tendency to constitutively produce high concentrations of H_2O_2. Therefore, the observed increased levels of ·OH-modified DNA bases in cancerous tissues could be a result of either increased susceptibility to or increased production of ·OH. Alternatively, it is possible that some preceding genetic or epigenetic event decreased the rate or activity of DNA repair enzymes; and the increased levels of ·OH-modified DNA bases are due to decreased repair, rather than increased production, of ·OH-modified DNA bases. Finally, it is possible that the observed increases in ·OH-modified DNA bases were a result, rather than a cause, of malignant transformation. This latter possibility is unlikely, however, because a recent study has shown that elevations in ·OH-induced DNA base modifications can be detected in tissues that show no histological evidence of malignancy (51), and large amounts of ·OH-modified DNA bases have been detected in the urine of normal humans (52,53). At any rate, regardless of the specific mechanism(s) responsible for increased levels of ·OH-modified DNA bases in a cell, it is possible that these modified DNA bases could lead to errors in replication or repair, and ultimately contribute to malignant transformation.

In regard to the potential carcinogenic activity of ·OH-modified DNA bases, several studies have attempted to directly assess the effects of ·OH-modified DNA bases on the fidelity of DNA replication. Specifically, one *in vitro* study (54), utilizing single-stranded oligonucleotide templates and *Escherichia coli* DNA polymerase I (Klenow fragment), demonstrated that 8-hydroxydeoxyguanosine (the major DNA base modification detected in leukocyte-damaged DNA) incorrectly pairs with deoxyguanosine, deoxythymidine, or deoxyadenosine with almost the same frequency as it correctly pairs with deoxycytidine. Moreover, 8-hydroxydeoxyguanosine also caused misreplication of pyrimidine nucleotides that were on its immediate 5′ or 3′ side. In contrast, another *in vitro* study (55), utilizing single-stranded oligonucleotides and a variety of DNA polymerases, demonstrated that 8-hydroxydeoxyguanosine pairs exclusively with deoxycytidine or deoxyadenosine, and no misreplications of adjacent nucleotides were detected. In addition, Wood *et al.* and Moriya *et al.* (56,57) have shown that 8-hydroxydeoxyguanosine pairs with either deoxycytidine or deoxyadenosine in bacteria when it is incorporated into single-stranded templates.

The mispairing ability of another major ·OH-induced DNA base product, 8-hydroxyadenine, has also been assessed utilizing single-stranded oligonucleotide templates and either *E. coli* DNA polymerase

I (Klenow fragment) or Taq DNA polymerase *in vitro* (58); however, no mispairing of this base product has been observed to date. Finally, cytosine glycol has been shown to mispair with deoxyadenosine in single-stranded bacteriophage DNA in *E. coli* (59), and the minor DNA base product, thymine glycol, has been shown to infrequently mispair with deoxyguanosine when it is incorporated into single- but not double-stranded DNA templates in *E. coli* (60). Thymine glycol has also been shown to inhibit DNA synthesis *in vitro* in most sequences (61–64), although certain local contexts allow DNA polymerases to bypass thymine glycol (63).

We are currently assessing the ability of ·OH-modified DNA bases to cause DNA mispairing in double-stranded DNA in mammalian cells, and we are also assessing the individual ability of these DNA modifications to contribute to the malignant transformation of cells. These studies should significantly improve our understanding of the carcinogenic potential of each of the ·OH-induced DNA base modifications.

In addition to the aforementioned studies, we also performed studies (64a) to determine if leukocyte-derived, ·OH-induced DNA damage could cause oncogene activation. These studies were undertaken because oncogene activation is one of the two major types of genetic damage that has been detected in cancer cells (the other is tumor suppressor gene inactivation). Specifically, we determined whether treatment of normal human K-*ras* or c-*raf* protooncogenes with leukocyte- or chemically generated H_2O_2 plus Fe^{2+} would convert these protooncogenes to activated oncogenes that can malignantly transform cells. These particular protooncogenes were chosen because normal K-*ras* and c-*raf* protooncogenes are believed to play a crucial role in signal transduction and cell growth. In addition, the fact that K-*ras* and c-*raf* can be converted to transforming oncogenes by different molecular mechanisms also made them desirable candidates for study. Specifically, previous studies have shown that normal *ras* protooncogenes can be converted to activated oncogenes by point mutations which result in amino acid substitutions primarily at codons 12, 13, or 61 *in vivo*, or at codons 12, 13, 59, 61, 63, 116–119, or 146 *in vitro;* these activated *ras* oncogenes, when transfected into NIH 3T3 mouse fibroblast cells, cause the cells to become malignantly transformed (65). Similarly, previous studies have shown that normal c-*raf* protooncogenes can be converted to activated oncogenes by strand breaks which result in deletions of the N-terminal regulatory domain of the encoded c-*raf* protein, and these truncated c-*raf* oncogenes also efficiently maligantly transform NIH 3T3 mouse fibroblast cells (66,67).

Accordingly, we treated normal K-*ras* or c-*raf* protooncogenes, contained in a mammalian expression vector, with phorbol myristate acetate

(PMA)-stimulated leukocytes or chemically generated H_2O_2, in the presence or absence of Fe^{2+}, and, after transfecting these constructs into NIH 3T3 cells, analyzed the cells for the development of transformed foci. Transformed foci were subsequently subcloned, and DNA from these subcloned foci was amplified by the polymerase chain reaction (PCR) and sequenced. Approximately 25–30% of the dishes transfected with K-*ras* or c-*raf* DNA that had been treated with PMA-stimulated leukocytes or purine and xanthine oxidase developed transformed foci. No transformed foci occurred in the absence of Fe^{2+} or in the presence of Fe^{2+} alone. Sequence analysis of our K-*ras* transformants revealed mutations predominantly at codons 12 and 61, although a few mutations occurred at other sites, including codons 13, 18, 117, and 146. Notably, each of these mutations has also been occasionally detected in human and/or rodent carcinomas.

In the majority of our K-*ras* transformants, mutations involved G→T and G→A transitions, and this same predominance of G→T and G→A transversions was observed in a review of several large studies of human lung and colon cancers (68). Interestingly, although leukocyte-derived ·OH caused very efficient K-*ras* oncogene activation (25–30%), the ability of leukocyte-derived ·OH to cause H-*ras* oncogene activation, under identical experimental conditions, was extremely inefficient (<1%). These results are consistent with the very infrequent activation of H-*ras* in human epithelial carcinomas, in comparison to the relatively frequent activation of K-*ras* in these malignancies. Since the transforming activity of activated H-*ras* or K-*ras* oncogenes in NIH 3T3 cells is equivalent, it appears that ·OH preferentially damages K-*ras* as opposed to H-*ras* DNA. Further studies will be needed to define the nature of this selectivity. However, our current studies suggest that primary DNA sequence or secondary DNA structure may be important determinants of susceptibility to ·OH attack.

While it can be argued that studies utilizing naked protooncogene sequences can lead to erroneous conclusions (because of the absence of surrounding chromosomal structure, histones, and other cellular components, such as antioxidant enzymes), the fact that our isolated DNA system reflected the same selectivity for K-*ras* over H-*ras*, preference for codons 12 and 61, and predominance of G→T and G→A transversions that is observed in human carcinomas suggests that this system may be a useful and predictive model of human biology. Moreover, this model system offers the distinct advantage of allowing us to selectively assess the role of direct ·OH-induced DNA damage (in the absence of other ·OH-mediated effects) in carcinogenesis. In addition, comparisons between the types of mutations detected in this system with the mispairing profile of each of the ·OH-modified DNA bases should prove informative. Obviously, it will be important to correlate the results obtained from the aforementioned isolated DNA studies with genetic alterations detected in cells treated with leukocyte-derived ·OH, or epithelial cells isolated from human carcinomas that are associated with chronic inflammation. These studies are currently underway.

In summary, accumulating evidence suggests that leukocyte-derived ·OH-induced DNA damage may contribute to carcinogenesis. However, it is apparent from the foregoing discussion that much work remains to be done in order to determine the validity of this premise.

G. Cytotoxic Effects of Hypochlorous Acid

Hypochlorous acid, a highly reactive oxidant, attacks targets at the site of its production. It reacts in particular with various protein moieties (e.g., amino groups, sulfhydryls, methionines, tyrosines) (69,70). *In vivo*, inactivation of α_1-AT due to methionine sulfoxide formation of its active site (71) is thought to be mediated by HOCl. Because of its high reactivity, HOCl is likely to react with whatever protein moieties it encounters first, presumably plasma and plasma membrane proteins. In protein-free medium it is extremely toxic to target cells in concentration as low as 20 μM, where it inactivates various sulfhydryl-dependent transporter systems (glucose transporter, various amino acid transporters, Na^+K^+-ATPase) (72) and, generally speaking, causes a poorly defined "leakiness" to small molecules, resulting in cell swelling and eventually cell lysis. No specific pathways involved in cell lysis can be determined, and cell death appears to result from the combined effect on various independent targets.

Effects of HOCl at low concentrations are closely stimulated by the poorly cell-permeable sulfhydryl reagent *p*-chloromercuriphenylsulfonate. Since HOCl causes oxidation of plasma membrane sulfhydryls, these are a likely site of initial attack (72).

While HOCl can damage isolated DNA, cell death precedes DNA oxidation in whole cells, and the addition of myeloperoxidase inhibits H_2O_2-induced DNA strand breakage (72). One may speculate that myeloperoxidase converts a reasonable microbicidal agent (H_2O_2) to an outstanding one (HOCl) and at the same time diverts the genotoxic H_2O_2 into HOCl, which is extremely cytotoxic in a protein-free system but which is considerably less toxic in the *in vivo* situation (73).

References

1. R. G. Spragg, D. B. Hinshaw, P. A. Hyslop, I. U. Schraufstatter, and C. G. Cochrane, *J. Clin. Invest.* **76,** 1471–1476 (1985).
2. P. A. Hyslop, D. B. Hinshaw, W. A. Halsey, I. U. Schraufstatter, R. D. Sauerheber, R. G. Spragg, J. H. Jackson, and C. G. Cochrane, *J. Biol. Chem.* **263,** 1665–1675 (1988).
3. I. U. Schraufstatter, D. B. Hinshaw, P. A. Hyslop, R. G. Spragg, and C. G. Cochrane, *J. Clin. Invest.* **77,** 1312–1320 (1986).
4. D. A. Carson, S. Seto, and D. B. Wasson, *J. Exp. Med.* **163,** 746–748 (1986).
5. K. Ueda, *Annu. Rev. Biochem.* **54,** 73–100 (1985).
6. I. U. Schraufstatter, P. A. Hyslop, D. B. Hinshaw, R. G. Spragg, L. A. Sklar and C. G. Cochrane, *Proc. Natl. Acad. Sci. U.S.A.* **83,** 498–502 (1986).
7. A. Cohen and J. Barankiewicz, *Arch. Biochem. Biophys.* **258,** 498–503 (1987).
8. C. J. Skidmore, M. I. Davies, P. M. Goodwin, H. Halldorsson, P. J. Lewis, S. Shall, and A. A. Zia'ee, *Eur. J. Biochem.* **101,** 135–139 (1979).
9. J. L. Sims, S. L. Berger, and N. A. Berger, *Biochemistry* **22,** 5188–5191 (1983).
10. M. O. Bradley and L. C. Erickson, *Biochim. Biophys. Acta* **654,** 135–143 (1981).
11. A. C. M. Filho and R. Meneghini, *Biochim. Biophys. Acta* **847,** 82–89 (1985).
12. I. U. Schraufstatter, P. A. Hyslop, J. H. Jackson, and C. G. Cochrane, *J. Clin. Invest.* **82,** 1040–1050 (1988).
13. K. Brawn and I. Fridovich, *Arch. Biochem. Biophys.* **206,** 414–419 (1980).
14. J. H. Jackson, I. U. Schraufstatter, P. A. Hyslop, K. Vosbeck, R. Sauerheber, S. A. Weitzman, and C. G. Cochrane, *J. Clin. Invest.* **80,** 1090–1095 (1987).
15. J. H. Jackson, E. Gajewski, I. U. Schraufstatter, P. A. Hyslop, A. F. Fuciarelli, C. G. Cochrane, and M. Dizdaroglu, *J. Clin. Invest.* **84,** 1644–1649 (1989).
16. K. Frenkel, K. Chrzan, W. Troll, G. W. Teebor, and J. J. Steinberg, *Cancer Res.* **46,** 5533 (1986).
17. R. A. Floyd, J. J. Watson, J. Harris, M. West, and P. K. Wong, *Biochem. Biophys. Res. Commun.* **137,** 841 (1986).
18. C. Richter, J. W. Park, and B. N. Ames, *Proc. Natl. Acad. Sci. U.S.A.* **85,** 6465–6467 (1988).
19. O. I. Aruoma, B. Halliwell, and M. Dizdaroglu, *J. Biol. Chem.* **264,** 13024–13028 (1989).
20. G. Bellomo, S. A. Jewell, H. Thor, and S. Orrenius, *Proc. Natl. Acad. Sci. U.S.A.* **79,** 6842–6846 (1982).
21. P. A. Hyslop, D. B. Hinshaw, I. U. Schraufstatter, L. A. Sklar, R. G. Spragg, and C. G. Cochrane, *J. Cell. Physiol.* **129,** 356–366 (1986).
22. A. H. Wyllie, *Nature (London)* **284,** 555–556 (1980).
23. S. A. Jewel, G. Bellomo, H. Thor, S. Orrenius, and M. T. Smith, *Science* **217,** 1257–1259 (1982).
24. D. P. Jones, O. J. McConkey, P. Nicotera, and S. Orrenius, *J. Biol. Chem.* **264,** 6398–6403 (1989).
25. T. Lindahl, *Annu. Rev. Biochem.* **51,** 61–87 (1982).
26. S. S. Wallace, *Environ. Mol. Mutagen* **12,** 431–477 (1988).
27. S. A. Weitzman, and L. I. Gordon, *Blood* **76,** 655 (1990).
28. G. J. Devroede, W. F. Taylor, W. G. Sauer, R. J. Jackman, and G. B. Stickler, *N. Engl. J. Med.* **285,** 17 (1971).
29. A. J. Greenstein, D. B. Sachar, H. Smith, A. Pucillo, A. E. Papatestas, I. Kreel, S. A. Geller, H. D. Janowitz, and A. H. Aufses, Jr., *Gastroenterology* **77,** 290 (1979).

30. A. H. Cruickshank, E. M. McConnell, and D. G. Miller, *J. Clin. Pathol.* **16,** 573 (1963).
31. W. W. Lovell, R. E. King, and R. Alldredge, *South Afr. Med. J.* **50,** 266 (1957).
32. A. F. Kantor, P. Hartge, R. N. Hoover, and J. F. Fraumeni, *Cancer Res.* **48,** 3853 (1988).
33. J. R. Locke, D. E. Hill, and Y. Walzer, *J. Urol.* **133,** 1034 (1985).
34. A. K. Diehl, *J. Am. Med. Assoc.* **250,** 2323 (1983).
35. P. Correa, *Cancer Res.* **48,** 3554 (1988).
36. A. J. Cameron, B. J. Ott, and W. S. Payne, *N. Engl. J. Med.* **313,** 857 (1985).
37. B. B. Dahms, and F. C. Rothstein, *Gastroenterology* **86,** 318 (1984).
38. S. A. Weitzman, A. B. Weitberg, E. P. Clark, and T. P. Stossel, *Science* **227,** 1231 (1985).
39. L. Nassi-Calo, A. C. Mello-Filho, and R. Meneghini, *Carcinogenesis* **10,** 1055 (1989).
40. R. Zimmerman and P. Cerutti, *Proc. Natl. Acad. Sci. U.S.A.* **81,** 2085 (1984).
41. B. Halliwell and O. I. Aruoma, *FEBS Lett.* **281,** 9 (1991).
42. A. B. Weitberg, S. A. Weitzman, M. Destrempes, S. A. Latt, and T. P. Stossel, *N. Engl. J. Med.* **308,** 26 (1983).
43. S. A. Weitzman and T. P. Stossel, *J. Immunol.* **128,** 2770 (1982).
44. H. C. Birnboim, *Science* **215,** 1247 (1982).
45. J. G. Lewis and D. O. Adams, *Cancer Res.* **45,** 1270 (1985).
46. D. C. Malins and R. Haimanot, *Cancer Res.* **51,** 5430–5432 (1991).
47. D. Roy, R. A. Floyd, and J. G. Liehr, *Cancer Res.* **51,** 3882–3885 (1991).
48. D. C. Malins and R. Haimanot, *Biochem. Biophys. Res. Commun.* **173,** 614–619 (1990).
49. A. K. Costa and K. M. Ivanetich, *Carcinogenesis* **5,** 1629–1636 (1984).
50. T. P. Szatrowski and C. F. Nathan, *Cancer Res.* **51,** 794–798 (1991).
51. D. C. Malins and R. Haimanot, *Aquat. Toxicol.* **20,** 123–130 (1991).
52. R. Cathcart, E. Schwiers, R. L. Saul, and B. N. Ames, *Proc. Natl. Acad. Sci. U.S.A.* **81,** 5633 (1984).
53. R. Adelman, R. L. Saul, and B. N. Ames, *Proc. Natl. Acad. Sci. U.S.A.* **85,** 2706 (1988).
54. Y. Kuchino, F. Mori, H. Kasai, H. Inoue, S. Iwai, K. Miura, E. Ohtsuka, and S. Nishimuka, *Nature (London)* **327,** 77 (1987).
55. S. Shibutani, M. Takeshita, and A. P. Grollman, *Nature (London)* **349,** 431 (1991).
56. M. L. Wood, M. Dizdaroglu, E. Gajewski, and J. M. Essigman, *Biochemistry* **29,** 7024 (1990).
57. M. Moriya, C. Ou, V. Bodepudi, F. Johnson, M. Takeshita, and A. P. Grollman, *Mutat. Res.* **254(3),** 281–288 (1991).
58. W. Guschlbauer, A. Duplaa, A. Guy, R. Teoule, and G. V. Fazakerley, *Nucleic Acids Res.* **19,** 1753–1758 (1991).
59. R. C. Hayes, L. A. Petrullo, H. Huang, S. S. Wallace, and J. E. LeClerc, *J. Mol. Biol.* **201,** 239–246 (1988).
60. A. K. Basu, E. L. Loechler, S. A. Seadon, and J. M. Essigmann, *Proc. Natl. Acad. Sci. U.S.A.* **86,** 7677–7681 (1989).
61. P. Rouet and J. M. Essigman, *Cancer Res.* **45,** 6113–6118 (1985).
62. H. Ide, Y. W. Kow, and S. S. Wallace, *Nucleic Acids Res.* **13,** 8035 (1985).
63. R. C.. Hayes and J. E. LeClerc, *Nucleic Acids Res.* **14,** 1045 (1986).
64. J. M. Clark and G. P. Beardsley, *Nucleic Acids Res.* **14,** 737 (1986).
64a. J. H. Jackson, M. Vollenweider, C. J. Der, and C. Y. Kuo. submitted (1992).
65. M. Barbacid, *Annu. Rev. Biochem.* **56,** 779 (1987).
66. T. Tahira, M. Ochiai, K. Hayashi, M. Nagoo, and T. Sugimura, *Nucleic Acids Res.* **15,** 4809 (1987).
67. V. P. Stanton, D. W. Nichols, A. P. Laudono, and G. M. Cooper, *Mol. Cell. Biol.* **9,** 639 (1989).

68. J. L. Bos, *Cancer Res.* **49,** 4682–4689 (1989).
69. M. B. Grisham, M. M. Jefferson, D. F. Melton, and E. L. Thomas, *J. Biol. Chem.* **259,** 10404–10413 (1984).
70. H. Fliss, H. Weissbach, and N. Brot, *Proc. Natl. Acad. Sci. U.S.A.* **80,** 7160–7164 (1983).
71. C. G. Cochrane, R. G. Spragg, and S. D. Revak, *J. Clin. Invest.* **71,** 754–761 (1983).
72. I. U. Schraufstatter, K. Browne, A. Harris, P. A. Hyslop, J. H. Jackson, O. Quehenberger, and C. G. Cochrane, *J. Clin. Invest.* **85,** 554–562 (1990).
73. S. J. Weiss, *N. Engl. J. Med.* **320,** 365–369 (1989).

CHAPTER 3

Cytosolic Components of NADPH Oxidase: Identity, Function, and Role in Regulation of Oxidase Activity

Paul G. Heyworth, Paola Peveri, and John T. Curnutte

Department of Molecular and Experimental Medicine
The Scripps Research Institute
La Jolla, California 92037

I. Introduction

The superoxide-generating NADPH oxidase that drives the respiratory burst of the immune system's phagocytic cells (neutrophils, eosinophils, monocytes, macrophages) represents a powerful but double-edged sword. On the one hand it plays a critical role in nonspecific host defense, where superoxide (O_2^-) and its metabolites, hydrogen peroxide, hydroxyl radical, and hypohalous acids, are essential in the killing and

Cellular and Molecular Mechanisms of Inflammation, Volume 4

digestion of bacteria, fungi, and parasites. On the other hand, there is abundant evidence that inopportune activation of the oxidase can lead to severe tissue damage by these highly reactive oxygen derivatives (see Chapters 1, 7, and 8 in this volume).

The resting neutrophil consumes very little oxygen, relying largely on nonmitochondrial energy sources. Within seconds of contact with opsonized microorganisms and a wide range of both physiological and nonphysiological soluble stimuli, the consumption of oxygen increases by over 100-fold. NADPH oxidase catalyzes the one-electron reduction of oxygen to O_2^-:

$$\text{NADPH} + 2O_2 \rightarrow \text{NADP}^+ + \text{H}^+ + 2O_2^-$$

Superoxide is converted to hydrogen peroxide (either spontaneously or by superoxide dismutase), hydroxyl radical, and hypochlorous acid (by myeloperoxidase in the presence of chloride), all of which are powerful antimicrobial agents (1). The importance of the phagocyte respiratory burst in host defense is made very apparent by the consequences of gene mutations affecting one or another of the different components of the NADPH oxidase system, resulting either in the absence of any gene product or in the synthesis of defective proteins (2). The syndrome caused by these mutations is called chronic granulomatous disease (CGD) and is characterized by a total absence (or, in a few instances, very low levels) of O_2^- production by the phagocytes of affected individuals. Consequently, patients with CGD are highly susceptible to life-threatening bacterial and fungal infections from birth.

How does the cell cope with the difficult logistical problem of having to generate rapidly large amounts of O_2^- and its derivatives, while also limiting their indiscriminate release? Not surprisingly, given the potential damage the system can cause, regulation of NADPH oxidase operates at several levels. First, the body can control the number of phagocytes circulating in the blood, by regulating the rate of myelopoiesis. In a healthy adult, the number of circulating neutrophils is in the range of 2000–3000/μl, while during infection this can increase to over 20,000/μl. Clearly, limiting the number of circulating cells reduces the risk of severe and indiscriminate tissue damage. Second, at the level of the plasma membrane there are a number of receptors, each of which is highly specific for ligands that in many cases are both chemoattractants and (usually at higher concentrations) stimulators of the respiratory burst. These stimuli are present at the sites of inflammation and include chemotactic peptides [e.g., formylmethionylleucylphenylalanine (FMLP)], the complement fragment C5a, platelet-activating factor, and interleukin-8. Third, NADPH oxidase is controlled at the level of the diverse signal transduction pathways that operate between the cell surface receptors and the final processes, as yet poorly understood, that regulate the assembly and catalytic activity of the enzyme.

The final tier of regulation involves the apparent physical separation of the various protein components of NADPH oxidase. Of the components that have been purified, characterized, and cloned, two are integral membrane proteins (gp91-*phox* and p22-*phox*, the 91- and 22-kDa subunits of cytochrome b_{558}; *phox* for *ph*agocyte *ox*idase component) and two are found in the cytosol of fractionated neutrophils (p47-*phox* and p67-*phox*). The subcellular localization of the putative flavoprotein component of the NADPH oxidase is uncertain, but it is likely to be in the membrane; two of the low molecular mass GTP-binding proteins that have been implicated in the regulation of oxidase activity are found in the cytosol of resting neutrophils and macrophages. Only when all of these components are assembled together on the plasma membrane do they form a fully active catalytic complex. In addition to providing a quarternary level of regulation, the multicomponent structure of NADPH oxidase, together with the dual localization of components, may also permit the assembly of alternate functional units that have distinct catalytic properties (e.g., a high K_m for NADPH). These would have the effect of keeping the oxidase closer to the precipice of activation and provide a molecular basis for the phenomenon of priming.

In this chapter, we present an early 1992 mechanistic view of the role of the cytosolic components described above and discuss how they may function as essential elements of NADPH oxidase. This view is based largely on recent work both in our laboratory and elsewhere, with human neutrophils from normal subjects and CGD patients. We have not attempted an extensive review of the burgeoning literature on this subject, and for recent informative reviews readers are referred to Refs. 2–8.

II. Concept of Multiple NADPH Oxidase Components

The respiratory burst of phagocytosing cells was initially described as a nonmitochondrial, azide-insensitive increase in oxygen consumption. In guinea pig cells a cytosolic NADH oxidase was the main candidate for the respiratory burst enzyme, while in human cells a particulate NADPH oxidase was considered the primary enzyme. NADPH oxidase was conceived of as a membrane-bound, single-subunit flavoprotein capable of catalyzing the one-electron reduction of oxygen to O_2^-.

This tidy, but incomplete, picture, in which CGD was considered to be an X-linked disease caused by the absence of NADPH oxidase, was complicated by two observations. First, there were a number of reports of females with CGD who apparently inherited the disease in an autosomal recessive manner (2). Thus, the phenotype of absent O_2^- production could result from mutations affecting at least two distinct proteins, one encoded on the X chromosome and the other on an autosome. Second, a low-potential cytochrome *b* with a midpoint potential of −245 mV (termed cytochrome b_{-245} or cytochrome b_{558}) was identified in neutrophils and postulated to be a component of NADPH oxidase, based on its absence in X-linked CGD patients. It was noteworthy that most patients with autosomal recessive disease were found to have normal levels of cytochrome b_{558} (9), although several with cytochrome deficiency were eventually identified (10). Weening *et al.* established that the X-linked/cytochrome *b*-negative (X^-), autosomal recessive/cytochrome *b*-positive (A^+), and autosomal recessive/cytochrome *b*-negative (A^-) forms of the disease were genetically distinct by complementation studies, in which respiratory burst activity was restored in heterokaryons formed by the fusion of monocytes from patients with different types of CGD (10). Based on these studies, it appeared that oxidase function was dependent on at least three distinct proteins.

The molecular basis of this genetic heterogeneity became apparent with two important discoveries. One was that cytochrome b_{558} is a heterodimeric protein consisting of a 91-kDa heavily glycosylated subunit (termed gp91-*phox*) and a nonglycosylated 22-kDa subunit (termed p22-*phox*) (11,12). It was subsequently determined that X-linked cytochrome *b* deficiency was caused by mutations in the gene for gp91-*phox* (13), while autosomal recessive cytochrome deficiency was due to abnormalities in the p22-*phox* gene (14). The second discovery, which provided an explanation for the A^+ form of CGD, was made at about the same time by several laboratories. They reported that NADPH oxidase could be activated in a cell-free system by lipid-perturbing agents such as arachidonic acid, provided that both membrane and cytosolic fractions from unstimulated neutrophils were simultaneously present. It was quickly learned that patients with cytochrome *b* deficiency, whether X-linked or autosomal recessive, had defects in the membrane fraction (15), while patients with A^+ CGD had abnormalities in the cytosolic compartment (16).

The concept that different genetic forms of CGD are associated with different types of subcellular defects is illustrated by the experiment summarized in Table I. The plasma membranes from patients with cytochrome *b* deficiency (either X^- or A^-) are devoid of activity even when

TABLE I

Cell-Free Activation of NADPH Oxidase in CGD[a]

	Superoxide production ($nmol\ O_2^-/min/10^7$ cell eq. membrane)			
	Source of plasma membranes			
Source of cytosol	Normal	X^-	A^-	A^+
Normal	73.2	0.1	0.1	67.3
X^-	68.7	0.1	0	65.2
A^-	75.9	0	0	70.6
A^+	0.9	0	0	0.1

[a] Neutrophil subcellular fractions from a normal donor and from three CGD patients (each with a different genetic form of the disease) were mixed in various combinations in a cell-free activation system for NADPH oxidase. Superoxide production was initiated by the addition of sodium dodecyl sulfate (SDS). CGD subtypes are abbreviated according to the mode of inheritance (X, X-linked; A, autosomal recessive) and the presence ($^+$) or absence ($^-$) of cytochrome b_{558} in neutrophils from the patient. [Reprinted from Curnutte (2) with permission.]

combined with normal cytosol in the cell-free activation system. In contrast, their cytosols function normally, as made evident by the high levels of oxidase activity seen when they are combined with normal plasma membranes, as shown in the second column of Table I. A^+ CGD patients, on the other hand, have normal plasma membrane activities (line 1, last column) but have severely defective cytosol (line 4, second column).

A fourth type of CGD was subsequently identified utilizing the cell-free activation system. Earlier studies had shown that the extent of oxidase activation in the cell-free system was proportional to the 2.5-power of the cytosol concentration, a result suggesting there were at least three (possibly nonidentical) cytosolic oxidase components (17). It was hypothesized that the cytosolic defect observed in A^+ CGD patients might be due to more than one type of defect. Therefore, cytosols from different CGD patients were combined in the cell-free activation system. In the original report by Curnutte *et al.*, no complementation was observed among the seven patients studied (16). In a subsequent report by Nunoi and colleagues, one patient was identified whose cytosol complemented that obtained from a group of other A^+ patients (18). An example of this type of cytosolic complementation is shown in Table II. Cytosols from patients 1 and 2 failed to complement each other while each is

TABLE II

Complementation between Cytosols from Patients with Different Forms of Cytosol-Deficient Autosomal Recessive CGD[a]

Superoxide production (nmol O_2^-/min/10^7 cell eq. membrane)				
	Cytosol 2			
Cytosol 1	Normal	Patient 1	Patient 2	Patient 3
Buffer	74.4	1.3	0	0
Patient 1		4.2	0.9	52.2
Patient 2			0	34.1
Patient 3				0

[a] Neutrophil cytosols from a normal donor and three patients with autosomal recessive/cytochrome *b*-positive CGD were mixed in the combinations shown and assayed for O_2^- production in the cell-free NADPH oxidase activation assay, in the presence of normal membranes. Patients 1 and 2 were subsequently shown to be deficient in p47-*phox* while patient 3 was deficient in p67-*phox*.

able to complement that obtained from patient 3. To date, only two complementation groups have been identified among the cytosol-defective forms of CGD (19).

The first clue to the identity of the cytosolic oxidase components was provided in a 1985 report that showed defective phosphorylation of a 44-kDa protein in phorbol ester-stimulated neutrophils from several A^+ CGD patients (20). In 1988, Clark and colleagues (21) raised an antiserum against partially purified human neutrophil cytosol that recognized several proteins, including one at 67 kDa and another at 47 kDa. The latter was subsequently shown to be identical to the 44-kDa phosphoprotein. When analyzed with this antiserum, the cytosols from 22 of 25 A^+ CGD patients had undetectable levels of the 47-kDa protein, while the remaining 3 were missing the 67-kDa species (19). At approximately the same time, four cytosolic oxidase components were resolved by preparative isoelectric focusing (22). Two of these components, one with a p*I* of approximately 6 and the other with a p*I* around 9.5, restored activity to cytosols from CGD patients missing the 67-kDa and 47-kDa proteins, respectively. The other two components have not yet been identified.

As can be seen from the discussion above, the concept that NADPH oxidase is composed of multiple subunits was driven by careful studies on the heterogeneous nature of CGD. The finding that CGD is caused by deficiencies or defects in gp91-*phox*, p22-*phox*, p47-*phox*, or p67-*phox*, provides the strongest evidence to date that these proteins are essential for oxidase activity and likely to represent actual subunits of the enzyme. (The functional roles of the cytosolic oxidase components will be considered in greater detail in Sections VI–IX.) This finding also forms the basis for the current classification scheme for CGD (Table III), in which the disease is subclassified according to the mutant oxidase component.

A shorthand designation for the various types of CGD is also shown in Table III under the heading "Subtype." The first letter in this nomenclature represents the mode of inheritance [X-linked (X) or autosomal recessive (A)] while the number indicates the *phox* component which is genetically affected. The superscript symbol indicates whether the level of protein of the affected component is undetectable ($^{\circ}$), substantially diminished ($^{-}$), or normal ($^{+}$) as measured by immunoblot analysis. Within each of the four major subtypes, the majority of patients have undetectable levels of the affected component. A few individuals have been reported to have normal levels of a nonfunctional cytochrome b_{558} due to point mutations in the gene for either gp91-*phox* (23,24) or p22-*phox* (25) (referred to as X91^{+} and A22^{+}, respectively). Finally, there is a small minority of patients who are said to have "variant CGD," in that their neutrophils have low levels of NADPH oxidase activity associated with residual levels of cytochrome *b*. To date, all the mutations identified in these patients have been in the gp91-*phox* gene (J. T. Curnutte, 1992, unpublished results). These variant patients generally have levels of respiratory burst activity that are 3–20% of normal. Variant CGD forms involving p47-*phox* and p67-*phox* have yet to be reported.

III. Primary Structure and Properties of the Cytosolic Components

A. Cloning, Amino Acid Sequence, and Properties of p47-*phox*

As discussed above, two cytosolic components of NADPH oxidase, p47-*phox* and p67-*phox*, have been unequivocally identified. The expression of these proteins appears to be restricted to cells of myeloid (and to a much lesser degree, lymphoid) origin. Their cDNAs have been cloned and sequenced within the past 3 years. Some of the properties of p47-*phox* and p67-*phox* discussed below are summarized in Table IV, and,

TABLE III

Classification of Chronic Granulomatous Disease[a]

Component affected	Inheritance	Subtype[b]	Cytochrome *b* spectrum	NBT score (% positive)	Frequency (% of cases)	Immunoblot levels[c]				Activity in cell-free system	
						gp91	p22	p47	p67	Membrane	Cytosol
gp91-*phox*	X	$X91^{\circ}$	0	0	50	0	0–trace	N	N	0	N
		$X91^{-}$	Low	80–100 (weak)	3	Low	Low	N	N	Trace	N
		$X91^{+}$	N	0[d]	3	N	N	N	N	0–trace	N
p22-*phox*	A	$A22^{\circ}$	0	0	5	0	0	N	N	0	N
		$A22^{+}$	N	0	1	N	N	N	N	0	N
p47-*phox*	A	$A47^{0}$	N	0	33	N	N	0	N	N	0
p67-*phox*	A	$A67^{0}$	N	0	5	N	N	N	0	N	0

[a] Abbreviations X, X-linked inheritance; A, autosomal recessive inheritance; N, normal level; 0, undectable level; NBT, nitroblue tetrazolium. [Reprinted from Curnutte (2) with permission.]

[b] In this nomenclature, the first letter represents the mode of inheritance [X-linked (X) or autosomal recessive (A)] while the number indicates the *phox* component which is genetically affected. The superscript symbols indicate whether the level of protein of the affected component is undetectable (°), diminished ($^{-}$), or normal ($^{+}$) as measured by immunoblot analysis.

[c] Defined by immunoblotting with component-specific antibodies.

[d] In one case (24), all of the cells were weakly positive.

TABLE IV

Properties of the Phagocyte Respiratory Burst Oxidase Components[a]

Property	gp91-*phox*	p22-*phox*	p47-*phox*	p67-*phox*
Synonyms	β chain, heavy chain	α chain, light chain	NCF-1, SOC II, C4	NCF-2, SOC III, C2
Amino acids	570	195	390	526
Molecular weight (kDa)				
Predicted	65.0	20.9	44.6	60.9
As seen by PAGE	91	22	47	67
Glycosylation	Yes (N-linked)	No	No	No
Phosphorylation	No	No	Yes	No
p*I*	9.7	10.0	9.5	5.8
mRNA	4.7 kb	0.8 kb	1.4 kb	2.4 kb
Gene locus	CYBB, Xp21.1	CYBA, 16q24	NCF1, 7q11.23	NCF2, 1q25
Exons/span	13/30 kb	6/8.5 kb	9/18 kb	?
Cellular location in resting neutrophil	Specific granule membrane, plasma membrane	Specific granule membrane, plasma membrane	Cytosol, cytoskeleton	Cytosol, cytoskeleton
Level in neutrophil (pmol/10^6 cells)	3.3–5.3	3.3–5.3	3.3	1.2
Tissue specificity	Myeloid	mRNA in all cells tested; protein only in myeloid cells	Myeloid	Myeloid
Functional domains	Carboxy terminus may bind cytosolic oxidase components; heme-binding domain (?)	Heme-binding domain (?)	6–9 potential serine phosphorylation sites; cytoskeleton binding sites	Cytoskeleton binding sites
Homologies	None known	Polypeptide I of cytochrome-*c* oxidase (weak homology)	SH3 domain of *src*; p67-*phox*	SH3 domain of *src*; p47-*phox*

[a] Abbreviations: *phox*, *pha*gocyte *ox*idase component; NCF, neutrophil cytosol factor; SOC, soluble oxidase C, component PAGE, polyacrylamide gel electrophoresis; SH3, *src* homology domain 3. [Reprinted with permission from Curnutte (2).]

for the sake of completeness, related properties of the cytochrome b_{558} subunits, gp91-*phox* and p22-*phox*, are also included.

Two groups working independently cloned p47-*phox*, but the predicted amino acid sequences were substantially different in the C-terminal third of the molecule (26,27). Minor nucleotide sequencing errors were identified by both groups and a consensus reached on a correct sequence (28,29) (Fig. 1). Recombinant p47-*phox* restored activity to cytosol from A47° CGD patients. The cDNA for p47-*phox* contains an open reading frame encoding a protein with a predicted molecular mass of 44,632 Da. This agrees well with the approximate molecular mass of 47 kDa normally estimated from SDS-PAGE, and even better with the originally reported value of 44 kDa (20). The C-terminal region of the molecule is extremely rich in basic residues (of the final 100 residues 25 are either arginine or lysine), contributing significantly to the basic isoelectric point of the molecule (p*I* 9.5). This same region is also rich in serine residues, many of which are in close proximity to basic residues and thus favorable sites for phosphorylation by protein kinase C (30). This feature of the molecule was not unexpected as p47-*phox* was initially identified as a heavily phosphorylated protein that was absent in one form of CGD, and it was later shown to be phosphorylated at multiple sites on activation of O_2^- production. The tyrosine at residue 97 is also a potential site of phosphorylation (31) although there is no evidence that this occurs. The phosphorylation of p47-*phox* is discussed in more detail in Section IV.

Two regions of the p47-*phox* sequence, each approximately 50 residues long, exhibit homology with a well-conserved motif [known as *src*-homology (SH) region 3] present in a diverse group of proteins, including members of the *src* family of protooncogenes, α-spectrin, *ras* GTPase-activating protein (*ras* GAP), phospholipase C-γ, yeast actin-binding protein (ABP1p), myosin-I, and p67-*phox* (32). A common feature of these proteins is their ability to interact, physically or functionally, with the cytoskeleton, and in many cases directly with actin.

B. Cloning, Amino Acid Sequence, and Properties of p67-*phox*

The p67-*phox* cDNA encodes a 526-amino acid protein (Fig. 2) with a predicted molecular mass of 60,900 Da, a value significantly smaller than the 67 kDa estimated from SDS-PAGE (33). This difference may be a reflection of the structure of the protein; a large mid segment of the sequence (residues 154–371) is rich in proline (13.3%), a property known to lead to anomalous electrophoretic migration. The C-terminal

10 20 30
M G D T F I R H I A L L G F E K R F V P S Q H Y V Y M F L V

40 50 60
K W Q D L S E K V V Y R R F T E I Y E F H K T L K E M F P I

70 80 90
E A G A I N P E N R I I P H L P A P K W F D G Q R A A E N R

100 110 120
Q G T L T E **Y** C S T L M S L P T K I S R C P H L L D F F K V

130 140 150
R P D D L K L P T D N Q T K K P E T Y L M P K D G K S T A T

160 170 180
D I T G P I I L Q T Y R A I A D Y E K T S G S E M A L S T G

190 200 210
D V V E V V E K S E S G W W F C Q M K A K R G W I P A S F L

220 230 240
E P L D S P D E T E D P E P N Y A G E P Y V A I K A Y T A V

250 260 270
E G D E V S L L E G E A V E V I H K L L D G W W V I R K D D

280 290 300
V T G Y F P S M Y L Q K S G Q D V S Q A Q R Q I K R G A P P

310 320 330
R R **S S** I R N A H S I H Q R **S** R K R L **S** Q D A Y R R N **S** V R

340 350 360
F L Q Q R R R Q A R P G P Q S P G S P L E E E R Q T Q R **S** K

370 380 390
P Q P A V P P R P **S** A D L I L N R C **S** E **S** T K R K L A **S** A V

FIGURE 1

Amino acid sequence of p47-*phox*. The two SH3 domains are underlined. The serine residues (S) in bold type are potential sites of phosphorylation by protein kinase C. Tyrosine 97 (bold type) is also a potential site for phosphorylation.

10 20 30
M S L V E A I S L W N E G V L A A D K K D W K G A L D A F S

40 50 60
A V Q D P H S R I C F N I G C M Y T I L K N M T E A E K A F

70 80 90
T R S I N R D K H L A V A Y F Q R G M L Y Y Q T E K Y D L A

100 110 120
I K D L K E A L I Q L R G N Q L I D **Y** K I L G L Q F K L F A

130 140 150
C E V L Y N I A F M Y A K K E E W K K A E E Q L A L A T S M

160 170 180
K S E P R H S K I D K A M E C V W K Q K L Y E P V V I P V G

190 200 210
K L F R P N E R Q V A Q L A K K D Y L G K A T V V A S V V D

220 230 240
Q D S F S G F A P L Q P Q A A E P P P R P K T P E I F R A L

250 260 270
E G E A H R V L F G F V P E T K E E L Q V M P G N I V F V L

280 290 300
K K G N D N W A T V M F N G Q K G L V P C N Y L E P V E L R

310 320 330
I H P Q Q Q P Q E E S S P Q S D I P A P P S S K A P G K P Q

340 350 360
L S P G Q K Q K E E P K E V K L S V P M P Y T L K V H Y K Y

370 380 390
T V V M K T Q P G L P Y S Q V R D M V S K K L E L R L E H T

400 410 420
K L S Y R P R D S N E L V P L S E D S M K D A W G Q V K N Y

430 440 450
C L T L W C E N T V G D Q G F P D E P K E S E K A D A N N Q

460 470 480
T T E P Q L K K G S Q V E A L F S Y E A T Q P E D L E F Q E

490 500 510
G D I I L V L S K V N E E W L E G E C K G K V G I F P K V F

520
V E D C A T T D L E S T R R E V

FIGURE 2

Amino acid sequence of p67-*phox*. The two SH3 domains (see text) are underlined. Tyrosine 109 (shown in bold type) is a potential site for phosphorylation.

domain of p67-*phox* is particularly rich in acidic residues, and the protein consequently has a predicted p*I* of 5.8. Like p47-*phox*, p67-*phox* has two SH3 regions, one in the central section of the primary sequence and a second close to the C-terminal end. Tyrosine 109 may be a potential site of phosphorylation, as there is an arginine seven residues N-terminal to it and an intervening acidic residue (Asp^{108}) (31). There is no evidence to date, however, that this protein is phosphorylated.

C. Mutations in the p47-*phox* Gene

In the monocytes from all A47° CGD patients reported to date, the p47-*phox* mRNA transcripts have appeared normal in abundance and size. Therefore, at least in the patients studied, the absence of p47-*phox* does not result from a failure of transcription. The majority of these patients are homozygous for a mutation in which two nucleotides, a G and a T, are deleted from a GTGT tandem repeat at the beginning of exon 2 (Fig. 3 and Table V) (34). This deletion predicts a frame shift resulting in an incorrect amino acid sequence from residue 26 onward and a premature stop codon after amino acid residue 50. Three patients followed at Scripps Clinic were heterozygous for this deletion and had a missense mutation in the other allele, leading to a single amino acid substitution (Thr^{53}→Ala in one patient and Lys^{135}→ Glu in the other two; see Table V) (35). Northern blots probed with p67-*phox* cDNA have also shown the presence of normal sized mRNA (33), but no mutations in this gene have yet been reported.

IV. Phosphorylation of p47-*phox*

The cytosolic oxidase component now known as p47-*phox* was originally identified as a 44-kDa protein that became heavily phosphorylated when normal neutrophils were stimulated with phorbol myristate acetate (PMA), but was absent from A^{+} CGD neutrophils (20). On one-dimensional gel electrophoresis, phosphorylation of the protein was apparently normal in X^{-} CGD, indicating that the absence of phosphorylation was not a secondary phenomenon due to the general failure of NADPH oxidase in CGD. Several studies [reviewed by Heyworth and Badwey (36)] showed that phosphorylation of p47-*phox*

	Exon 1			Exon 2								
	CAC	TAT	.....	GTG	TAC	ATG	TTC	...	GAG	TTC	CAT	AAA
Normal	his	tyr		val	tyr	met	phe	...	glu	phe	his	lys
	23	24		25	26	27	28	...	49	50	51	52
	CAC	TAT	.....	GTA	CAT	GTT	CCT	...	GTT	CCA	TAA	---
CGD	his	tyr		val	his	val	pro	...	val	pro	stop	---
	23	24		25	26	27	28	...	49	50	---	---

FIGURE 3

GT dinucleotide deletion responsible for some cases of p47-*phox*-deficient CGD. The GT deletion at the beginning of exon 2 is underlined. [Reprinted with permission from Curnutte (2).]

occurred when the neutrophil respiratory burst was stimulated by a wide range of agents. The kinetics of NADPH oxidase activation corresponded well with the kinetics of phosphorylation, further implying a close relationship between the two phenomena. The lack of p47-*phox* phosphorylation in CGD is now known to result directly from an absence of the protein (rather than a primary defect in the protein kinase), and is confined to the A47° subtype of the disease. However, in other forms of CGD, the extent of phosphorylation of p47-*phox* appears to be abnormal (see below).

Early studies demonstrated that phosphorylated p47-*phox* was present in both the cytosol and membrane fractions of normal, PMA-activated neutrophils (37,38). Its association with the membrane was subsequently shown to depend on the presence of cytochrome b_{558}, since in cytochrome-deficient CGD neutrophils phosphorylated p47-*phox* was confined to the cytosol (39). In neutrophil membranes from heterozygous carriers of X^- CGD, which on average have half the normal level of cytochrome b_{558}, intermediate levels of phosphorylated p47-*phox* were present after stimulation. Using two-dimensional gel electrophoresis, Okamura *et al.* (40,41) demonstrated that phosphorylated p47-*phox* appears as a chain of at least six spots, with p*I* values ranging from around 10 to 7. This indicates that the protein is phosphorylated at multiple sites, since the addition of each phosphate group increases the negative charge of the protein, thus lowering its p*I*. In cytochrome-deficient forms of CGD (X91° and A22°) the two most acidic (i.e., the most highly phosphorylated) spots were missing

TABLE V

Summary of p47-*phox* Mutations in Nine Patients with A47 CGD[a]

Patient/sex	Mutation type	O_2^-	p47-*phox* Protein	p47-*phox* mRNA	Nucleotide change	Amino acid change	CGD type	Ref.
1–3/M	Deletion/frameshift (homozygous)	NR	0	N	Deletion of G-95 and T-96 at beginning of exon 2	Frameshift with substitution of 25 incorrect amino acids (residues 26–50) before premature stop codon	A47°	34
4–6/2M, 1F	Deletion/frameshift (homozygous)	0	0	N	Same as patients 1–3	Same as patients 1–3	A47°	35
7/F	(1) Deletion/frameshift (2) Missense	0–1%	0	N	(1) Same as patients 1–3 (2) A-179→G	(1) Same as patients 1–3 Thr-53→Ala	A47°	35
8, 9/M	(1) Deletion/frameshift (2) Missense	0–1%	0	N	(1) Same as patients 1–3 (2) A-425→G	(1) Same as patients 1–3 Lys-135→Glu	A47°	35

[a] Nucleotide residues are numbered as per Casimir *et al.* beginning with the 5′ end of the p47-*phox* cDNA (34). N, Normal in appearance; NR, not reported; O, undetectable. [Reprinted from Curnutte (8) with permission.]

(Table VI) (40,42). Since phosphorylated p47-*phox* is confined to the cytosol in these patients, this observation suggested that the final phosphorylation steps only occur once the protein is associated with the membrane. A recent report, which indicates that p47-*phox* undergoes phosphorylation at as many as eight sites, reached the same conclusion (43). The observation that phosphorylation of p47-*phox* in $X91^+$ and $A67^\circ$ CGD neutrophils was normal at all sites (Table VI) (42,44) is consistent with the normal translocation of p47-*phox* in these forms of the disease (see Section V).

Phosphorylation of p47-*phox* appears to be confined to serine residues (40), but the physiological kinase(s) responsible is unknown. The ability of PMA, a known activator of protein kinase C, to cause phosphorylation of the protein suggests a role for this kinase. Indeed, partially purified p47-*phox* is a substrate for protein kinase C (38), a finding consistent with the serine- and arginine-rich nature of the carboxy-terminal region of the protein. The possible role of protein kinase C in activation of O_2^- generation, and other aspects of p47-*phox* phosphorylation, are reviewed in detail elsewhere (36).

The precise role of protein phosphorylation in NADPH oxidase activation has yet to be determined. It is interesting to speculate, given the highly basic nature of the carboxy-terminal region of p47-*phox*, that the

TABLE VI

Multiple Phosphorylation of p47-*phox* in Normal and CGD Neutrophils[a]

	Phosphorylated form of p47-*phox* at p*I*[b]					
Source of neutrophils	10	9.5	8.7	7.8	7.3	6.8
Normal control	+	+	+	+	+	+
CGD subtype						
$X91^\circ$	+	+	+	+	−	−
$X91^+$	+	+	+	+	+	+
$A22^\circ$	+	+	+	+	−	−
$A47^\circ$[c]	−	−	−	−	−	−
$A67^\circ$	+	+	+	+	+	+

[a] For definition of CGD subtypes, see Table III. [Reprinted from Smith and Curnutte (5) with permission.]
[b] p*I* values are approximate; + indicates the presence and − the absence of each phosphorylated form of p47-*phox*. As the protein becomes more highly phosphorylated, the p*I* becomes more acidic.
[c] In all patients studied to date with p47-deficient CGD, this protein is undetectable, hence the failure to see phosphorylation.

change in charge accompanying phosphorylation allows the protein to interact with other positively charged oxidase components (see Table IV for their p*I* values). However, it is important to point out that activation of O_2^- generation in intact cells has been demonstrated in the absence of detectable phosphorylation of p47-*phox* (45). This is perhaps analogous to the cell-free NADPH oxidase system, in which ATP is not required and p47-*phox* exists in its p*I* 10 form. Conversely, under the same conditions, it appears p47-*phox* can be phosphorylated with no concurrent generation of O_2^- (46). Phosphorylation of p47-*phox* on its own is therefore neither sufficient, nor always necessary, for NADPH oxidase activation.

V. Translocation of p47-*phox* and p67-*phox*

The observations described in the previous section strongly supported the emerging idea that translocation of cytosolic components to the membrane was an essential step in oxidase activation, although the possibility could not be excluded that the dual localization of phosphorylated p47-*phox* represented two pools of the protein. Conclusive proof that both p47-*phox* and p67-*phox* translocate to the plasma membrane during activation of O_2^- generation in intact neutrophils was provided by Clark *et al.* (47). Protein immunoblots of cellular fractions from neutrophils disrupted by sonication in relaxation buffer (a high-potassium, low-sodium, calcium-free buffer designed to mimic cytoplasmic conditions) (48) were probed with a polyclonal antiserum which recognizes both components. The two proteins were confined to the cytosolic fraction of resting cells, while in stimulated cells they were also detected in the particulate fraction.

The translocation studies were extended to neutrophils from patients with different forms of CGD (49). In patients with cytochrome-negative forms of the disease, whether X-linked or autosomal in origin (X91° or A22°), there was no translocation of either p47-*phox* or p67-*phox* from the cytosol to the membrane (Table VII, lines 2 and 4). This was consistent with the lack of phosphorylated p47-*phox* in membranes from stimulated cytochrome-negative CGD neutrophils and suggests that cytochrome b_{558}, or a closely linked factor, acts as a membrane docking site for the cytosolic components. Antibodies to peptides corresponding to the carboxy-terminal domain of gp91-*phox*, as well

TABLE VII
Translocation to the Membrane of p47-*phox* and p67-*phox* in Stimulated Normal and CGD Neutrophils

Source of neutrophils	Translocation of cytosolic component to membrane fraction[a]	
	p47-*phox*	p67-*phox*
Normal control	Yes	Yes
CGD subtype		
X91°	No	No
X91⁺	Yes	Yes
A22°	No	No
A47°	N/A	No
A67°	Yes	N/A

[a] Based on data presented by Heyworth *et al.* (49). Neutrophils were stimulated for 5 min with PMA. p47- and p67-*phox* were detected on protein immunoblots with a polyclonal antiserum which recognized both components. For definition of CGD subtypes see Table III. N/A, Not applicable (component absent in this subtype of CGD).

as the peptides themselves, blocked O_2^- production in a cell-free NADPH oxidase activation system, suggesting that this region of the cytochrome subunit is involved in the interaction (50). Translocation of both p47-*phox* and p67-*phox* was normal in $X91^+$ CGD, in which cytochrome *b* is present but does not function due to a single amino acid substitution (49).

In p67-*phox*-deficient CGD, there was apparently normal translocation of p47-*phox* from the cytosol to the membrane, whereas in the absence of p47-*phox*, p67-*phox* was not detected in the membrane fraction of stimulated cells (Table VII, lines 5 and 6). Thus, translocation of the cytosolic components depends not only on the presence of cytochrome b_{558}, but also on p47-*phox*, suggesting that this protein mediates the membrane association. The dependence of p67-*phox* translocation on the presence of p47-*phox* also suggests that these components may exist in a complex. However, it is possible that p67-*phox* translocates independently of p47-*phox* to a site formed by the interaction of p47-*phox* and the cytochrome.

VI. Cytosolic Oxidase Components Exist as Complexes in the Unstimulated Cell

We recently investigated the possibility raised by earlier chromatographic studies (51,52) and the translocation experiments described above, namely, that the cytosolic components of NADPH oxidase exist as one or more preformed complexes in the unstimulated cell (53). Neutrophil cytosol from normal individuals and that from patients with p47-*phox*- and p67-*phox*-deficient CGD were subjected to Sephacryl S-300 gel filtration chromatography. Column fractions were assessed for their ability to substitute for whole cytosol in a cell-free O_2^--generating system. Individual components and partial complexes were identified by the ability of column fractions to complement (i) a suboptimal amount of normal cytosol; (ii) p47-*phox*-deficient cytosol; and (iii) p67-*phox*-deficient cytosol. As described above (Section II), p47-*phox*- and p67-*phox*-deficient CGD cytosols are complementary in the cell-free system, with each cytosol providing the component absent from the other. When used individually in the presence of column fractions they provide a sensitive means of detecting low levels of the component in which they are deficient.

Normal cytosol consistently separated into two peaks of activity (Table VIII). One peak (designated peak A) eluted with an apparent molecular mass of 260 kDa and appeared to contain all the cytosolic components necessary for activation of NADPH oxidase, as it could effectively substitute for whole cytosol in the cell-free system. A second peak (designated B), with an apparent molecular mass of 53 kDa, was only clearly detected when the fractions were assayed in the presence of a threshold amount of normal cytosol that provided at least a small amount of all the oxidase components required for activation. Peak A fractions complemented both p47-*phox*- and p67-*phox*-deficient CGD cytosols, with the maximal activity in each case coeluting exactly with the peak of activity seen when fractions were assayed on their own. Peak B fractions only complemented p47-*phox*-deficient cytosol. Protein immunoblots of column fractions, probed with antibodies raised to synthetic peptides corresponding to internal sequences of p47-*phox* and p67-*phox*, confirmed that p67-*phox* was confined to peak A fractions, while p47-*phox* was distributed equally between peaks A and B. Peak A therefore appeared to represent a relatively stable complex of all the proteins necessary for NADPH oxidase activation, including p47-*phox* and p67-*phox*, but not necessarily limited to these two.

Cytosol from p67-*phox*-deficient CGD patients produced a very different chromatographic activity profile. Peak B was normal, but peak A was

TABLE VIII
Properties of Cytosolic NADPH Oxidase Complexes

Property	Complex of cytosolic oxidase components		
	Complex A	Complex A′	Complex B
Apparent molecular mass (kDa)[a]	260	212	53
Constituents			
p47-*phox*	Yes	No	Yes
p67-*phox*	Yes	Yes	No
Present in cytosol from			
Normal controls	Yes	No	Yes
p47-deficient CGD	No	Yes	No
p47-deficient CGD carriers	Yes	No	No
p67-deficient CGD	No	No	Yes
p67-deficient CGD carriers	Decreased	No	Yes
Mixture of p47- and p67-deficient CGD	No	Yes	Yes

[a] From gel filtration chromatography on Sephacryl S-300.

totally absent from this cytosol. No activity was detected in the region of peak A, either with a suboptimal amount of normal cytosol or with p47-*phox*-deficient cytosol included in the reaction mixtures (Table VIII). These results suggest that, in the absence of p67-*phox*, the 260-kDa complex does not form, either because p67-*phox* forms the bulk of the complex or because it has an important role in maintaining complex integrity. Results with cytosol from carriers of p67-*phox* deficiency, who would be expected to have about half the normal level of p67-*phox*, support this hypothesis, in that they showed diminished levels of peak A but normal levels of peak B.

Neither peak A nor peak B were detected when p47-*phox*-deficient cytosol was subjected to gel filtration chromatography. Instead, there was a single unique peak (designated A′), with a molecular mass of approximately 212 kDa, that was associated with the presence of p67-*phox* based on protein immunoblots and positive complementation of fractions with p67-*phox*-deficient cytosol. After chromatography of cytosol from a carrier of p47-*phox*-deficient CGD, the activity and molecular mass of peak A were normal, but peak B was severely diminished under all assay conditions. In the cell-free oxidase activation assay, cytosol from this carrier had normal activity, suggesting that the pool of p47-*phox* associated with peak B in normal cytosol may represent a reservoir of excess protein. These results are summarized in Table VIII.

When estimating protein molecular mass by gel filtration there are always potential pitfalls that must be considered, such as the aberrant behavior of nonglobular proteins. Even so, the observation that the high molecular mass complex in p47-*phox*-deficient cytosol elutes at 212 kDa rather than 260 kDa (a difference of 48 kDa) strongly suggests that the normal peak A complex contains a single unit of p47-*phox*. It has been estimated that neutrophils contain two to three times as much p47-*phox* as p67-*phox* (Table IV) (54). As all of the p67-*phox* and about half of the p47-*phox* appears to be associated with the peak A complex (from semiquantitative immunoblots), then this complex must contain approximately equal amounts of the two proteins. Therefore, if there is a single unit of p47-*phox* in the complex there must also be only one unit of p67-*phox*. This would leave over 140 kDa of mass unaccounted for and suggests, as mentioned above, that the single unit of p67-*phox* is vital for integrity of the peak A complex. So far attempts to identify the other components of peak A have proved unsuccessful, partly due to the apparent instability of the complex on subsequent chromatography. Somewhat unexpectedly, we found that p47-*phox* is not alone in contributing to the oxidase-stimulating activity of peak B. The fractions in this region from an experiment using p47-*phox*-deficient CGD cytosol, while having very little activity in the presence of a threshold amount of cytosol, did synergize strongly with peak A from normal cytosol. At present the nature of this approximately 50-kDa species is unknown, but it may represent a dimeric form of the low molecular mass GTP-binding protein, *rac*2, or a complex of *rac*2 and one of its effector proteins [e.g., rho GDP-dissociation inhibitor (GDI)]. Protein immunoblotting has localized *rac*2 exclusively to the fractions in the region of peak B (P. G. Heyworth, P. Peveri, and J. T. Curnutte, 1992, unpublished observation). The role of *rac*2 in the regulation of NADPH oxidase activity is discussed below in Section VIII.

VII. Cytoskeletal Involvement in NADPH Oxidase

There is now overwhelming evidence, both direct and circumstantial, for the involvement of the cytoskeleton in NADPH oxidase activity. The studies of Quinn and co-workers (55) provided an elegant demonstration of the association between the O_2^--generating enzyme complex and cytoskeletal elements in a heavy plasma membrane fraction isolated from

PMA-activated neutrophils. This fraction was heavily enriched in actin and fodrin, and contained nearly all of the membrane-bound flavin as well as the O_2^--generating activity. Interestingly, it contained only about 25% of the total cellular cytochrome b_{558}. (This final observation agreed with previous evidence and suggests that at any given moment there is a large pool of the cytochrome not involved in oxygen reduction). The actin and O_2^--generating activity remained associated with each other even after detergent extraction of the heavy plasma membrane fraction, and both were found in the detergent-insoluble pellet fractions.

Similar results have been reported by Woodman *et al.* (56), who also found, using protein immunoblotting, that p67-*phox* was associated with the cytoskeletal (detergent-insoluble) fraction, while p47-*phox* was in the detergent-soluble fraction, irrespective of the activation state of the oxidase. This raises the possibility that although p47-*phox* is clearly required for activation of NADPH oxidase, it may not be a component of the enzymatically active complex. However, in sharp contrast, Nauseef and colleagues (57) have shown that more than half of the p47-*phox* became associated with the cytoskeletal pellet when neutrophils were stimulated with PMA and solubilized in 1% Triton X-100. Under the same disruption conditions, all the p67-*phox* was present in the cytoskeletal fraction of both resting and PMA-stimulated cells. As described above (Section V), when neutrophils were disrupted in relaxation buffer, both p47-*phox* and p67-*phox* were found exclusively in the cytosolic fraction of resting neutrophils, and a portion (~10%) of each protein was localized in the membrane fraction of stimulated neutrophils.

Although there are apparent inconsistencies between some of these observations on the subcellular localization of p47-*phox* and p67-*phox*, their interaction with cytoskeletal elements, and their presence in high molecular mass, cytosolic complexes, it is possible to form an hypothesis that unifies these findings. Rather than being dispersed throughout the cytosol, p47-*phox* and p67-*phox* are probably linked to the submembranous cytoskeleton and therefore in close proximity to the membrane components of the oxidase with which they most interact. Translocation would thus represent an increase in the affinity of these proteins, held in a preformed complex in the cytoskeletal matrix, for the oxidase components in the plasma membrane. When neutrophils are disrupted in relaxation buffer (by sonication or nitrogen cavitation), the intact complex containing p47-*phox* and p67-*phox* dissociates from the cytoskeleton. All the p67-*phox* and about half the p47-*phox* are in the complex, with the remaining p47-*phox* apparently in a monomeric uncomplexed form. (The role of this free p47-*phox* is unclear, but it is possible that it dissociates from an even larger complex.) Disruption of unstimulated neutrophils with Triton X-100, on the other hand, produces a soluble fraction containing all the p47-*phox* and a pellet containing cytoskeletal elements and p67-*phox*. Under these conditions, it would appear that the bonds between p47-*phox* and p67-*phox* are preferentially broken by the detergent, while the association between p67-*phox* and the cytoskeleton remains intact. Activation of NADPH oxidase prior to disruption serves to strengthen the binding of p47-*phox* to p67-*phox* and/or cytoskeletal proteins, and to promote association of p47-*phox*, p67-*phox*, and possibly other components with the membrane.

Neither the nature of the interaction between the cytosolic NADPH oxidase components and cytoskeletal proteins, nor the identities of the cytoskeletal proteins involved, are clear at present. However, the presence in both p47-*phox* and p67-*phox* of two domains (each ~50 residues) with homology to the *src* family of nonreceptor tyrosine kinases (SH3 regions) probably provides a clue. SH3 regions are also present in a wide variety of proteins, as mentioned in Section III, all of which are known to interact with the cytoskeleton, and many of which directly interact with actin (32). Figure 4 shows the SH3 regions of p47-*phox* and p67-*phox* aligned with the SH3 regions of several other proteins, with homologous and highly conserved amino acids indicated. Taking into account both identical residues and conservative substitutions, levels of homology between the SH3 regions of the cytosolic oxidase components and the other proteins are as high as 62% (e.g., between the second SH3 region of p67-*phox* and ABP1 of yeast). So far there is no direct evidence that interaction of p47-*phox* and p67-*phox* with the cytoskeleton, be it constitutive or stimulus-dependent, is mediated through the SH3 regions.

VIII. GTP-Binding Proteins Involved in NADPH Oxidase

A. Nucleotide Requirement of NADPH Oxidase

Over recent years a body of evidence has developed implicating adenine and/or guanine nucleotides in NADPH oxidase activation. First, ATP, but not its nonhydrolyzable analog adenylyl imidodiphosphate (AppNHp), is essential for activation of NADPH oxidase in electropermeabilized human neutrophils. This finding is consistent with the observation discussed above (Section IV) that p47-*phox* is phosphorylated at multiple sites on activation of intact cells by PMA and that this modification appears to be essential for activation (rather than just being a conse-

```
                    * * *   *             *   * *         * *   * *   * * *     *     *                 *     *     * *   * * *
p47-phox       163  A I A D Y E K T S G S E - M A L S T G D - V V E K S E K S E S G W W F C Q M K - - A K R G W I P A S F L E
p47-phox       233  A I K A Y T A V E G D E - V S L L E G E - A V E V I H K L L D G W W V I R   K D D - V T G Y F P S M Y L Q
p67-phox       247  V L F G F V P E T K E E - L Q V M P G N - I V F V L K K G N D N W A T V M F N - - G Q K G L V P C N Y L E
p67-phox       464  A L F S Y E A T Q P E D - L E F Q E G D - I I L V L S K V N E E W L E G E C K - - G K V G I F P K V F V E
GAP            286  A I L P Y T K V P D T D E I S F L K G D - M F I V H N E L K D G W M W V T N L R T D E Q G L I V E D L V E
α-spectrin     974  A L Y D Y Q E K S P R E - V T M K K G D - I L T L L N S T N K D W W K V E - V N D R Q - G F V P A A Y V K
ABP1           539  A E Y D Y D A A E D N E - L T F V E N D K I I - N I E F V D D D W W L G E L E K D G S K G L F P S N Y V S
myoIB          983  A L Y D F A A E N P D E - L T F N E G A - V V T V I N K S N P D W W E G E L - - N G Q R G V F P A S Y V E
myoI Dict.    1060  A L Y D Y D A S S T D E - L S F K E G D - I I F I V Q K D N G G W T Q G E L K - S G Q K G W A P T N Y L Q
c-src           88  A L Y D Y E S R T E T D - L S F K K G E - R L Q I V N N T E G D W W L A H S L T T G Q T G Y I P S N Y V A
```

FIGURE 4

The SH3 domains of p47-*phox* and p67-*phox* aligned with those of other proteins. GAP, GTPase-activating protein; α-spectrin, human nonerythroid α-spectrin; ABP1, yeast actin-binding protein; myoIB, *Acanthamoeba* myosin IB; myoI Dict., *Dictyostelium* myosin I; c-*src*, human *src*-like nonreceptor tyrosine kinase. Letters in bold type represent residues where the level of homology (identical plus highly conserved amino acids) is at least 70% within this group of ten SH3 domains; the columns are also marked by asterisks. Numbers refer to the first amino acid in each sequence.

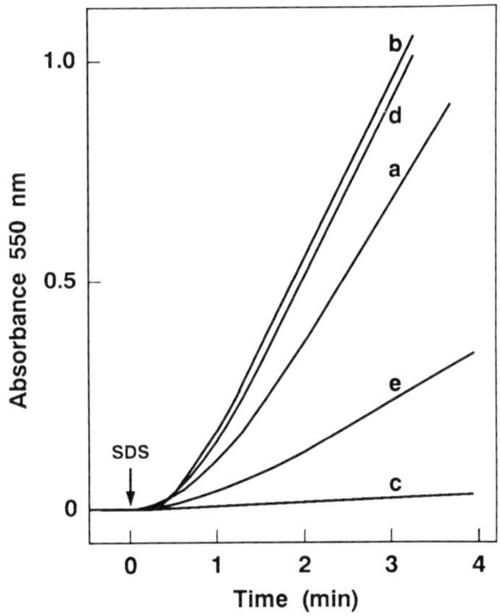

FIGURE 5

Time courses of O_2^- production using untreated (a and b) or dialyzed (c, d, and e) neutrophil cytosol in a cell-free activation system. At the beginning of a 3-min preincubation period, reaction mixtures were supplemented with the following: a, buffer; b, 10 μM GTPγS; c, buffer; d, 10 μM GTPγS; e, 100 μM ATP. NADPH oxidase activation was initiated by the addition of 40 μM SDS. The maximal rates of O_2^- production were as follows (in nmol O_2^-/min/10^7 cell eq. membrane): a, 42.8; b, 53.9; c, 1.3; d, 53.9; e, 14.9. GTPγS completely restored activity of the dialyzed cytosol. [Reprinted from Peveri *et al.* (60) with permission.]

quence of it). In cell-free NADPH oxidase activation systems, the role of protein phosphorylation remains unclear. Although one group has demonstrated a requirement for ATP in such a system, other investigators using similar systems have found no such requirement. Second, several groups have shown that GTP, or its nonhydrolyzable analog GTPγS, can cause a 2- to 4-fold enhancement in O_2^- production in cell-free systems (51,58,59). The problem with these experiments is that they involved the addition of exogenous nucleotides of unknown purity to reaction mixtures already rich in both endogenous nucleotides and the enzymes capable of interconverting them.

Using extensive dialysis and charcoal treatment to remove endogenous nucleotides from human neutrophil cytosol, we recently reexamined the role of GTP in the cell-free system (60). Figure 5 (trace a) shows

TABLE IX

Guanine and Adenine Nucleotide Concentrations in Neutrophil Cytosol[a]

	Nucleotide concentration (μM)			
Cytosol treatment	GTP	GDP	GMP	ATP
None	21.4 ± 4.2	2.56 ± 0.14	<0.2	548.1 ± 35.7
Dialyzed	0.13 ± 0.02	1.01 ± 0.04	<0.2	2.72 ± 0.50
Dialyzed/charcoal	0.08 ± 0.02	0.67 ± 0.05	<0.1	0.86 ± 0.14

[a] The nucleotide concentrations in the cytosols from three different normal donors were determined by anion-exchange HPLC. Each cytosol was divided into three aliquots. Of these three, two were dialyzed overnight at 4°C and one was kept at 4°C for the same length of time. One of the dialyzed samples was then treated with charcoal as described (60). The GMP peak could not always be clearly distinguished from other nucleotide peaks, and its concentration, therefore, could not always be precisely determined. Results are expressed as means ± SD of the data obtained with the cytosol of the three donors. [From Peveri *et al.* (60) with permission.]

a normal time course of O_2^- production initiated with 40 μM SDS in a cell-free activation reaction containing undialyzed cytosol. The potentiation of NADPH oxidase activity achieved with 10 μM GTPγS is shown in trace b. In this instance, the enhancement was approximately 25%. No effect was seen when 100 μM ATP was used (not shown). When cytosol was extensively dialyzed, activity was almost completely lost (trace c), but it could be fully restored by the addition of 10 μM GTPγS (trace d). GTP and guanylyl imidodiphosphate (GppNHp) were equally as effective, whereas 100 μM ATP could only partially restore activity to the dialyzed cytosol (trace e) and AppNHp was ineffective. Although low in activity, ATP (but not AppNHp) was able to act synergistically with 10 μM GMP or GDP (either of which alone did not support O_2^- production in dialyzed cytosol) to restore oxidase activity to the level achieved with GTP alone. When a suboptimal concentration of GTP (0.1 μM) and 100 μM ATP were used in combination, the effect was only additive.

Taken together, these results suggested that phosphate transfer from ATP to GDP or GMP, with the formation of GTP, could account for the oxidase activity observed in dialyzed cytosol in the presence of ATP. They also predicted that GMP and GDP levels in dialyzed cytosol would be high enough to allow the ATP-dependent generation of GTP to reach the levels required for oxidase activation. Anion-exchange high-performance liquid chromatography (HPLC) analysis of dialyzed cytosols confirmed this prediction (Table IX); the concentration of GDP was

TABLE X

Nucleotide Reconstitution of NADPH Oxidase Activation in the Cell-Free System Using Charcoal-Treated Dialyzed Cytosol[a]

	O_2^- production (nmol O_2^-/min/10^7 cell eq. membrane) using	
Nucleotide added (μM)	Dialyzed cytosol	Charcoal-treated dialyzed cytosol
None	0.6 ± 0.1	0
GTPγS (10)	42.7 ± 2.0	33.7 ± 1.8
GTP (10)	26.0 ± 2.7	17.3 ± 1.3
ATP (100)	8.1 ± 2.1	1.2 ± 0.2
ATP (100) + GDP (10)	24.9 ± 2.6	17.6 ± 1.5
ATP (100) + GMP (10)	27.4 ± 0.8	16.5 ± 2.8

[a] Each reaction contained 1.0 × 10^7 cell eq./ml of either dialyzed or charcoal-treated dialyzed cytosol. Reaction mixtures containing charcoal-treated dialyzed cytosol also included membranes that were incubated with charcoal as described (60). Nucleotides were added to the reaction mixtures at the beginning of the 3-min preincubation to give the final concentrations shown. Results are expressed as means ± SD of three experiments, each using cytosol from a different donor. [From Peveri *et al.* (60) with permission.]

1 μM, which if converted to GTP by ATP would support intermediate rates of O_2^- production similar to those seen when ATP alone was added to dialyzed cytosol (see trace e, Fig. 5).

As evident from Table IX, GDP was much more difficult to remove by dialysis than either GTP or ATP, presumably because more of it is bound with high affinity to cytosolic proteins (neutrophil cytosol is known to be rich in GTP-binding proteins). In an attempt to reduce the levels of nucleotides still further, dialyzed cytosol was treated with activated charcoal, analyzed by HPLC, and then assayed for its ability to support oxidase activation. The levels of all measured nucleotides were further decreased by this charcoal treatment (Table IX). Under these conditions, there was no O_2^- production in the absence of added nucleotides. In contrast to the previous experiments using dialyzed-only cytosol, the addition of 100 μM ATP now resulted in barely detectable levels of activity (Table X). However, when either GMP or GDP was added in combination with ATP, activity was restored to the rate seen with GTP alone, indicating that ATP is active only when small amounts of GMP or GDP are available for conversion to GTP. Such a conversion was directly demonstrated by HPLC analysis of nucleotides in complete reaction mixtures, where, following a 5-min incubation (during which O_2^- production was measured), over 75% of GDP or GMP (initially at 10 μM) was converted to GTP in the presence of ATP. The rate of O_2^- production paralleled the final concentration of GTP achieved.

Taken together, these experiments show that ATP is neither necessary nor sufficient for activation of NADPH oxidase in the cell-free system. The apparent stimulatory effect of ATP is due to the presence of ATP-dependent enzymes in neutrophil cytosol capable of interconverting guanine nucleotides (e.g., guanylate kinase and nucleoside diphosphate kinase). Such interconversions have been demonstrated experimentally, as described above. These results do not, however, preclude a role for ATP in NADPH oxidase activation in *intact* cells. Two pathways of activation may exist, one that is ATP-dependent and functional only in intact cells (e.g., protein phosphorylation) and another that does not require ATP and is operative in both intact cells and cell-free systems. What clearly emerges from these experiments is that there is an absolute requirement for GTP (or one of its analogs) for NADPH oxidase activation in the cell-free system. Kinetic studies in this system indicated that GTP is required at or before the rate-limiting step, and that a catalytic complex cannot assemble without it. It was also apparent that GTP itself did not represent one of the kinetically distinct components of neutrophil cytosol. Superoxide generation increases as the 2.5-power of the cytosol concentration, and this value did not change over a 1000-fold range of GTP concentrations.

B. Low Molecular Mass GTP-Binding Proteins Implicated in the Regulation of NADPH Oxidase

What is the molecular mediator of the GTP requirement, and is it one of the elusive cytosolic components of NADPH oxidase? The ability of nonhydrolyzable guanine nucleotides (GTPγS and GppNHp) not only to replace GTP but to exceed it in activity suggests the involvement of one or more GTP-binding proteins in NADPH oxidase activation. Furthermore, inhibition of protein isoprenylation with compactin during dimethyl sulfoxide (DMSO)-induced differentiation of HL-60 cells blocked the ability of the cells to generate O_2^- when stimulated with PMA or FMLP (61). As discussed below, posttranslational prenylation is an important modification of many GTP-binding proteins.

Recent reports suggest that the GTP effect on NADPH oxidase is, at least in part, mediated through a cytosolic component (62). With this in mind, we recently purified and identified a low molecular mass GTP-binding protein from human neutrophil cytosol on the basis of its ability both to bind [^{35}S]GTPγS and to enhance O_2^- generation in the presence of threshold amounts of normal cytosol (63). After purification to near homogeneity by a combination of anion-exchange, gel filtration, and hydrophobic interaction chromatography, the protein (designated G_{ox}) migrated on SDS-PAGE as a single band with a molecular mass of 21 to 22 kDa. The known cytosolic NADPH oxidase components, p47-*phox* and p67-*phox*, as assessed by protein immunoblotting, were separated from G_{ox} at an early stage in the purification. Purified G_{ox} was electrophoretically transferred to nitrocellulose, digested with trypsin, and the amino acid sequences of four peptide fragments determined and compared to the sequences of other GTP-binding proteins. The sequences of all four peptides were identical to stretches of the amino acid sequence predicted from the cDNA encoding *rac*2, a member of the rho family of low molecular mass GTP-binding proteins, previously cloned and identified as being myeloid cell-specific, but of unknown function (64). Within the sequences of the four peptides there were three amino acid residues which differed from the predicted primary structure of *rac*1, a very closely related protein having 92% homology with *rac*2 (Fig. 6, Table XI). In addition, an antibody to a peptide corresponding to the C-terminal region of *rac*2 bound to G_{ox} on protein immunoblots, whereas an antibody to the equivalent peptide of *rac*1 did not. When added to a cell-free NADPH oxidase system containing a threshold amount of cytosol (sufficient to provide at least a small amount of all the components required) 22 pmol of purified *rac*2 caused a 2.5-fold enhancement of the basal level of O_2^- production (Table XII). This augmentation was concentration-dependent and was seen with either intact membrane vesicles or with deoxycholate-solubilized membranes.

*rac*2 is not the only low molecular mass GTP-binding protein that has been implicated in NADPH oxidase activation. rap1A (also known as Krev1), a member of the *ras* family of proteins with about 50% homology to human K-*ras* (Table XI, Fig. 6), is found in the human neutrophil membrane physically associated with the gp91-*phox* and p22-*phox* subunits of cytochrome b_{558} (65). The biological function of rap1A is unknown, but Bokoch and colleagues recently showed that its association with cytochrome b_{558} is modulated by its phosphorylation state (66). Phosphorylation by cAMP-dependent protein kinase at Ser^{180}, near the C terminus of the protein, greatly diminished the ability of rap1A to form a complex with the cytochrome. In another report, a truncated, recombinant form of rap1A (lacking residues 167–184) restored NADPH oxidase activity to cytosol immunodepleted with a monoclonal antibody which recognizes the conserved GTP-binding site of low molecular mass

```
                          10                  20                  30
rac1    M Q A I K C V V V G D G A V G K T C L L I S Y T T N A F P G
        * * * * * * * * * * * * * * * * * * * * * * * * * * * * * *
rac2    M Q A I K C V V V G D G A V G K T C L L I S Y T T N A F P G
        *       *   * *   *   *   * * *     *                 *
rap1A   M R E Y K L V V L G S G G V G K S A L T V Q F V Q G I F V E

                          40                  50                  60
rac1    E Y I P T V F D N Y S A N V M V D G K P V N L G L W D T A G
        * * * * * * * * * * * * * * * * *   * * * * * * * * * * * *
rac2    E Y I P T V F D N Y S A N V M V D S K P V N L G L W D T A G
          *   * *     *   *       *   * *           *       * * * *
rap1A   K Y D P T I E D S Y R K Q V E V D C Q Q C M L E I L D T A G

                          70                  80                  90
rac1    Q E D Y D R L R P L S Y P Q T D V F L I C F S L V S P A S F
        * * * * * * * * * * * * * * * * * * * * * * * * * * * * *
rac2    Q E D Y D R L R P L S Y P Q T D V F L I C F S L V S P A S Y
          *           *   *               *         *
rap1A   T E Q F T A M R D L Y M K N G G G F A L V Y S I T A Q S T F

                         100                 110
rac1    E N V R A K W Y P E V R H H C P - N T P I I L V G T K L D L
        * * * * * * *   * * *   * * * *       * * * * * * * * * * * *
rac2    E N V R A K W F P E V T H H C P - S T P I I L V G T K L D L
                                              *   * * * *   *   * *
rap1A   N D L Q D L R E Q I L R V K D T E D V P M I L V G N K C D L

       120                 130                 140
rac1    R D D K D T I E K L K E K K L T P I T Y P Q G L A M A K E I
        * * * * * * * * * * * * * * *   * * * * * * * * *   * * * *
rac2    R D D K D T I E K L K E K K L A P I T Y P Q G L A L A K E I
          *
rap1A   E D E - - - - - - - - - - - - - R V V G K E Q G Q N L A R Q

       150                 160                   170
rac1    G A - V K Y L E C S A L T Q R G L K T V F D E A I R A V L -
              * * * * * * * * * * * * * * * * * * * * * * * * * *
rac2    D S - V K Y L E C S A L T Q R G L K T V F D E A I R A V L -
                  * * *   * *                   *         *
rap1A   W C N C A F L E S S A K S K I N V N E I F Y D L V R Q I N R

               180                 190
rac1    - - C P P P V K K R K R K C L L L
            * *   *         * *   *   * *
rac2    - - C P Q P T R Q Q K R A C S L L
                            *     *   * *
rap1A   K T P V E K K K P K K K S C L L L
                                ↑
```

GTP-binding proteins (67). Full-length baculovirus-expressed rap1A had no detectable stimulatory activity in a similar system (63).

In elicited guinea pig macrophages, Pick and colleagues have identified a cytosolic oxidase component distinct from p47-*phox* termed $\sigma1$ (68). The active components of $\sigma1$ have recently been identified as *rac*1 and rhoGDI (Table XI) (69). The addition of partially purified recombinant *rac*1 (in the GTPγS-bound form) and purified $\sigma1$ enhanced O_2^- production approximately 3-fold in a macrophage cell-free oxidase activation system in which $\sigma1$-depleted cytosol was employed (69). The activity of either native or recombinant *rac*2 was not tested in this system.

The predicted amino acid sequences of *rac*1, *rac*2, and rap1A are shown aligned in Fig. 6, with important functional domains marked. The C-terminal CAAX domain (underlined; where C is cysteine, A is an aliphatic residue, and X is almost any amino acid) and the regions associated with guanine nucleotide binding (boxed) are highly conserved throughout the *ras* superfamily of proteins (70). The cysteine of the CAAX domain is the site of posttranslational covalent modifications which attach either 15- or 20-carbon isoprenoid groups that are important in the subcellular localization of the molecule. In the case of these three proteins, a 20-carbon geranylgeranyl group is attached, followed by proteolytic cleavage of the AAX residues and methylation of the terminal cysteine residue. In Fig. 6, the dashed underline (*rac* residues 31–44) indicates the putative effector region thought to be the site of interaction of *ras* proteins with their respective GTPase-activating proteins (GAP). The sequences of *rac*1 and *rac*2 in this region are identical, indicating that they may be regulated by the same GAP.

Table XI summarizes additional properties of *rac*1, *rac*2, and rap1A as well as those for the effector protein rho GDI which copurified with

FIGURE 6

Alignment of predicted amino acid sequences of three low molecular mass GTP-binding proteins (*rac*1, *rac*2, and rap1A) that have been implicated in the regulation of phagocyte NADPH oxidase activity. The numbering of residues refers to *rac*1 and *rac*2. Homology with *rac*2 is indicated by asterisks. Four domains and two single, highly conserved residues involved in guanine nucleotide binding are boxed. The dashed underline (residues 31–44) indicates the putative GAP-binding region, and the solid line indicates the domain involved in posttranslational covalent modification and membrane attachment. The serine indicated by the arrow near the C terminus of rap1A is phosphorylated by cAMP-dependent protein kinase.

TABLE XI

Properties of the Low Molecular Mass GTP-Binding Proteins and the Effector Protein Implicated in Phagocyte NADPH Oxidase Activation

Property	GTP-Binding proteins			Effector protein, rho GDI[a]
	*rac*1	*rac*2	rap1A/Krev 1	
Amino acids	192	192	184	204
Molecular mass (kDa)				
Predicted	21.4	21.4	20.9	23.4
By PAGE	22	22	22	26
p*I*[b]	8.5	7.6	6.5	4.9
mRNA	1.1 kb, 2.4 kb	1.45 kb	1.6 kb	1.9 kb
Cellular location[c]	Cytosol	Cytosol	Membrane	Cytosol
Tissue specificity	Myeloid and other	Myeloid	Widespread	Widespread
Covalent modification	Isoprenylation	Isoprenylation	Isoprenylation phosphorylation	
Homology	92% with *rac*2 58% with rho ~30% with *ras*	92% with *rac*1 58% with rho ~30% with *ras*	<30% with *rac*1/2 <30% with rho ~50% with *ras*	Weak with *ras* GAP

[a] Rho GDI, GDP dissociation inhibitor for rho proteins.
[b] Calculated from the amino acid sequences (see text for references).
[c] For resting cells; subcellular localization may vary with activation state of the cell and method of cellular disruption.

TABLE XII

Enhancement of Superoxide Generation in the Cell-Free NADPH Oxidase Assay by the Low Molecular Mass GTP-Binding Protein *rac*2

Addition to reaction mixture[a]	Rate of O_2^- generation (nmol/min/10^7 cell eq. membrane)			
	Exp. 1	Exp. 2	Exp. 3	Exp. 4
None	6.68	4.24	3.27	4.02
*rac*2	17.90	14.00	7.80	11.22
*rac*2 buffer	8.29	7.80	2.50	6.06
Increase (-fold)	2.4	2.5	2.6	2.3

[a] *Rac*2 purified from neutrophil cytosol, or an equivalent volume of buffer, was added to NADPH oxidase reaction mixtures containing a threshold amount of neutrophil cytosol and membrane vesicles (Exp. 1) or deoxycholate-solubilized membranes (Exp. 2–4). [For full details see Knaus et al. (63), from which this table was reprinted, with permission.]

*rac*1 (see above). Of particular interest is the highly specific expression of *rac*2 mRNA in cells of myeloid origin (monocytes, neutrophils). *rac*1 and rap1A mRNA, on the other hand, are expressed in a number of different cell types. This may indicate that *rac*2 has some special function in phagocytic cells. Also of note is the predicted isoelectric point (p*I*) for *rac*2 of 7.6 In earlier work from our group, preparative isoelectric focusing of neutrophil cytosol resulted in four peaks of NADPH oxidase-enhancing activity with approximate pI values of 3.1, 6.0, 7.1, and 9.5 (22). Two of these components, with p*I* values of 6.0 and 9.5, have been identified as p67-*phox* and p47-*phox*, respectively. The p*I* of 7.1 reported for one of the unidentified components is similar to the p*I* calculated for *rac*2.

At present it is unclear whether the identification of *rac*2 as a regulator of O_2^- generation in human neutrophils, and of *rac*1 as having a similar role in guinea pig macrophages, represents a species difference or can be accounted for by the difference in cell type.It is possible that both of these highly homologous proteins have an important role in the regulation of NADPH oxidase activation in the same cell. The greatest divergence between the sequences of *rac*1 and *rac*2 occurs between residues 180 and 190 (see Fig. 6), a region that is hypervariable throughout the *ras* superfamily and that has been implicated in the interaction with at least two effector proteins, namely,

GDP dissociation inhibitor (GDI) and GDP dissociation stimulator (GDS). Variability between *rac*1 and *rac*2 within this region suggests that they are controlled by different effector proteins and may therefore have subtly different functions.

It is worth noting at this point that other members of the rho family, to which *rac*1 and *rac*2 are very closely related, have been implicated in the organization of the cytoskeleton (71). Given the apparent involvement of the cytoskeleton in NADPH oxidase activity, and the potential of *rac* proteins to become inserted into the membrane by virtue of their C-terminal isoprenoid groups, it is interesting to speculate that these proteins may, in some way, regulate the association between cytoskeletal proteins and the cytosolic and membrane-bound oxidase components.

Irrespective of their identity and exact physiological function, it is likely that any NADPH oxidase-related, GTP-binding protein operates in the manner outlined in Fig. 7, based on current knowledge of how

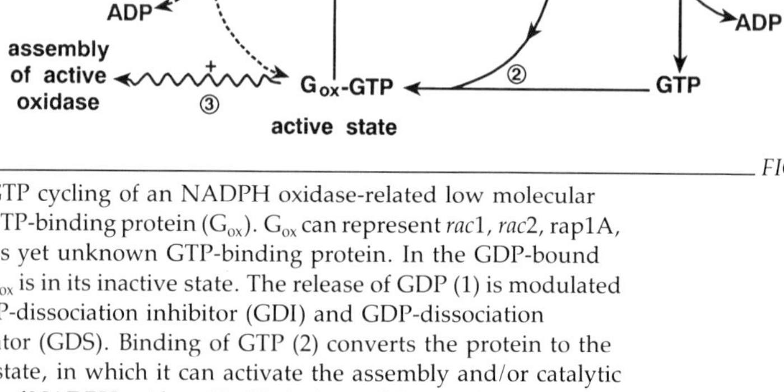

FIGURE 7

GDP/GTP cycling of an NADPH oxidase-related low molecular mass GTP-binding protein (G_{ox}). G_{ox} can represent *rac*1, *rac*2, rap1A, or an as yet unknown GTP-binding protein. In the GDP-bound form G_{ox} is in its inactive state. The release of GDP (1) is modulated by GDP-dissociation inhibitor (GDI) and GDP-dissociation stimulator (GDS). Binding of GTP (2) converts the protein to the active state, in which it can activate the assembly and/or catalytic activity of NADPH oxidase (3). Hydrolysis of GTP to GDP (4) causes G_{ox} to revert to its inactive form. By analogy with other low molecular mass GTP-binding proteins, this step is likely to be regulated by a GTPase-activating protein (GAP). Freed GDP can be phosphorylated by nucleoside diphosphate kinase (NDPK) to GTP (5). There is also recent evidence that GDP bound to GTP-binding proteins can be phosphorylated by NDPK (6), although in this scheme this step is entirely speculative.

low molecular mass GTP-binding proteins function (71). In response to a stimulus, GDP is released from G_{ox} (step 1) which is now free to bind GTP (step 2). [*Ras*-like proteins typically have similar affinities for GDP and GTP, but GTP is present at much higher concentrations (~10-fold; see Table IX) and is therefore preferentially bound (71)]. GDP dissociation is modulated by GDI and GDS. The former prevents dissociation and thus renders G_{ox} inactive while the latter has the opposite effects. GTP binding is associated with a conformational change which in some way transduces the signal to associated proteins, thus activating NADPH oxidase (step 3). The G_{ox}–GTP complex remains active until GTP is hydrolyzed by the intrinsic GTPase activity of G_{ox}, which is probably stimulated by a GAP (step 4). Recent reports indicate that nucleoside diphosphate kinase, which can convert free GDP to GTP in the presence of ATP (or another nucleoside triphosphate) (step 5), can also phosphorylate bound GDP, thereby directly activating GTP-binding proteins (72) (step 6).

IX. Other Potential NADPH Oxidase Components

Despite the enormous advances that have been made recently in our understanding of the phagocyte NADPH oxidase, particularly with regard to the characterization of the cytosolic components of the system, it is still impossible to ascribe specific functions to them. It appears unlikely that either p47-*phox* or p67-*phox* is the elusive flavoprotein component, since the predicted amino acid sequences do not contain FAD-binding motifs, and neither protein has been found to contain (or bind) FAD, in either its native or recombinant form (33). Indeed it is not even clear whether the flavoprotein and the NADPH-binding component are one and the same molecule, but in view of the close proximity that is necessary for NADPH to reduce the flavin, it seems likely that a single component will play both roles (see Chapter 1). Alternatively, it is possible that these functions are separate and that the cytosolic components serve to bring the NADPH binding site into close alignment with the flavoprotein in the membrane. Two candidate proteins for these functions have so far been identified. One is a 32-kDa cytosolic protein, recently reported to be the NADPH-binding subunit of the oxidase, based on its ability to bind NADPH 2′,3′-dialdehyde and to translocate to the membrane on neutrophil stimulation (73). Whether this protein binds FAD, or whether it associates with a flavoprotein, has not been established. The other is a 45-kDa protein identified by Cross and colleagues (74) that is equally distributed between the cytosol and membrane. This protein contains flavin and is readily labeled with diphenylene iodonium, but it has not been established whether it binds NADPH. Further studies will be required to characterize fully the nature and function of these candidate oxidase components.

Finally, an intriguing recent report suggests that components of NADPH oxidase may serve an additional function (75). The respiratory burst is associated with a substantial rise in metabolic proton generation (76). A fraction of the protons are removed by an Na^+/H^+ exchanger, but, in addition, an H^+ (equivalent) conductance, activated by protein kinase C (concurrently with activation of NADPH oxidase), plays an important role (77). Compared to normal neutrophils, proton conductance in X91° and A47° CGD cells was greatly diminished, suggesting that full assembly of NADPH oxidase is required for activation of the proton conductance in the membrane (75). This raises the possibility that the complete oxidase itself provides the pathway for proton extrusion, or that one or more components or closely associated proteins fulfill this role.

References

1. S. J. Weiss, *N. Engl. J. Med.* **320,** 365–376 (1989).
2. J. T. Curnutte, *Immunodef. Rev.* 3(2), 149–172 (1992).
3. F. Morel, J. Doussiere, and P. V. Vignais, *Eur. J. Biochem.* **201,** 523–546 (1991).
4. A. R. Cross and O. T. G. Jones, *Biochim. Biophys. Acta* **1057,** 281–298 (1991).
5. R. M. Smith and J. T. Curnutte, *Blood* **77,** 673–686 (1991).
6. R. A. Clark, *J. Infect. Dis.* **161,** 1140–1147 (1990).
7. B. M. Babior, *Adv. Enzymol.* **65,** 49–95 (1992).
8. J. T. Curnutte, *in* "Hematologic Disorders of Infancy and Childhood" (D. G. Nathan, ed.), in press, 1992.
9. A. W. Segal, A. R. Cross, R. C. Garcia, N. Borregaard, N. Valerius, J. F. Soothill, and O. T. G. Jones, *N. Engl. J. Med.* **308,** 245–251 (1983).
10. R. S. Weening, L. Corbeel, M. de Boer, R. Lutter, R. van Zwieten, M. N. Hamers, and D. Roos, *J. Clin. Invest.* **75,** 915–920 (1985).
11. C. A. Parkos, R. A. Allen, C. G. Cochrane, and A. J. Jesaitis, *J. Clin. Invest.* **80,** 732–742 (1987).
12. A. W. Segal, *Nature* (*London*) **326,** 88–92 (1987).
13. M. C. Dinauer, S. H. Orkin, R. Brown, A. J. Jesaitis, and C. A. Parkos, *Nature* (*London*) **327,** 717–720 (1987).
14. M. C. Dinauer, E. A. Pierce, G. A. P. Bruns, J. T. Curnutte, and S. H. Orkin, *J. Clin. Invest.* **86,** 1729–1737 (1990).

15. J. T. Curnutte, *J. Clin. Invest.* **75,** 1740–1743 (1985).
16. J. T. Curnutte, R. L. Berkow, R. L. Roberts, S. B. Shurin, and P. J. Scott, *J. Clin. Invest.* **81,** 606–610 (1988).
17. B. M. Babior, R. Kuver, and J. T. Curnutte, *J. Biol. Chem.* **263,** 1713–1718 (1988).
18. H. Nunoi, D. Rotrosen, J. I. Gallin, and H. L. Malech, *Science* **242,** 1298–1301 (1988).
19. R. A. Clark, H. L. Malech, J. I. Gallin, H. Nunoi, B. D. Volpp, D. W. Pearson, W. M. Nauseef, and J. T. Curnutte, *N. Engl. J. Med.* **321,** 647–652 (1989).
20. A. W. Segal, P. G. Heyworth, S. Cockcroft, and M. M. Barrowman, *Nature (London)* **316,** 547–549 (1985).
21. B. D. Volpp, W. M. Nauseef, and R. A. Clark, *Science* **242,** 1295–1297 (1988).
22. J. T. Curnutte, P. J. Scott, and L. A. Mayo, *Proc. Natl. Acad. Sci. U.S.A.* **86,** 825–829 (1989).
23. M. C. Dinauer, J. T. Curnutte, H. Rosen, and S. H. Orkin, *J. Clin. Invest.* **84,** 2012–2016 (1989).
24. B. L. Schapiro, P. E. Newburger, M. S. Klempner, and M. C. Dinauer, *N. Engl. J. Med.* **325,** 1786–1790 (1991).
25. M. C. Dinauer, E. A. Pierce, R. W. Erickson, T. J. Muhlebach, H. Messner, S. H. Orkin, R. A. Seger, and J. T. Curnutte, *Proc. Natl. Acad. Sci. U.S.A.* **88,** 11231–11235 (1991).
26. K. J. Lomax, T. L. Leto, H. Nunoi, J. I. Gallin, and H. L. Malech, *Science* **245,** 409–412 (1989).
27. B. D. Volpp, W. M. Nauseef, J. E. Donelson, D. R. Moser, and R. A. Clark, *Proc. Natl. Acad. Sci. U.S.A.* **86,** 7195–7199 (1989).
28. K. J. Lomax, T. L. Leto, H. Nunoi, J. I. Gallin, and H. L. Malech, *Science* **246,** 987 (1989).
29. B. D. Volpp, W. M. Nauseef, J. E. Donelson, D. R. Moser, and R. A. Clark, *Proc. Natl. Acad. Sci. U.S.A.* **86,** 9563 (1989).
30. P. J. Kennelly and E. G. Krebs, *J. Biol. Chem.* **266,** 15555–15558 (1991).
31. T. Hunter and J. A. Cooper, *Annu. Rev. Biochem.* **54,** 897–930 (1985).
32. C. A. Koch, D. Anderson, M. F. Moran, C. Ellis, and T. Pawson, *Science* **252,** 668–674 (1991).
33. T. L. Leto, K. J. Lomax, B. D. Volpp, H. Nunoi, J. M. G. Sechler, W. M. Nauseef, R. A. Clark, J. I. Gallin, and H. L. Malech, *Science* **248,** 727–730 (1990).
34. C. M. Casimir, H. N. Bu-Ghanim, A. R. F. Rodaway, D. L. Bentley, P. Rowe, and A. W. Segal, *Proc. Natl. Acad. Sci. U.S.A.* **88,** 2753–2757 (1991).
35. S. J. Chanock, D. M. Barrett, J. T. Curnutte, and S. H. Orkin, *Blood* **78,** 165a (Abstr.) (1991).
36. P. G. Heyworth and J. A. Badwey, *J. Bioenerg. Biomembr.* **22,** 1–26 (1990).
37. T. Hayakawa, K. Suzuki, S. Suzuki, P. C. Andrews, and B. M. Babior, *J. Biol. Chem.* **261,** 9109–9115 (1986).
38. I. J. M. Kramer, A. J. Verhoeven, R. L. van der Bend, R. S. Weening, and D. Roos, *J. Biol. Chem.* **263,** 2352–2357 (1988).
39. P. G. Heyworth, C. F. Shrimpton, and A. W. Segal, *Biochem.* **260,** 243–248 (1989).
40. N. Okamura, J. T. Curnutte, R. L. Roberts, and B. M. Babior, *J. Biol. Chem.* **263,** 6777–6782 (1988).
41. J. A. Badwey, J. T. Curnutte, J. M. Robinson, C. B. Berde, M. J. Karnovsky, and M. L. Karnovsky, *J. Biol. Chem.* **259,** 7870–7877 (1984).
42. N. Okamura, S. E. Malawista, R. L. Roberts, H. Rosen, H. D. Ochs, B. M. Babior, and J. T. Curnutte, *Blood* **72,** 811–816 (1988).

43. D. Rotrosen and T. L. Leto, *J. Biol. Chem.* **265,** 19910–19915 (1990).
44. N. Okamura, B. M. Babior, L. A. Mayo, P. Peveri, R. M. Smith, and J. T. Curnutte, *J. Clin. Invest.* **85,** 1583–1587 (1990).
45. J. A. Badwey, J. M. Robinson, P. G. Heyworth, and J. T. Curnutte, *J. Biol. Chem.* **264,** 20676–20682 (1989).
46. J. Ding and J. A. Badwey, *J. Biol. Chem.* **267,** 6442–6448 (1992).
47. R. A. Clark, B. D. Volpp, K. G. Leidal, and W. M. Nauseef, *J. Clin. Invest.* **85,** 714–721 (1990).
48. N. Borregaard, J. M. Heiple, E. R. Simons, and R. A. Clark, *J. Cell Biol.* **97,** 52–61 (1983).
49. P. G. Heyworth, J. T. Curnutte, H. Rosen, W. M. Nauseef, B. D. Volpp, D. W. Pearson, and R. A. Clark, *J. Clin. Invest.* **87,** 352–356 (1991).
50. D. Rotrosen, M. E. Kleinberg, H. Nunoi, T. Leto, J. I. Gallin, and H. L. Malech, *J. Biol. Chem.* **265,** 8745–8750 (1990).
51. T. G. Gabig, D. English, L. P. Akard, and M. J. Schell, *J. Biol. Chem.* **262,** 1685–1690 (1987).
52. J. T. Curnutte, R. Kuver, and P. J. Scott, *J. Biol. Chem.* **262,** 5563–5569 (1987).
53. P. G. Heyworth, J. O. Tolley, R. M. Smith, and J. T. Curnutte, *Blood* **76,** 183a (Abstr.) (1990).
54. T. L. Leto, M. C. Garrett, H. Fujii, and H. Nunoi, *J. Biol. Chem.* **266,** 19812–19818 (1991).
55. M. T. Quinn, C. A. Parkos, and A. J. Jesaitis, *Biochim. Biophys. Acta* **987,** 83–94 (1989).
56. R. C. Woodman, J. M. Ruedi, A. J. Jesaitis, N. Okamura, M. T. Quinn, R. M. Smith, J. T. Curnutte, and B. M. Babior, *J. Clin. Invest.* **87,** 1345–1351 (1991).
57. W. N. Nauseef, B. D. Volpp, S. McCormick, K. G. Leidal, and R. A. Clark, *J. Biol. Chem.* **266,** 5911–5917 (1991).
58. R. Seifert, G. Schultz, and W. Rosenthal, *FEBS Lett.* **205,** 161–165 (1986).
59. E. Ligeti, J. Doussiere, and P. V. Vignais, *Biochem. J.* **27,** 193–200 (1988).
60. P. Peveri, P. G. Heyworth, and J. T. Curnutte, *Proc. Natl. Acad. Sci. U.S.A.* **89,** 2494–2498 (1992).
61. G. M. Bokoch and V. Prossnitz, *J. Clin. Invest.* **89,** 402–408 (1992).
62. B. G. J. M. Bolscher, S. W. Denis, A. J. Verhoeven, and D. Roos, *J. Biol. Chem.* **265,** 15782–15787 (1990).
63. U. G. Knaus, P. G. Heyworth, T. Evans, J. T. Curnutte, and G. M. Bokoch, *Science* **254,** 1512–1515 (1991).
64. J. Didsbury, R. F. Weber, G. M. Bokoch, T. Evans, and R. Snyderman, *J. Biol. Chem.* **264,** 16378–16382 (1989).
65. M. T. Quinn, C. A. Parkos, L. Walker, S. H. Orkin, M. C. Dinauer, and A. J. Jesaitis, *Nature (London)* **342,** 198–200 (1989).
66. G. M. Bokoch, L. A. Quilliam, B. P. Bohl, A. J. Jesaitis, and M. T. Quinn, *Science* **254,** 1794–1796 (1991).
67. E. A. Eklund, M. Marshall, J. B. Gibbs, C. D. Crean, and T. G. Gabig, *J. Biol. Chem.* **266,** 13964–13970 (1991).
68. E. Pick, T. Kroizman, and A. Abo, *J. Immunol.* **143,** 4180–4187 (1989).
69. A. Abo, E. Pick, A. Hall, N. Totty, C. G. Teahan, and A. W. Segal, *Nature (London)* **353,** 668–670 (1991).
70. A. Valencia, P. Chardin, A. Wittinghofer, and C. Sander, *Biochemistry* **30,** 4637–4648 (1991).
71. H. Haubruck and F. McCormick, *Biochim. Biophys. Acta* **1072,** 215–229 (1991).
72. P. A. Randazzo, J. K. Northup, and R. A. Kahn, *Science* **254,** 850–853 (1991).

73. T. Umei, B. M. Babior, J. T. Curnutte, and R. M. Smith, *J. Biol. Chem.* **266,** 6019–6022 (1991).
74. C. M. Yea, A. R. Cross, and O. T. G. Jones, *Biochem. J.* **265,** 95–100 (1990).
75. A. Nanda, S. Grinstein, and J. T. Curnutte, *FASEB J.* **6,** A1428 (Abstr.) (1992).
76. L. M. Henderson, J. B. Chappell, and O. T. G. Jones, *Biochem. J.* **246,** 325–329 (1987).
77. A. Nanda and S. Grinstein, *Proc. Natl. Acad. Sci. U.S.A.* **88,** 10816–10820 (1991).

CHAPTER 4

Generation of Reactive Species by Vascular Endothelium

Rafael Radi,[1,2*] Peter C. Panus,[1,4] James A. Royall,[3] Andrés Paler-Martínez,[1,5] and Bruce A. Freeman[1,2,3]

Departments of Anesthesiology,[1] Biochemistry,[2]
Pediatrics,[3] Pharmacology,[4] and Microbiology[5]
University of Alabama at Birmingham
Birmingham, Alabama 35233

I. Introduction

Endothelial cells are critical sources and targets of reactive species in the intravascular compartment. These reactive species include superoxide (O_2^-), hydrogen peroxide (H_2O_2), hydroxyl radical (·OH), and nitric oxide (·NO, endothelial-derived relaxation factor). The rates of production of reactive species by vascular endothelium can be exacerbated during diverse pathophysiological conditions including hyperoxia, inflammatory processes, and ischemia–reperfusion. Both *in vitro* and *in vivo* experiments demonstrate that vascular endothelium is exquisitely sensitive to the toxic effects of reactive oxygen species. Exposure of endothelium to reactive species derived from exogenous sources (i.e.,

* Permanent address: Department of Biochemistry, Faculty of Medicine, University of the Republic, Montevideo, Uruguay CP11800.

xenobiotics), to increased intracellular rates of free radical production (i.e., hyperoxia), or to activated neutrophils results in altered endothelial cell metabolic homeostasis, increased membrane permeability, changes in cell function, and, in some cases, cell death.

Because of their transient and reactive nature, reactive oxygen and nitrogen-centered species are difficult to detect and quantify, presenting a challenge to investigators attempting to define their role in vascular biology and medicine. Herein, we review recent investigations from our laboratory directed toward obtaining a detailed understanding of the metabolism of vascular endothelial-derived reactive species.

II. Identification of Sources and Quantities of Reactive Oxygen Species in Endothelium

Identification and quantitation of reactive species in the biological milieu is not a trivial endeavor, if one considers that these species (1) are intrinsically unstable under physiological conditions, (2) rapidly react with different cellular or extracellular targets, and/or (3) are efficiently enzymatically metabolized. As a consequence, cellular steady-state concentrations of H_2O_2 and O_2^- are very low, normally in the submicromolar range. This presents a challenge in devising and applying detection systems for these reactive species which will effectively compete with other target molecule reactions and efficient cellular antioxidant scavenging systems. In the following sections we summarize the methods we have applied or developed to directly assess the intracellular production and extracellular release of reactive oxygen species in vascular endothelial cells. We also discuss critical aspects and new concepts of endothelial metabolism of reactive species.

A. Nonrespiratory Oxygen Consumption

An initial approach to quantifying intracellular production of O_2^- and H_2O_2 is to measure cellular oxygen consumption in the presence of inhibitors of the mitochondrial electron transport chain. Under normal conditions, more than 95% of cellular oxygen consumption occurs at cytochrome-*c* oxidase, the terminal cytochrome of the respiratory chain, where dioxygen is tetravalently reduced to two molecules of H_2O. Most of the remaining non-cytochrome-*c* oxidase-dependent oxygen consumption corresponds to the partial reduction of oxygen to O_2^- and H_2O_2

TABLE I

Endothelial Cell Oxygen Consumption in the Absence and Presence of Mitochondrial Respiratory Chain Inhibitors[a]

Condition	O_2 Consumption (nmol O_2/min/mg protein)	*n*
Control	22.0 ± 6.0	16
Myxothiazole (0.33 μM)	0.4 ± 0.2*†	4
Antimycin A (0.033 μM)	1.0 ± 0.6*†	4
KCN (200 μM)	6.3 ± 2.2*	8

[a] Dose–response studies of bovine endothelial cell O_2 consumption by respiratory inhibitors showed that the concentrations employed resulted in maximal inhibition of O_2 consumption. *, Significantly different from control; †, significantly different from the KCN-treated group (Reproduced from Ref. 1).

by a multitude of cellular sources. This respiratory inhibitor-resistant oxygen consumption can be studied in the presence of different mitochondrial inhibitors such as cyanide, antimycin A, and myxothiazole. Cyanide blocks cellular respiration by competitive binding to the heme of cytochrome a_3, thus interfering with electron transfer from iron to oxygen. However, cyanide is not a specific inhibitor because it binds to other heme proteins as well. Myxothiazole and antimycin A block mitochondrial respiration at the ubiquinone–cytochrome *b* region, thus are more specific and potent electron transport inhibitors than cyanide. We prefer to calculate cytochrome-*c* oxidase-resistant oxygen consumption based on myxothiazole-resistant respiration, because antimycin A can artifactually increase the amount of mitochondrial ubisemiquinone available for reduction of O_2 to O_2^-.

In normoxia, endothelial cell oxygen consumption under noninhibitory conditions was 22.0 nmol/min/mg protein (Table I) (1). Myxothiazole, antimycin A, and cyanide decreased O_2 consumption by 98, 95, and 71%, respectively. Inhibitor-resistant cellular respiration represents only an approximate measure of cell O_2^- and H_2O_2 production, for two reasons. First, the presence of the inhibitor can increase the extent of reduction of the mitochondrial respiratory chain and cellular electron-transferring molecules (i.e., NADH, $FADH_2$), thus resulting in potentially greater rates of mitochondrial O_2^- generation. Second, intracellular dismutation of O_2^- to O_2 and H_2O_2, followed by metabolism of H_2O_2 via catalase and peroxidases, can result in a 4-fold underestimation of actual cellular O_2^- generation. Even with these limitations, mitochondrial inhibitor-resistant cellular respiration provides useful data not only for comparing with other approaches for the quantitation of the generation of reactive oxygen species, but also when initially examining the influence of conditions expected to modify cellular rates of oxygen radical production.

Oxygen radical production from cells will approximately follow a second-order rate equation:

$$dO_2/dt = k[O_2][R\cdot] \quad (1)$$

Thus, if the concentrations of either O_2 or the reduced autoxidizable cell components (R·) increase, there will be a proportional increase in reactive oxygen species production. For instance, hyperoxia increases mitochondrial inhibitor-resistant respiration and H_2O_2 production by rat lungs and isolated mitochondria as a linear function of oxygen concentration (2).

B. Spin Trapping of Superoxide

Intracellular O_2^- production by cultured porcine aortic endothelium was demonstrated by electron paramagnetic resonance (EPR) spectroscopy, using cells incubated with the spin trap 5,5-dimethyl-1-pyrroline 1-oxide (DMPO) (Fig. 1) (3). With this technique, an initially unstable free radical reacts with the spin trap (in our case O_2^- reacting with DMPO) to form a long-lived nitroxide free radical adduct that gives a characteristic EPR signal at room temperature. The hyperfine splitting of the adduct provides information regarding the chemical nature of the short-lived free radical. Spin trapping of O_2^- was enhanced by incubation of cells with redox-active menadione, and it occurred both intra- and extracellularly, as concluded from the differential locations of the spin adduct (3). The O_2^--derived DMPO-OOH adduct partially spontaneously decomposed to DMPO-OH, forming ·OH as a by-product in this process. DMPO-OH was also formed from reduction of DMPO-OOH by cellular glutathione peroxidase activity. In these studies, we had no evidence for a direct cellular production of ·OH yielding DMPO-OH. During exposure of endothelial cells to menadione, the enhanced O_2^- levels led to the secondary formation of lipid radicals as well, which were detected using the spin trap phenyl-*N*-*tert*-butylnitrone (3).

Also, using EPR spectroscopy, we observed that exogenously generated O_2^- and H_2O_2, formed by exposure of cultured endothelial cells to xanthine plus xanthine oxidase (XO), reacts with cells to increase membrane protein rotational and translational mobility (4). This was analyzed using the thiol-reactive spin label 4-maleimido-2,2,6,6-tetramethyl-1-piperindinyloxy (4-Mal-TEMPO), which predominantly

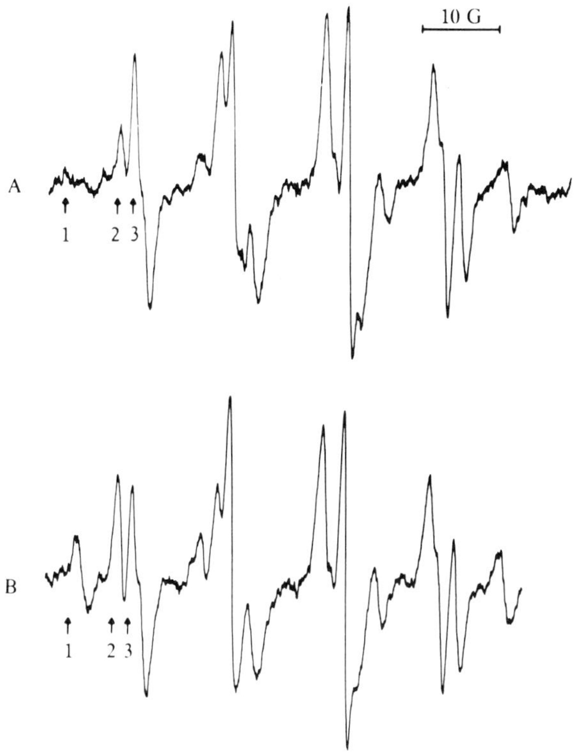

FIGURE 1

EPR spectra obtained when endothelial cells were incubated with menadione (0.1 m*M* in 0.14 *M* dimethyl sulfoxide) in the presence of the spin trap DMPO. Of interest is the observation that this spectrum is a composite of three different spin-trapped adducts: 2,2,5-trimethyl-1-pyrrolidinyloxyl (DMPO-CH_3, peak 1), 5-hydroxy-2,2-dimethyl-1-pyrrolidinyloxyl (DMPO-OH, peak 2), and 5-hydroperoxy-2,2-dimethyl-1-pyrrolidinyloxyl (DMPO-OOH, peak 3). The spectra were obtained under identical conditions except that scan B was initiated 10 min after the reaction commenced. (Reproduced from Ref. 3.)

reacts with protein thiols. Western blot analysis with an antibody to the spin label showed that two membrane proteins of 30 and 45 kDa mass bound the majority of the label. EPR spectroscopy indicated the membrane disorder parameter by showing respective peak amplitudes of the low- (S) and high-field (W) anisotropic interactions of the protein-bound nitroxide. In the absence of exogenously generated O_2^-, analysis of the EPR spectra from spin-labeled endothelial cells gave a *W/S* ratio of 2.80

± 0.02 at 25°C in Hanks' balanced salt solution (HBSS). On exposure of cells to XO-derived O_2^- and H_2O_2, the *W/S* ratio increased irreversibly as a function of time (Fig. 2). Native superoxide dismutase (SOD) but not catalytically inactive SOD partially inhibited *W*/S ratio changes, confirming that O_2^- played a key role in causing protein mobility changes. A recent reexamination of the data showed that 70% of XO-derived reactive species affected endothelial cell membrane properties in a manner resistant to exogenously administered SOD and catalase, with only SOD having a minimal protective effect. This was our first observation suggesting an intimate interaction between XO and the endothelial cell

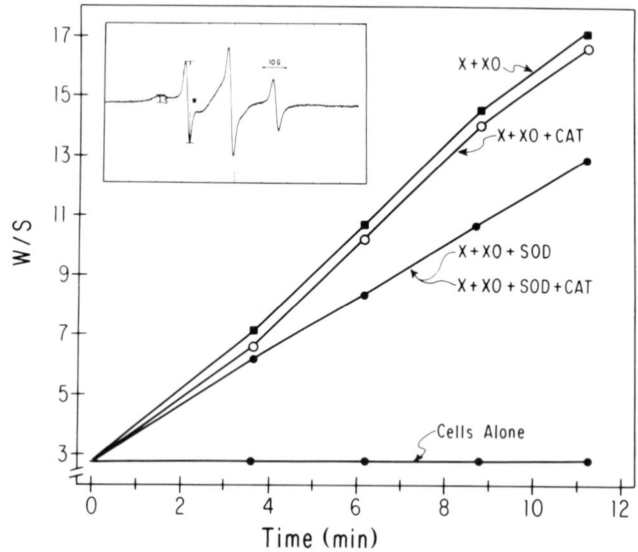

FIGURE 2

Effect of a superoxide-generating system on the *W*/S ratio of 4-Mal-TEMPO-labeled endothelial cells. Cultured endothelial cells were spin-labeled with 4-Mal-TEMPO, and the *W/S* ratio was determined. Spin-labeled cells in the presence of XO (2.5 mU/ml) and 0.5 m*M* xanthine (X) in HBSS buffer, pH 7.4; the superoxide generation rate from this concentration of xanthine oxidase plus xanthine was 1 nmol O_2^-/min/ml. O, Spin-labeled cells in the presence of the xanthine oxidase/xanthine system with the addition of catalase (CAT). ●, Spin-labeled cells in the presence of the xanthine oxidase/xanthine system with the addition of superoxide dismutase (SOD) or SOD plus CAT. The stable *W/S* ratio of control cells without additions is shown for comparison (●). The inset shows the EPR spectrum of cells treated with xanthine plus xanthine oxidase for 10 min. (Reproduced from Ref. 4.)

surface, now relevant because of the emerging concept of the induction of remote tissue injury by circulating XO, which can bind with high affinity to cell surface glycosaminoglycans (see Table VIII) (5).

C. Detection of Superoxide by Cytochrome c^{3+} Reduction

The reduction of cytochrome c^{3+} by O_2^- is the most commonly used method for the measurement of superoxide production in biological systems due to its simplicity, sensitivity, and low cost. The extracellular release of O_2^- has been spectrophotometrically monitored at 550 nm by ourselves and others via the SOD-inhibitable reduction of cytochrome c^{3+} (3). We have used both succinoylated and native cytochrome c^{3+} to quantitate O_2^- in cellular studies. Native cytochrome c^{3+} is positively charged at pH 7.4, and it can bind avidly to anionic cell surfaces. This protein–cell surface association may result in O_2^- independent cytochrome *c* reduction by membrane-bound reductases. Thus, cytochrome–cell membrane interactions can be minimized using succinoylated cytochrome *c*, which has most of the positive charge of the native protein blocked and is not utilized as an electron acceptor by reductases (6). An important limitation of cytochrome *c* succinoylation is the reduced sensitivity of O_2^- detection, since the rate of cytochrome *c* reaction with O_2^- is one-tenth that of the native protein.

We have observed that porcine and bovine endothelial cell monolayers and detached cell suspensions often have a basal rate of cytochrome c^{3+} reduction which is not inhibited by SOD, indicating that under basal conditions there was no detectable O_2^- diffusion out of the cell (Table II). After augmentation of O_2^- formation by porcine aortic endothelial cells by menadione, there was a significantly greater rate of cytochrome c^{3+} reduction, which was SOD-inhibitable, thus indicating the formation of O_2^-. When O_2^- was detected extracellularly after menadione exposure, it was due to the diffusion of menadione radical out of the cell followed by extracellular reoxidation to form O_2^-, rather than O_2^- directly diffusing across the plasma membrane. When endothelial cells were exposed to 95% oxygen, intracellular detection of O_2^- by DMPO was greater, but the rate of extracellular cytochrome c^{3+} reduction was less. This is consistent with a more efficient intracellular reoxidation of menadione semiquinone in hyperoxia, since the fate of the semiquinone in hyperoxia depends on the oxygen tension. Thus, less menadione radical diffused extracellularly, with cytochrome c^{3+} reduction rates consequently decreasing.

TABLE II

Reduction of Succinoylated Cytochrome *c* by Endothelial Cell Suspensions[a]

Addition	Cytochrome *c* reduced (nmol/min/mg protein)
None	0.42
Superoxide dismutase	0.42
Menadione	2.64
Menadione + superoxide dismutase	0.39
95% oxygen	0.39
95% oxygen + menadione	1.72

[a] Porcine aortic endothelial cells were suspended (0.18 mg of protein/ml) in HBSS plus 100 μM succinoylated cytochrome *c* (oxidized form) after removal from flasks by scraping. Succinoylated cytochrome c reduction was measured at 25°C in ambient air-saturated buffer, unless otherwise specified. Conditions: superoxide dismutase, 20 μg/ml; menadione, 0.1 m*M*; 95% O_2, buffer plus cells were bubbled with 100% oxygen to adjust oxygen in solution to 1.075 m*M* (95% of saturation). Each value represents the average of triplicate determinations using the same cell suspension. (Adapted from Ref. 3.)

We have tried unsuccessfully to detect extracellular release of O_2^- from bovine aortic endothelial cells using either native or succinoylated cytochrome c^{3+}. Experiments were carried out in 25-cm^2 flasks (3–4 × 10^6 cells) maintained in Hanks' balanced salt solution and compared to control flasks having no cells. Surprisingly, we observed that native cytochrome *c* reduction was greater in the cell-free flasks (Fig. 3). Moreover, SOD did not affect either the cell-independent or cell-dependent rate of cytochrome *c* reduction. This can be due to several factors, including the ability of cytochrome *c* to be directly reduced by several substances, such as ascorbate and ferrous ions (7). In the cellular system, there was no detectable O_2^- release. Intracellularly formed O_2^- could be prevented from reacting with the extracellular cytochrome *c* after rapid consumption via competing reactions with cytoplasmic target molecules or SOD, which reacts with superoxide about 10^3 times faster than cytochrome *c*. In the presence of cells, the compound responsible for reducing cytochrome *c* may be bound, metabolized, or oxidized by cells, thus prevented from reacting with cytochrome *c*. Another consideration is that native reduced cytochrome *c* can be reoxidized by membrane oxidases, resulting in a slower rate of cytochrome *c* reduction in the presence of cells. Because of multiple

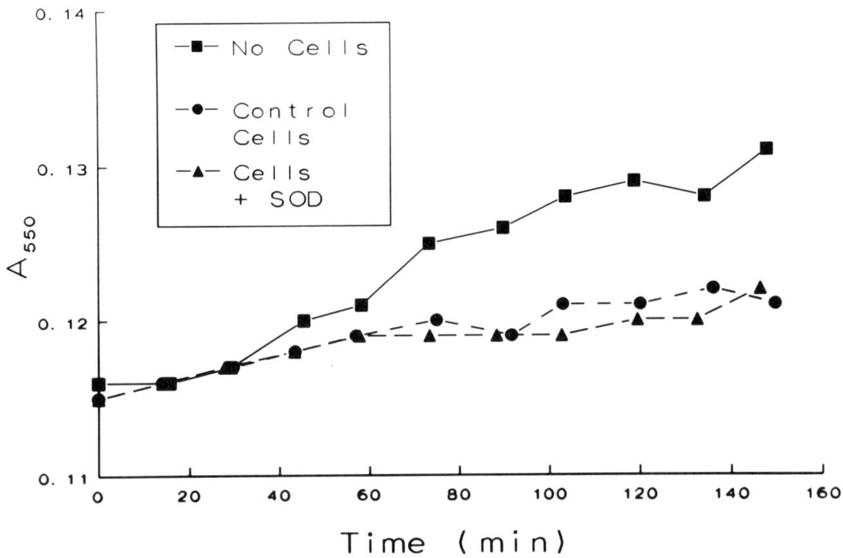

FIGURE 3

Endothelial cell superoxide release measured by cytochrome *c* reduction. Bovine aortic endothelial cell monolayers in 25-cm^2 flasks were incubated with 5 ml of 0.1 m*M* oxidized cytochrome *c* in HBSS supplemented with 10 m*M* potassium phosphate (pH 7.4). Aliquots were removed approximately every 30 min and the absorbance read at 550 nm before returning to the flasks. Bovine Cu/Zn superoxide dismutase (300 U/ml) was added to some flasks to measure SOD-insensitive cytochrome *c* reduction.

confounding variables, studies of cellular O_2^- release should also include additional controls for these phenomena.

This inability to detect extracellular O_2^- release by endothelial cell cytochrome *c* reduction differs from several previously published results. These investigations used cells derived from rat pulmonary artery or bovine aorta and pulmonary artery. The assay systems in many cases are different, and this may explain some of the discrepant results. For example, in one study of XO-dependent cell O_2^- release, only 1 ml of cytochrome c^{3+} solution was added to a 25-cm^2 cell surface area (8), an extremely small volume. The use of dry gases can cause evaporation, with concomitant significant increases in osmolarity which can affect cellular metabolism in diverse ways. Also, this system was an end point assay, where the cells were incubated with cytochrome c^{3+} in Hanks' balanced salts before collecting the supernatant for spectrophotometric analysis. This approach would miss any changes in rates of cell O_2^- release or possible O_2^- production by medium components. In spite of this, the observed XO-derived and O_2^--dependent reduction of approximately 0.5 n*M* cytochrome *c* present in a 1.0 ml reaction volume added to a T-25 flask having about 3×10^6 cells for 4 hr meant a change in absorbance at 550 nm of approximately 0.0001. We conclude that cytochrome *c* can be a useful method for the measurement of O_2^- production, but it may often not be sensitive or specific enough to detect extracellular release of O_2^- by endothelial cells.

In summary, our data support the concept that, despite the fact that O_2^- has the capability to cross cell membranes (9), most intracellularly generated endothelial cell O_2^- is consumed by either spontaneous or enzymatically catalyzed dismutation or via direct reaction with target molecules before a significant amount is released to the extracellular milieu.

D. Aminotriazole-Mediated Inactivation of Catalase

Rates of intracellular generation of H_2O_2 have been estimated from the kinetic analysis of aminotriazole-mediated inactivation of endogenous catalase (10). Catalase catalyzes the decomposition of $2H_2O_2$ to O_2 and $2H_2O$. The reaction mechanism of catalase has two basic steps, the first being the formation of the reactive intermediate, "compound I," after the reaction of catalase with the first H_2O_2. Catalase compound I then reacts with a second H_2O_2, yielding (in a normal catalytic cycle) free catalase, O_2, and $2H_2O$ as below.

$$\text{Catalase} + H_2O_2 \xrightarrow{k_1} \text{compound I} \tag{2}$$

$$\text{Compound I} + H_2O_2 \xrightarrow{k_2} \text{catalase} + O_2 = 2H_2O_2 \tag{3}$$

The rate of catalase compound I formation depends on the intracellular rate of H_2O_2 generation, decomposition, target molecule reactions, and diffusion of H_2O_2 to react with catalase. Aminotriazole can react with compound I to irreversibly inactivate catalase. Because aminotriazole is added in excess of the local H_2O_2 concentration, catalase compound I will preferentially react with aminotriazole to form the inactive enzyme rather than reacting with a second H_2O_2 molecule to complete the normal catalytic cycle.

$$\text{Compound I} + \text{aminotriazole} \xrightarrow{k_{AT}} \text{inactive complex} \tag{4}$$

The rate of formation of compound I will be proportional to the peroxisomal levels of H_2O_2 found in the region of catalase.

$$d\,\text{compound I}/dt = k_1[\text{CAT}][\text{H}_2\text{O}_2] \qquad (5)$$

From this, the rate of cell catalase inactivation by aminotriazole will approximate a linear function of the endogenous H_2O_2 concentration vicinal to catalase. Thus, catalase activity in the presence of aminotriazole will decay exponentially, and a pseudo-first-order rate constant of catalase inactivation (k_{cat}) can be defined (Fig. 4). By derivation of the steady-state rate equations of compound I formation and catalase inactivation, H_2O_2 can be estimated by

$$[\text{H}_2\text{O}_2] = k_{\text{cat}}/k_1 \qquad (6)$$

where k_1 is the second-order rate constant for the reaction of catalase with H_2O_2 to form compound I, that is, $1.7 \times 10^7\ M^{-1}\ \text{sec}^{-1}$.

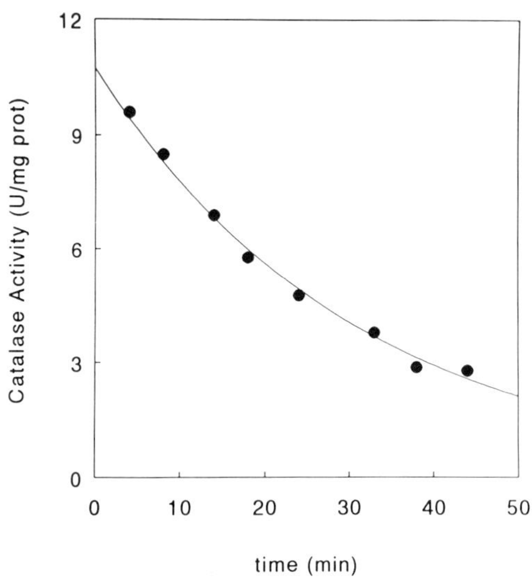

FIGURE 4

Catalase inactivation by aminotriazole for determination of intracellular H_2O_2 concentration. Bovine endothelial cells were incubated for stated times with 10 m*M* of 3-amino-1,2,4-triazole in phenol red-free M199 before removal of excess aminotriazole by washing with HBSS. Cells were then scraped into 1 ml of 0.1% Triton X-100, 50 m*M* potassium phosphate, 0.1 m*M* EDTA, pH 7.4, and sonicated for catalase assay. Catalase activity was monitored spectrophotometrically by the consumption of H_2O_2 at 240 nm.

Endothelial cell catalase is at least in part located in peroxisomes. Thus, aminotriazole-mediated catalase inactivation will report the steady-state concentration of H_2O_2 in or near the peroxisome. An increase in intracellular H_2O_2 concentration can be reflected in this region, since H_2O_2 freely diffuses to and crosses membranes. A faster rate of aminotriazole-mediated catalase inactivation will occur if either increased peroxisomal H_2O_2 production occurs or the H_2O_2 gradient between cytosol and peroxisomes is increased. Still, cellular peroxidases (e.g., glutathione peroxidase) and direct reactions of H_2O_2 with target molecules can scavenge some H_2O_2 before it reaches peroxisomal catalase.

We have also recently detected catalase in the matrix of mitochondria isolated from rat heart, but not lung (11). It is probable that there is a species-, organ-, and cell-specific distribution of this key enzyme of oxidant detoxification. Recent observations show that mitochondrial cytochrome *c* plays an important role in catalyzing hydroperoxide-dependent lipid peroxidation, and that the matrix catalase offers critical defense against this injurious process (12). Thus, in some cases, the use of aminotriazole to indicate cell H_2O_2 generation can also reflect the microenvironment near mitochondrial catalase as well. Under basal conditions, we estimated the intracellular steady-state concentration of H_2O_2 to be about 30 p*M* in bovine aortic endothelial cells (10).

E. Hydrogen Peroxide-Mediated Oxidation of *P*-Hydroxyphenylacetic Acid

Extracellular H_2O_2 release from endothelial cells occurs constitutively and was measured using the horseradish peroxidase-catalyzed, H_2O_2-mediated oxidation of *p*-hydroxyphenylacetic acid (PHPA) (13). This sensitive and reliable assay for H_2O_2 is advantageous because a fluorescent product is formed rather than lost (as with the scopoletin assay for H_2O_2), resulting in minimal background interference. In this reaction, H_2O_2 mediates the oxidative dimerization of PHPA to a fluorescent product after combining with horseradish peroxidase (HRP) to form the reactive compound I intermediate [Eq. (7)].

$$\text{HRP} + H_2O_2 \rightarrow \text{HRP–compound} \tag{7}$$

$$\text{PHPA} + \text{HRP–compound I} \rightarrow (\text{PHPA})_2 + 2H_2O + \text{HRP} \tag{8}$$

A key technical consideration of this assay is that $(\text{PHPA})_2$ fluorescence is affected by pH changes in the physiological pH range. For instance, from pH 7.0 to 8.0 there is a 7-fold increase in fluorescence yield by $(PHPA)_2$ (13). Cell culture media also often contain HCO_3^- which is lost as CO_2, causing alkalinization of the reaction medium that will result in artifactually greater fluorescence. Thus, fluorescence measurements for different samples must be carried out at the same pH to obtain reliable results for H_2O_2 release by vascular endothelium. We detected a basal rate of extracellular H_2O_2 release of 4–14 pmol/min/10^6 cells by bovine aortic endothelium depending on growth conditions (Table III) (14). (*Note:* 10^6 cells typically have 7 μg DNA and 70 μg protein for data conversion calculations.) This extent of H_2O_2 release represents a significant proportion of the cytochrome-*c* oxidase-independent O_2 consumption by these cells.

F. Fluorometric Assay of Xanthine Dehydrogenase + Oxidase Activity

The oxygen radical-producing enzyme xanthine oxidase (XO) has been proposed to be a key source of reactive oxygen species in vascular endothelium. Xanthine oxidase catalyzes the oxidation of hypoxanthine and xanthine to uric acid with the concomitant generation of O_2^- and H_2O_2.

TABLE III

Contribution of Extracellular Hydrogen Peroxide Release to Total and Nonmitochondrial Oxygen Consumption by Endothelial Cells[a]

	Culture medium	
Measurement	DMEM (pmol/min/10^6 cells)	M199 (pmol/min/10^6 cells)
Total O_2 consumption	855 ± 451(4)	1539 ± 408(4)
Myxothiazole-resistant O_2 consumption	67 ± 22(4)	25 ± 17(4)
Extracellular H_2O_2 release	14.0 ± 4.3(6)	4.2 + 1.3(6)

[a] Bovine endothelial cells were cultured in serum-containing medium with either Dulbecco's modified Eagle's medium (DMEM) or M199. Consumption of O_2 was mesaured polarographically with suspended cells removed from flasks by scraping in the presence or absence of 0.33 μM myxothiazole. Extracellular H_2O_2 release was measured fluorometrically via horseradish peroxidase-dependent oxidation of p-hydroxyphenylacetic acid. The values in parentheses represent n. Information represents a summary of previously published information (13,14).

$$\text{Hypoxanthine} \xrightarrow{O_2 \;\rightarrow\; O_2^- \text{ or } H_2O_2} \text{xanthine} \xrightarrow{O_2 \;\rightarrow\; O_2^- \text{ or } H_2O_2} \text{uric acid} \quad (9)$$

Xanthine oxidase is a biochemically modified form of xanthine dehydrogenase (XDH), the predominant from of the enzyme in normal tissues. The dehydrogenase form uses NAD^+ rather than O_2 as an electron acceptor, thus not producing reactive oxygen species. Sulfhydryl oxidation or limited proteolysis of XDH will result in the generation of the oxidase form of the enzyme. We observe endothelial cell XDH and XO to exist in both the dehydrogenase form and the oxidase form (see Tables IV and V).

We measure XO activity in cultured endothelial cells fluorometrically by the allopurinol-inhibitable oxidation of pterin to a fluorophore, isoxanthopterin (Fig. 5) (15). This approach has a 20-fold greater sensitivity than high-performance liquid chromatography (HPLC) analyses and more than 50-fold sensitivity over the spectrophotometric assays for XDH + XO activity, both based on detection of uric acid formation at 295 nm. Cell lysates are prepared in the presence of protease inhibitors, thiol reductants, and under cold temperatures to prevent the artifactual conversion of XDH to XO during cell manipulation and enzyme activity analysis. Methylene blue is used as electron acceptor to measure XDH activity, thus avoiding interference from NADH fluorescence (Fig. 5).

III. Xanthine Oxidase in Vascular Endothelium

A. Tissue Distribution of Xanthine Dehydrogenase + Oxidase

There is currently an ongoing evolution in concepts about tissue localization of XDH + XO and its specific role in oxidant tissue injury. The liver and the intestine have the greatest tissue-specific activity of XDH + XO, with vascular endothelium throughout the body also reported to be enriched in XDH + XO activity relative to other cell types (16,17). Immunocytochemical localization with antibodies to XDH + XO have demonstrated the presence of XDH + XO in hepatocytes, Kupffer cells, and endothelial cells lining several vascular beds throughout the body (18,19).

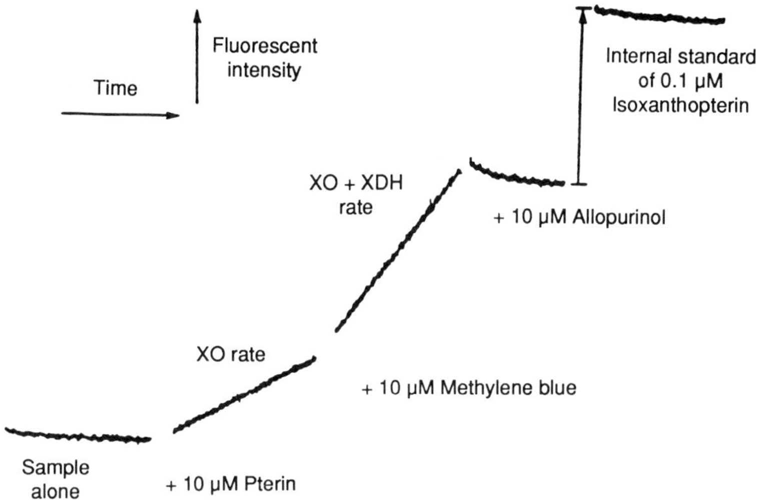

FIGURE 5

Measurement of vascular endothelial XDH and XO in human brain with a fluorometric assay using pterin as substrate. After the reaction was terminated with allopurinol, isoxanthopterin (from 0.1 to 1 μM depending on the sensitivity setting of the fluorometer) was added to serve as an internal standard to calibrate the assay. (Reproduced from Ref. 15).

Recently, the important observation that immunoglobulins, namely, IgG and IgA, routinely copurify with XDH + XO was published (20). These investigators showed that a variety of antisera raised against putatively pure XDH + XO and used by others for immunolocalization studies also cross-reacted with IgG, IgA, and IgM. This raises the strong possibility that immunohistochemical localization studies showing XDH + XO location in endothelium may also be artifactually detecting immunoglobulin presence. Also, this can explain why some tissues with no detectable XDH + XO by biochemical analysis activity demonstrated positive "XDH + XO" staining by immunocytochemical analysis. Because of this potential pitfall in the study of the free radical biochemistry and cell biology of xanthine oxidase, we recommend a final enzyme purification step with a folate affinity column (21).

Cellular localization of tissue XDH + XO may also be attempted by isolating specific cell types and biochemically assaying for XDH + XO activity. A potential problem with this approach is that several cell types lose expression of XDH + XO activity during primary culture (22–24). Freshly isolated pulmonary type II alveolar epithelial cells lost 50% of total XDH + XO activity within the first 12 hr after isolation (22), with liver cell cultures demonstrating similar rates of loss of cellular XDH + XO activity (23). Thus, lack of expression of XDH + XO activity in cultured cells does not necessarily negate the possibility of XDH + XO presence *in vivo*.

B. Cell Culture Conditions and Enzyme Activity

The study of XDH + XO activity in endothelial cells is significant because of the role these cells play in regulating both vascular homeostasis and responses to injury and the key contributions of reactive oxygen species to these processes. Endothelial cells cultured from vessels of different species demonstrated variable levels of cellular XDH + XO activity (Table IV). Rat endothelial cells contained the greatest XDH + XO specific activity of all species studied, while rabbit and bovine endothelial cells had similar XDH + XO specific activities.

We have been unable to detect XDH + XO activity in cultured human umbilical vein endothelium or human aortic endothelium. Separate histo-

TABLE IV

Xanthine Dehydrogenase + Oxidase Activity of Aortic Endothelium Isolated and Cultured from Different Species[a]

Species	Enzyme activity (μU XDH + XO/10^6 cells)	%XO
Bovine	1.7 ± 0.4(4)	51 ± 13
Rat	7.9 ± 3.3(4)	40 ± 8
Rabbit	1.0 ± 0.4(3)	31 ± 10
Porcine	0 ± 0.0	—
Human	0 ± 0.0	—

[a] Endothelial cells were isolated from vessels and cultured as follows: bovine aortic cells, M199, 5% fetal calf serum, 5% iron-supplemented calf serum, and 10 μM thymidine; rat aortic cells, DMEM, 10% calf serum, and 2 mM glutamine; rabbit aortic cells, M199 with 10% fetal calf serum; porcine aortic cells, M199 and 10% fetal calf serum; and human umbilical vein cells, M199, 15% fetal calf serum, 10 μg/ml heparin, and 10 μM thymidine. Cells were harvested and cell lysate XDH + XO activity was determined spectrofluorometrially as previously described (15). The percentage of total XDH + XO activity in the XO form is reported as the percent oxidase (%XO). The values in parentheses represent n.

chemical evidence suggests the enzyme is present in human vascular endothelium, so we are pursuing this issue further in order to obtain a cell model which is more reflective of human metabolism and pathophysiology. The finding of XDH + XO activity in cultured rabbit endothelial cells (Table IV) and in freshly isolated rabbit type II alveolar cells was surprising, since rabbit tissues generally contain low XDH + XO activities (25–27). Similar to rabbit, hamster also has a very low XDH + XO activity. Thus, XO-derived oxygen products, which were thought not to play a significant role in oxygen-mediated tissue dysfunction in rabbit and hamster, have been observed to participate in the disruption of normal cell function in both rabbit alveolar type II cells and cultured hamster mixed lung cells (28,29). In summary, low net tissue activities of XDH + XO activity do not necessarily reflect the damaging potential that XO can have, when concentrated in specific cell types making up some fraction of that tissue. Also, some species very high in XDH + XO activity (e.g., rat) may not serve as appropriate models for reflection of oxidant metabolic properties of human vascular tissue.

C. Modulation of Cellular Xanthine Dehydrogenase + Oxidase

The XDH + XO activity in cultured endothelial cells can be modulated by *in vitro* conditions. For example, growth of bovine aortic endothelial cells in Dulbecco's modified Eagle's (DMEM)-based media yielded the greatest XDH + XO activity, while cells cultured in M199 had the least (Table V).

TABLE V

Influence of Culture Medium on Endothelial Cell Xanthine Dehydrogenase + Oxidase Activity[a]

Culture medium	Enzyme activity (μU XDH + XO/10^6 cells)	%XO
M199	0.62 ± 0.15	64 ± 7%
Ham's F12/DMEM	1.1 ± 0.14	54 ± 8%
DMEM	8.9 ± 2.9	59 ± 6%

[a] Bovine aortic endothelial cells were cultured as follows: M199, as described in Table IV; Ham's F12/DMEM (1:1), 10% fetal calf serum and 1% nonessential amino acids; and DMEM, 10% heat-inactivated calf serum, 2 m*M* glutamine, and 2 ng/ml fibroblast growth factor was included. XDH + XO activity was determined as in Table IV. *N* = 6 for all determinations.

The biochemical mechanism explaining these differences in cellular XDH + XO activity was at least partially due to (1) the presence of an XDH + XO inhibitor in DMEM which caused enzyme induction over extended periods of time and (2) greater concentrations of xanthine and hypoxanthine present in M199 and DMEM/Ham's F12 which could support generation of O_2^- and H_2O_2 and lead to enzyme autoinactivation. In explanation, we note that folic acid is in a greater concentration in DMEM than other media. A photolytic breakdown product, 6-pterin aldehyde, which is almost always present in folic acid preparations, is a potent inhibitor of XDH + XO (30). Enzyme kinetic studies and HPLC analysis demonstrated the presence of approximately 325 n*M* of 6-pterin aldehyde in DMEM. This XDH + XO inhibitor–enzyme induction phenomenon has been noted in other tissues as well, with augmentation of liver XDH + XO occurring as a response to chronic allopurinol administration (31).

It has been long recognized that XO can catalytically inactivate itself via reaction of self-generated oxidants. This seems to be the case for cells grown in purine-containing media. Hypoxanthine and xanthine is absent in DMEM and calf serum, but present in fetal calf serum, M199, and Ham's F12 nutrient mixture. Hypoxanthine and xanthine concentrations are highest in serum-supplemented Ham's F12/DMEM (23 and 4.7 μM, respectively), followed by M199 which contains 6.4 and 4.3 μM, respectively. The augmentation of cellular XDH + XO activity by 6-pterin aldehyde in the DMEM/Ham's F12 media was apparently partially overcome by the inhibitory effects of hypoxanthine and xanthine present in the media as well. These data show that careful consideration should be given to culture conditions before defining the presence and biological roles of XDH + XO. Even though many studies of tissue oxidant injury suggests a beneficial role of XDH + XO inhibitors, the possibility of subsequent enzyme induction should be realized. Also, pathological processes such as chronic hypoxia or ischemia–reperfusion could influence tissue purine levels, XO autoinactivation, and extents of subsequent oxidant production by XO.

Tissue XDH + XO activity can be altered *in vivo* by both environmental and humoral influences, with cultured endothelial cell XDH + XO responses often mimicking those observed *in vivo*. For example, pulmonary XDH + XO activity decreases during hyperoxic exposure (32). Similarly, bovine endothelial cells exposed to 48 hr of hyperoxia experienced almost complete loss of cell XDH + XO activity (Table VI). In contrast, 48 hr exposure to 3% O_2 resulted in an increase in cell XDH + XO activity. Hypoxic exposure of endothelial cells also resulted in a 6% increase in the proportion of XDH + XO as percent XO. The biochemical mechanisms regulating endothelial cell XDH + XO activity during hy-

TABLE VI

Modulation of Endothelial Cell Xanthine Dehydrogenase + Oxidase Activity by Oxygen Concentration

Condition	Enzyme activity (μU XDH + XO/10^6 cells)	%XO
Control	3.8 ± 0.5(6)	37 ± 7%
Hypoxia	20 ± 1.5(6)	43 ± 6%
Hyperoxia	0.03 ± 0.07(9)	100 ± 6%

[a] Endothelial cells were grown in M199 in 95% air, 5% CO_2 as described in Table IV. Prior to exposure, the medium was replaced and confluent cells exposed to 48 hr of hyperoxia (95% O_2, 5% CO_2) or hypoxia (3% O_2, 5% CO_2, 92% N_2), then compared to cells cultured for a similar period with 95% air, 5% CO_2. The cells were harvested and XDH + XO activity determined as in Table IV.

poxia and hyperoxia are unclear at present. We hypothesize that, in hyperoxia, XDH + XO is inactivated by excess rates of production of reactive oxygen species generated by diverse cellular loci. The increased XDH + XO activity by exposure of cultured endothelial cells to inhibitors of XDH + XO or hypoxia may be related to a feedback mechanism exerted at the transcriptional, translational, or postranslational level(s), via regulation of the rate of enzyme synthesis, degradation by purine metabolism intermediates or oxidant-responsive gene regulatory elements.

D. Contribution of Xanthine Oxidase to Net Cellular Superoxide and Hydrogen Peroxide Production

The contribution of XO-derived products to net non-cytochrome-*c* oxidase-dependent O_2 consumption can be estimated by comparison of oxygen consumption expected from V_{max} XO activity to myxothiazole-resistant O_2 consumption. Assuming the complete reduction of O_2^- and H_2O_2 to H_2O by antioxidant enzymes during the myxothiazole-resistant O_2 consumption, a maximum of 268 and 100 pmol O_2^- plus H_2O_2/min/10^6 cells (O_2 consumption multiplied by 4, discussed previously) can be produced by DMEM and M199 cultured cells, respectively (Table III). This prediction of cell O_2^- and H_2O_2 production is likely an overestimate, because covalent incorporation of O_2 into substrates such as arachidonic acid can still occur. Assuming no conversion of XDH to XO, the reduction of O_2 to O_2^- plus H_2O_2 by bovine endothelial cells cultured in DMEM and M199 would be 16 and 1.2 pmol/min/10^6 cells, respectively. The formation of O_2^- and H_2O_2 by XO was calculated from Table III, correcting for the rate of oxidation of xanthine by bovine XDH + XO being three times greater than pterin oxidation (15). Thus, the contribution of XO to overall cell O_2^- and H_2O_2 formation in DMEM and M199 cultured bovine endothelial cells would be 6 and 1%, respectively. If XDH becomes fully converted to XO, the contribution of XO-derived O_2^- and plus H_2O_2 would represent 10 and 2% of the total O_2^- and plus H_2O_2 formation in DMEM and M199 cultured cells when XO is functioning at V_{max}.

We do not observe a decrease in the rate of aminotriazole-mediated inactivation of catalase in cells following XO inhibition. Endothelial XO inhibition was induced by growth in tungsten or exposure to allopurinol (Table VII). This confirms that the XO contribution to net rates of H_2O_2 production in "unstressed" endothelial cells was not great enough to modify the H_2O_2 gradient between the cytosol and sites of catalase distribution.

The contribution of XO-derived H_2O_2 to extracellular H_2O_2 release was also examined in cultured bovine aortic endothelial cells. The rates of H_2O_2 release and myxothiazole-resistant respiration of DMEM cultured cells are greater than for M199 cultured cells (Table III). In separate investigations, the release of H_2O_2 was greatest in cultured rabbit endothelial cells, while the rate of release of H_2O_2 from cultured human umbilical vein endothelial cells having no detectable XO was similar to bovine endothelial cells cultured in M199 (33,34). Inhibition of cell XO did not affect rates of H_2O_2 release. Thus, there is no

TABLE VII

Influence of Xanthine Dehydrogenase + Oxidase Activity on Endothelial Cell Intracellular Hydrogen Peroxide Concentration[a]

Culture condition	Enzyme activity (μU XDH + XO/10^6 cells)	Intracellular H_2O_2 (pM)
M199	1.5 ± 0.5	18.45 ± 5.93
M199 + 50 μM tungsten	0.0	20.62 ± 0.52
DMEM	6.6 ± 2.6	24.28 ± 0.61
+0.1 mM allopurinol	ND	18.10 ± 2.33
+1.0 mM allopurinol	ND	15.87 ± 9.24
+0.1 mM xanthine	ND	22.39 ± 9.15

[a] Intracellular hydrogen peroxide concentration of bovine aortic endothelial cells as calculated for cells cultured in M199, DMEM, or M199 + 50 μM tungsten from rates of aminotriazole-mediated inactivation of catalase. Data represent means ± SD, n = 3. ND, Not determined. Data adapted from Ref. 14.

correlation between XO specific activity and rates of cell H_2O_2 release. The lack of XO involvement in basal rates of H_2O_2 release does not, however, rule out a role for XO in extracellular H_2O_2 release during pathologic conditions.

E. Influence of Lipopolysaccharide and Tumor Necrosis Factor on Endothelial Cell Xanthine Oxidase Activity and Oxidant Production

Acute injury to the vascular endothelium occurs with inflammation. Bacterial products such as endotoxin (LPS) can directly injure endothelial cells, with many of the pathologic effects of LPS mediated by cytokines, particularly tumor necrosis factor-α (TNF), released from LPS-stimulated macrophages. Cytokine-activated inflammatory cells can be triggered to have a respiratory burst yielding extensive amounts of reactive oxygen species. Inflammatory mediators can also have profound effects on endothelial cells including induction of adhesive glycoprotein expression and loss of cell barrier function. We have previously reported that TNF increases the permeability of cultured bovine aortic endothelial cell monolayers to macromolecules, with the maximum effect occurring after a 12-hr exposure to 1000 U/ml TNF (35). Some reports suggest that a key influence of TNF leading to changes in cell function is the stimulation of endogenous reactive oxygen species production, possibly via an XO-dependent mechanism (36,37). In bovine pulmonary artery endothelial cells, increased endogenous reactive oxygen species production was suggested based on a decrease in nitroblue tetrazolium reduction and a decrease in 2′,7′-dichlorofluorescein diacetate oxidation, after treatment of LPS-exposed cells with dimethyl sulfoxide and allopurinol (36). In rat pulmonary artery endothelial cells, exposure to TNF and several other inflammatory mediators resulted in the conversion of xanthine dehydrogenase to xanthine oxidase (37). To further investigate inflammatory mediator-induced influences on endogenous endothelial oxidant metabolism, we directly quantified rates of H_2O_2 production and metabolism in bovine aortic endothelial cells after exposure to TNF and LPS. Table VIII summarizes our results related to inflammatory mediator influences on H_2O_2 production and metabolism in bovine aortic endothelium (10).

Intracellular H_2O_2 was determined by kinetic analysis of aminotriazole-mediated inactivation of endogenous catalase. A basal intracellular H_2O_2 concentration of 32.8 ± 10.7 p*M* (mean $\pm$ SD, $n = 22$) was not changed by cell exposure to 1000 U/ml TNF for 1, 4, or 12 hr, nor was it changed by exposure to 1 μg/ml LPS for 1, 4, 6–8, or 12

TABLE VIII

Production and Metabolism of Hydrogen Peroxide in Bovine Aortic Endothelial Cells: Lack of Influence by Tumor Necrosis Factor or Lipopolysaccharide[a]

Measurement	Result	*N*
Intracellular H_2O_2 concentration	32.8 ± 10.7 p*M*	22
Extracellular H_2O_2 release rate	75 ± 12 pmol/min/mg protein	21
Pentose phosphate pathway activity	0.48 ± 0.18%	10
Catalase activity	5.72 ± 1.61 U/mg protein	22
Glutathione peroxidase activity		
H_2O_2 as substrate	8.13 ± 3.79 mU/mg protein	4
tert-Butyl hydroperoxide as substrate	34.6 ± 5.0 mU/mg protein	2
Xanthine dehydrogenase/oxidase		
Total activity	2.32 ± 0.75 μU/mg protein	12
%XO	47.1 ± 11.7%	
Intracellular purines		
Hypoxanthine	1.19 ± 1.04 nmol/mg protein	4
Xanthine	0.13 ± 0.17 nmol/mg protein	4
Uric acid	Nondetectable	4

[a] Values are means ± SD. Methods are described in the text. Percent pentose phosphate pathway activity indicates the percent of total glucose metabolism occurring via this pathway. Exposure of endothelial cells to 1000 U/ml TNF or to 1 μg/ml LPS had no significant effect on these parameters of endothelial cell H_2O_2 production and metabolism, following ANOVA and multiple comparison procedures. Data adapted from Ref. 10.

hr. Extracellular release of H_2O_2 was determined by oxidation of *p*-hydroxyphenylacetic acid. The control H_2O_2 release rate of 75 ± 12 pmol/min/mg cell protein (n = 21) was not altered by 2 to 6 hr exposure to 1000 U/ml TNF or 1 μg/ml LPS.

The glutathione peroxidase–reductase system is a key cytosolic antioxidant system and may metabolize intracellularly generated H_2O_2 before H_2O_2 concentrations become elevated at the peroxisome or before H_2O_2 diffuses extracellularly. Therefore, we measured the flux of glucose through the pentose phosphate pathway after LPS and TNF exposure of cells, along with the basal activity of glutathione peroxidase. With increased metabolism of hydroperoxides by the glutathione peroxidase–reductase system, increased flux of glucose via the pentose phosphate pathway is required for NADPH production. We found no evidence of increased H_2O_2 metabolism via this mechanism following cell exposure. For example, 1000 U/ml TNF or 1 μg/ml LPS for 6 hr did not increase the 0.48 ± 0.18% (n = 10) of total glucose metabolism that occurred via the pentose phosphate pathway under control conditions. The activity of glutathione peroxidase was relatively low, 8.13 ± 3.79 mU/mg protein (n = 4), when using H_2O_2 as substrate and 34.6 ± 5.0 mU/mg protein (n = 2) with *tert*-butyl hydroperoxide. Catalase activity was 5.72 ± 1.61 U/mg protein (n = 22). In summary, intracellular H_2O_2 concentration, as reflected by its relative rate of scavenging via catalase or by the glutathione peroxidase–reductase system, was not different from control cells after exposure to TNF or LPS. Because the conditions of these studies were similar to our previous work demonstrating increased endothelial permeability induced by cytokine exposure, we conclude that increased endogenous endothelial cell production of O_2^- or H_2O_2 is not causally related to direct inflammatory mediator-induced endothelial toxicity.

There is also a discrepancy between our conclusions, based on direct H_2O_2 measurements, and suggestions of others for an oxidant-mediated pathological role of inflammatory mediators via increased cell XO activity. A previous report was performed with inherently XO-rich rat pulmonary artery endothelial cells while our studies were carried out in bovine aortic endothelial cells (37). It should be noted that increased cell XO activity does not necessarily result in enhanced steady-state concentrations of H_2O_2 unless there is a concomitant increase in purine substrate supply. We carried out additional studies to evaluate inflammatory mediator influences on bovine endothelial cell XDH + XO activity as well as to quantify intracellular purine levels by HPLC. Basal intracellular XDH + XO activity was 2.32 ± 0.75 μU/mg protein (n = 12) with 47.1 ± 11.7% in the oxidase form. Intracellular purine levels (n = 4) of 1.19 ± 1.04 nmol hypoxanthine/mg protein, 0.13 ± 0.17 nmol xanthine/mg protein, and undetectable uric acid were consistent with a low level of cell XDH + XO activity. Exposure to 1000 U/ml TNF or 1 μg/ml LPS for 2–6 hr did not change cell XDH or XO activity or substrate concentrations which might alter cell H_2O_2 levels. The XDH + XO activity of the bovine aortic endothelial cells used in these experiments was approximately 10^3-fold lower than the reported rat pulmonary artery endothelial cell XDH + XO activity. Although direct comparisons between different studies is sometimes difficult, it seems that endothelial cells from different species, from different vessel sources, and when maintained under different conditions may express significant differences in basal and pathological cellular oxidant metabolism. These *in vitro* differences may be important when considering cultured cell systems as models of human pathological processes.

IV. Circulating Xanthine Oxidase and Interactions with Vascular Endothelium

A. Circulating Xanthine Oxidase in Pathology

It has become apparent that XO released by one organ can traverse the circulation and exert injury to remote vascular beds. For example, acute influenza virus infection of mice led to high levels of circulating XO, which ultimately resulted in pulmonary edema and death (38,39). Both lung edema and mortality were dramatically prevented by treatment of mice with allopurinol or a long circulating half-life derivative of SOD, conjugated to polymeric pyran. Hepatocellular damage (40), hemorrhagic shock (40), adult respiratory distress syndrome (41), and thermal injury to skin (42) will also result in the appearance of up to 5 mU/ml XO in plasma. The release of XO from tissues may also occur in the absence of metabolic disturbances, since up to 8% of plasma IgG from healthy humans is immunoreactive with XO and partially inhibitory to XO activity (43). The circulatory XO can serve as an intravascular locus of O_2^-, H_2O_2, and secondary toxic species which can (1) directly cause tissue injury, (2) deplete tissue antioxidants, or (3) activate secondary inflammatory responses by oxidizing plasma components to chemotactic products.

A number of proteins that gain access to the intravascular compartment will bind to the luminal surface of endothelial cells (44–46). The binding of proteins to cell surface glycosaminoglycans will concentrate them several thousand fold. This phenomenon occurs with XO and may have significant pathological implications.

B. Xanthine Oxidase–Endothelial Glycosaminoglycan Interactions

In vivo studies of ischemia–reperfusion phenomena and hemorrhagic shock showed much higher concentrations of circulating XO in heparinized animals, suggesting possible interactions of XO with endothelial cell surface glycosaminoglycans (GAGs). This possibility was investigated by incubating cultured bovine aortic endothelium with 1–5 mU/ml XO. After a 2-hr incubation followed by extensive washing, significant heparin-reversible XO binding was observed which could be detected by nitroblue tetrazolium staining of O_2^- and by radiosotopic or enzymatic analysis. The nitroblue tetrazolium staining of monolayers having bound XO was inhibited almost completely by allopurinol and partially inhibited by SOD. In one experiment, cells had an endogenous XO activity of 38±5 μU/mg protein, which increased to 120±16 μU/mg protein after a 2-hr incubation with 2.5 mU/ml XO and washing. Xanthine oxidase activity decreased to 83 μU/mg protein after 10 min of postincubation with 100 U/ml heparin, a 50% reduction in cell XO binding. We have also preliminarily observed that cells incubated with XO at 5°C have a greater extent of heparin-reversible XO binding, suggesting that at 37°C, more active endocytic mechanisms may sequester XO into a heparin-resistant compartment. A similar phenomenon has been observed for lipoprotein lipase interactions with endothelium.

When endothelial cells were incubated at 5°C with 50 μg/ml (68 mU/ml) XO, the heparin-reversible binding of XO at 5°C approached saturation at 100 μg XO/ml, with near maximal binding in 2 hr. Scatchard analysis showed complex binding kinetics with at least two affinity sites, confirming that XO can bind significantly to cell surface GAGs especially at concentrations experienced during *in vivo* pathologic conditions (Table IX).

In model studies using a Sepharose-6B-heparin affinity column as a cell surface-like matrix, we found that XO binds and elutes with a linear NaCl gradient at 150–200 m*M* NaCl. This suggests ionic interactions

TABLE IX

Binding of Xanthine Oxidase to Endothelial Cell Surface Glycosaminoglycans[a]

Measurement	Binding site 1	Binding site 2
K_d (mU/ml)	0.9	42
K_d (n*M*)	5	236
Molecules bound XO/cell	18,000	65,000
Amount (ng) bound XO/10^6 cells	4	14
	Cell XO activity μU XO · mg protein^{-1}	
Control	38 ± 5	
Post XO incubation	120 ± 16	
Post XO incubation + heparin	83 ± 3	

[a] For Scatchard analysis, ^{125}I-labeled XO purified from fresh bovine cream (0 to 100 μg/ml) was incubated at 5°C with confluent endothelial cell monolayers for 2 hr. Enzyme binding was determined from the heparin-reversible component (~85%) and was maximal by 2 hr. Cell XO activity assessment was performed after a 2-hr incubation with 2.5 mU/ml XO at 37°C.

between XO and heparin and confirms the affinity of this protein for GAGs. Consistent with this concept is the observation that heparin, a glycosaminoglycan which interferes with protein–GAG binding, significantly decreases endothelial cell injury produced by XO (47).

C. Kinetics Changes of Immobilized Xanthine Oxidase

The properties of XO bound to Sepharose-heparin were studied because immobilization of enzymes can alter their kinetic properties as compared with enzymes in solution. Immobilization can cause protein conformational and steric effects that affect binding of substrates and catalysis. Also, there are partitioning effects of substrate between solution and the site of immobilization, which can potentially influence substrate concentration near the enzyme compared with that in bulk solution. Finally, since substrate and product need to diffuse to or from the immobilization matrix, the rate of reaction may be controlled by the rate of substrate or product diffusion, a rare occurrence with free enzymes. Kinetics of XO bound to S-6B-H were studied spectrophotometrically in stirred cuvettes. We observed a K_{mapp} of 20–30 μM for GAG-bound XO compared with a K_m of 2–6 μM for XO in free solution when using xanthine as substrate in the presence of 50 mM potassium phosphate, pH 7.4 (48). These findings indicate that XO–GAG binding may alter XO kinetics, influencing the rate of production of reactive oxygen species at the cell surface and possibly affecting the percentage of univalent versus divalent reduction of O_2 by XO.

D. Plasma Reactions of Xanthine Oxidase-Derived Oxidants

Plasma XO is resistant to autoinactivation, with plasma components protecting the enzyme from self-generated oxidants (Fig. 6). In the presence of substrate, XO-induced substantial oxidation of plasma sulfhydryls but did not cause significant lipid peroxidation (Fig. 7) (49). This supports the concept that reactive oxygen species generated in the intravascular compartment often react preferentially with more hydrophilic target molecules. These results demonstrate that plasma protein sulfhydryl oxidation is a more sensitive marker of oxidative stress to the vascular compartment than lipid peroxidation. Also, lipid peroxidation products such as conjugated dienes and thiobarbituric acid material (in part malonyldialdehyde) are not always specific markers of free radical damage to complex biological systems. Both thiobarbituric acid-positive mate-

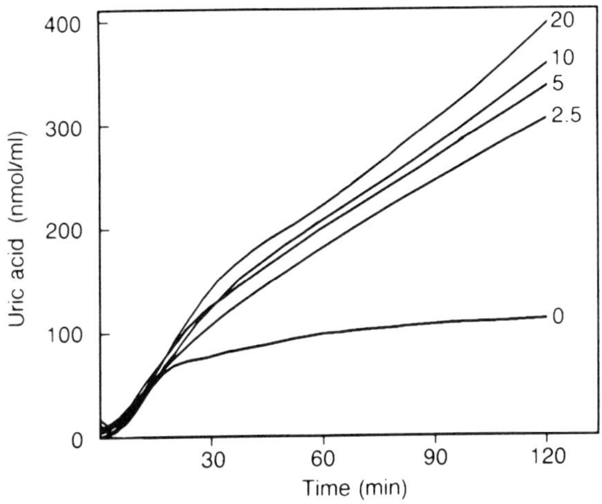

FIGURE 6

Influence of plasma on extended rates of uric acid production by xanthine oxidase. Reaction mixtures contained 5 mU/ml xanthine oxidase, 0.5 m*M* hypoxanthine, and 0, 2.5, 5, 10, or 20% plasma incubated in 0.1 *M* potassium phosphate, pH 7.4, as indicated. Reactions were conducted at 37°C for 120 min. [Reproduced from R. Radi, J. S. Beckman, K. M. Bush, and B. A. Freeman, Arch. Biochem. Biophys. **288,** 481–487 (1991).]

rial and conjugated dienes can alternatively represent (1) tissue release of compounds unrelated to free radical damage or (2) the increased rate of synthesis of leukotrienes or prostaglandins in response to oxidant-unrelated tissue injury (49).

Circulating levels of hypoxanthine plus xanthine in normal adults are low, 2–4 μM. Nevertheless, in certain physiopathological situations plasma hypoxanthine plus xanthine can approach 50–100 μM and be maintained at those levels for several days in the circulation (39,41). This substrate concentration will support near V_{max} XO activity and result in significant extents of oxygen radical production in the intravascular compartment. Plasma uric acid may serve to counter this potential oxidant stress in two ways. Human plasma possesses high concentrations of uric acid (200–500 μM) which can either act as an antioxidant or serve to inhibit XO activity (50). At the concentrations typically found in human plasma, uric acid inhibits XO activity by 40–50% (47). Thus, circulating uric acid may provide a feedback mechanism to partially attenuate intravascular generation of XO-derived O_2^- and H_2O_2. In summary, circulating or endothelial cell surface-associated XO has the poten-

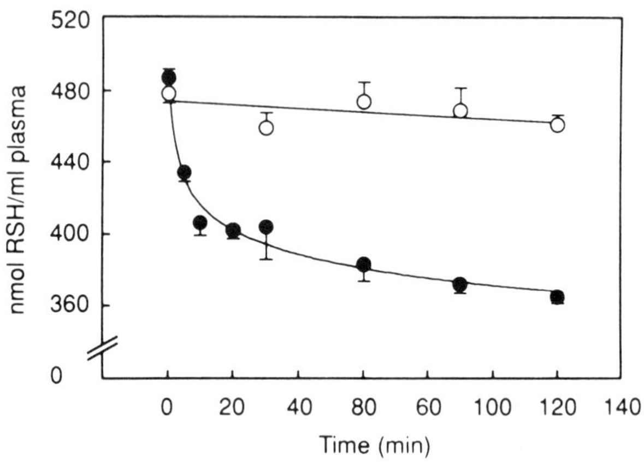

FIGURE 7

Time course of xanthine oxidase-mediated oxidation of sulfhydryls. Human plasma (90%, v/v) was incubated in the absence (O) or presence (●) of 5 mU/ml xanthine oxidase plus 0.5 ml xanthine in 0.1 *M* potassium phosphate, pH 7.4, 37°C. Aliquots of samples were periodically taken and reactions stopped with 33 μM allopurinol. Data represent means ± SD (n = 4). [Reproduced from R. Radi, J. S. Beckman, K. M. Bush, and B. A. Freeman, *Arch. Biochem. Biophys.* **288,** 481–487 (1991).]

tial to cause free radical damage to both plasma components and vascular endothelial cell targets (Fig. 8).

V. Nitric Oxide in Vascular Endothelium

A. Endothelial Production of Nitric Oxide

Endothelial cells produce and release dissolved nitric oxide (·NO), a gaseous vasodilatory free radical (51,52). Nitric oxide is synthesized by diverse cell types via O_2^- and NADPH-dependent oxidation of a guanidinium nitrogen of arginine via nitric oxide synthase [Eq. (10)].

$$\text{L-arginine} \xrightarrow[\text{nitric oxide synthetase}]{O_2,\ \text{NADPH}} \text{L-citrulline} + \cdot\text{NO} \tag{10}$$

Different biomolecules, some of them critical mediators of inflammatory responses, stimulate the endothelial synthesis of ·NO, which then causes vascular relaxation by stimulating smooth muscle guanylate cyclase (52). These molecules include acetylcholine, calcium ionophores, ATP, brady-

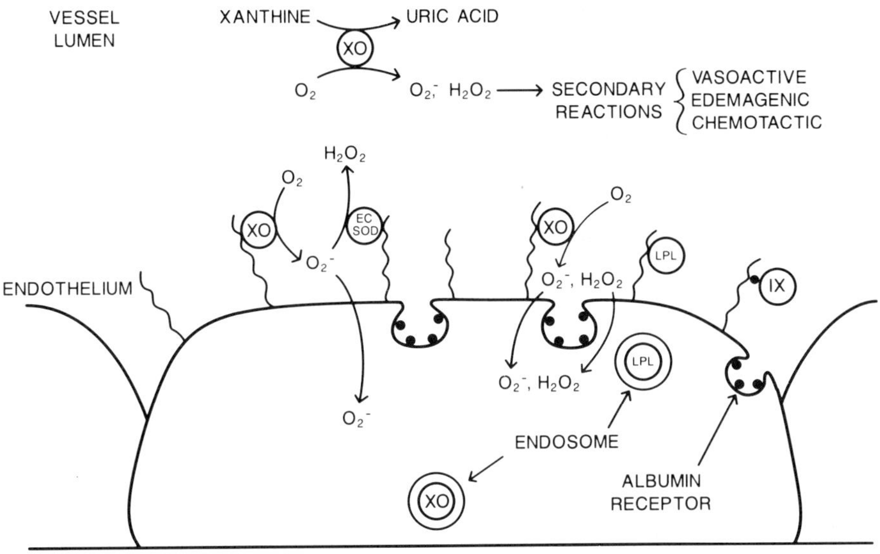

FIGURE 8

Interaction of circulating XO with vascular endothelial cell surface glycosaminoglycans, the intravascular compartment, and possible vascular endothelial XO uptake processes.

kinin, γ-interferon, TNF, and bacterial LPS (53–55). It has been estimated that a stimulated arteriole of 50 μm diameter could produce ·NO at a rate of 8 μM/min in the intraluminal space (56). *In vivo* injection of inhibitors of ·NO synthesis such as the L-nitroarginine methyl ester or *N*-monomethyl arginine causes a significant increase in vascular resistance and blood pressure, suggesting a constitutive endothelial production of ·NO.

The physiological half-life of ·NO is very short ($t_{1/2}$~5 sec), with more than one chemical pathway accounting for its disappearance (52). Nitric oxide can react with oxygen in aqueous solution to yield nitrogen dioxide (·NO_2) a reactive molecule that ultimately decomposes to stable products, NO_2^- (nitrite) and NO_3^- (nitrate). The observation that SOD stabilizes ·NO, thereby doubling its half-life, indicates that O_2^- participates in inactivation of the vasodilatory properties of ·NO (57).

B. Peroxynitrite: The Product of Superoxide and Nitric Oxide

We have observed that the reaction product of ·NO plus O_2^- is a potentially toxic reactive species rather than a benign product of ·NO inactivation. The reaction of O_2^- and ·NO is rapid (k_2 3.7 × 10^7 M^{-1} sec^{-1}), yielding peroxynitrite anion ($ONOO^-$) (56,58). Peroxynitrite anion becomes protonated at physiological pH to peroxynitrous acid (ONOOH, pK_a 6.8), which is an unstable species, decomposing with a half-life of less than a second in aqueous solution (56). Peroxynitrous acid can undergo homolysis to a molecule with ·OH-like reactivity and $·NO_2$ (nitrogen dioxide) or undergo intramolecular rearrangement to yield NO_3^- [Equation (11), Fig. 9].

$$O_2^- + \bullet NO \longrightarrow ONOO^- \overset{H^+}{\longleftrightarrow} ONOOH \longrightarrow \text{"}\bullet OH\text{"} + NO_2 \qquad ONOOH \longrightarrow NO_3^- + H^+ \tag{11}$$

C. Reactivity of Peroxynitrite

Peroxynitrite is an strong oxidizing agent as revealed by its reactivity toward different biomolecules including deoxyribose (56), unsaturated fatty acids of phospholipids (59), and protein or nonprotein sulfhydryls (60). Peroxynitrite can also attack molecular targets by more than one mechanism. For example, $ONOO^-$ directly reacts with sulfhydryl groups. We have reported that $ONOO^-$ reacts at 5000 M^{-1} sec^{-1} with cysteine and at 2100 M^{-1} sec^{-1} with the single thiol group of bovine

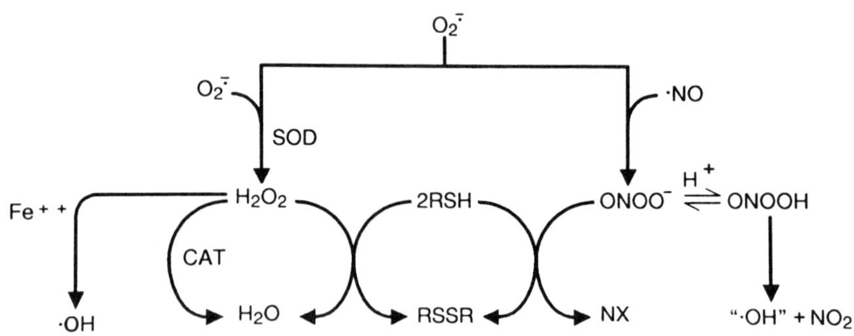

FIGURE 9

Potential mechanisms of O_2^--mediated cytotoxicity. The left-hand half of the scheme shows our current understanding of O_2^--mediated cytotoxicity, and the right-hand half shows recently revealed alternative mechanisms which can occur in the presence of ·NO. NX represents a yet unidentified nitrogen-containing species; CAT, catalase; SOD, superoxide dismutase. (Reproduced from Ref. 60.)

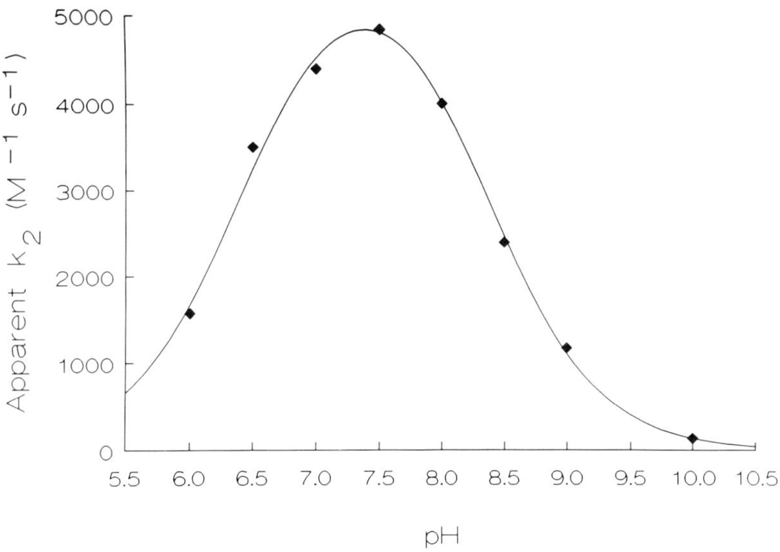

FIGURE 10

Rate constants for the reaction of peroxynitrite with cysteine as a function of pH. Peroxynitrite (60 μM) was added to 37.5 mM cysteine in 50 mM potassium phosphate at different pH values at 37°C. Apparent second-order rate constants were obtained as described in Ref. 60.

serum albumin, at pH 7.4 (Fig. 10) (60). These bimolecular rate constants are about 1000 times greater than the reaction of H_2O_2 with thiols. Alternatively, once ONOOH is formed, it decays (at least in part) via homolytic decomposition to an ·OH-like species and $\cdot NO_2$. Homolytic decomposition of ONOOH appears to account for the oxidation of deoxyribose (56) and phosphatidylcholine (PC) liposomes (59). Peroxidation of PC liposomes was assessed by oxygen consumption and the formation of conjugated dienes and thiobarbituric acid-positive material (Fig. 11).

Peroxynitrite-induced lipid peroxidation did not require the presence of iron in the reaction mixtures unlike other mechanisms of oxidant-induced lipid peroxidation (59). Still, the iron chelator desferrioxamine caused inhibition of ONOOH-mediated oxidation reactions by direct scavenging of ONOOH (56,59). This points out that part of the protective antioxidant function of desferrioxamine *in vivo* may be due to direct reaction with ONOOH, in addition to iron chelation.

While reaction of ·NO with FeS clusters and the concomitant release of Fe has been reported, and ·NO has been shown to be involved in enzyme

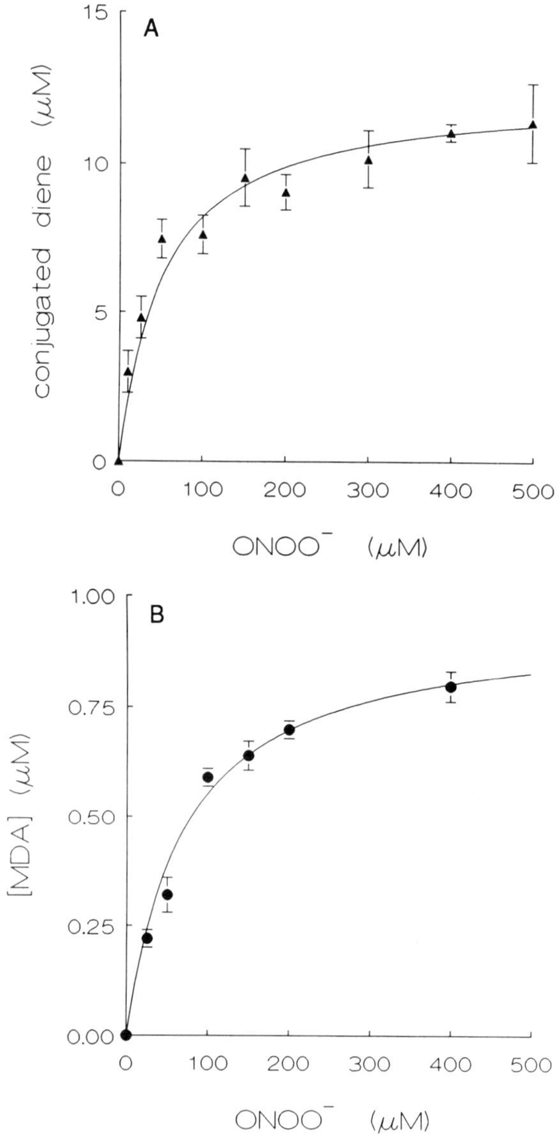

FIGURE 11

Yield of lipid peroxidation products as a function of peroxynitrite concentration. Peroxynitrite was added to phosphatidylcholine liposomes (2.6 μmol liposome lipid/ml) in 100 m*M* potassium phosphate, pH 7.4, 37°C, and reaction mixtures were incubated for 5 min. Aliquots were assayed for malonyldialdehyde (MDA) (A) and conjugated dienes (B). Data represent means ± SD (n = 4). (Reproduced from Ref. 59.)

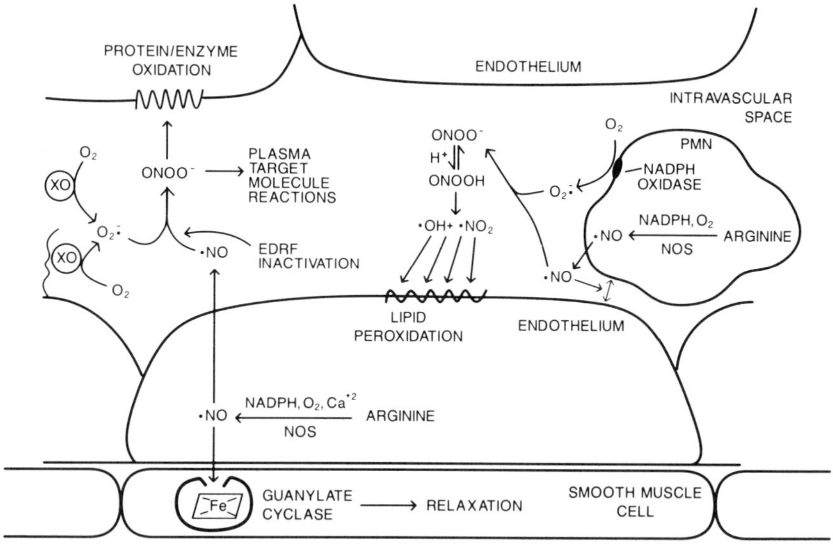

FIGURE 12

Production and reactions of O_2^- and ·NO in the intravascular compartment.

inhibition, macrophage-induced tumor cell killing, and the bactericidal activity of Kupffer cells, the mechanisms of action of ·NO have only been partially defined because of multiple possible reaction pathways (52). Pathophysiological dilemmas such as acute inflammation, immune complex-induced lung injury, sepsis, and ischemia–reperfusion increase the formation of both O_2^- and ·NO and may favor the formation of $ONOO^-$ (61–63). The protective effects of SOD observed in different organs and *in vivo* models of these pathological processes may be due in part to the inhibition of the formation of the toxic $ONOO^-$. In confirmation of this new concept, it has recently been proposed that $ONOO^-$ may be a major toxic intermediate in a variety of pathophysiological conditions including immunecomplex-stimulated pulmonary edema (63,64), glutamate toxicity to cortical neurons, (14), myocardial ischemia–reperfusion injury (62) and rejection of transplanted organs (65). Figure 12 depicts our conceptualization of possible mechanisms explaining these recent observations.

VI. Future Directions

New concepts have recently emerged concerning the generation of reactive species by vascular endothelium. A number of issues should be better developed to gain clearer insight into the role of free radicals in vascular homeostatic mechanisms and pathological processes. (A) Better define the interplay between endothelial and inflammatory cell-derived O_2^- and ·NO. The influence of disease processes such as sepsis and ischemia–reperfusion phenomena should be examined, as well as delineation of the relative contributions of specific vascular cells to net production of O_2^- and ·NO. The species-, organ- and vascular bed-specific O_2^- and ·NO metabolic characteristics should be defined as well. (B) Once mechanisms of $ONOO^-$ formation and reactions are better understood, further examine the role of $ONOO^-$ as a mediator of target molecule and cell injury. (C) The dynamics of circulating xanthine oxidase should be described in more detail, including defining the mechanism of release from source tissues, its fate and actions while circulating free in blood, and its actions following binding to vascular and interstitial cell glycosaminoglycans. (D) Characterize the cellular mechanisms that modulate XO activity in vascular endothelium from both an enzymological and gene expression perspective. Then, determine the contribution of XO to the net production of reactive oxygen species by endothelium derived from different vascular beds and species. (E) Examine the interactions between serum lipoprotein oxidation processes and endothelial or inflammatory cell-derived O_2^-, ·NO, $ONOO^-$ during the progression of atherosclerosis and associated abnormal vasoregulatory properties.

References

1. P. C. Panus, S. A. Wright, P. H. Chumley, R. Radi, and B. A. Freeman, *Arch. Biochem. Phys.* **294,** 695–702 (1992).
2. B. A. Freeman and J. D. Crapo, *J. Biol. Chem.* **258,** 10986–10992 (1981).
3. G. M. Rosen and B. A. Freeman, *Proc. Natl. Acad. Sci. U.S.A.* **81,** 7269–7273 (1984).
4. B. A. Freeman, G. M. Rosen, and M. J. Barber, *J. Biol. Chem.* **261,** 6590–6593 (1986).
5. B. A. Freeman, K. Whitfied, D. Gelman, and D. A. Parks, *Free Radical Biol. Med.* **9,** 94 (1990).
6. H. Kuthan, V. Ullrich, and R. W. Eastbrook, *Biochem. J.* **203,** 551–558 (1982).
7. W. F. Beyer and I. Fridovich, *Arch. Biochem. Biophys.* **285,** 60–63 (1991).
8. T. C. Rodell, J. C. Chronis, C. L. Ohnemus, D. J. Piermattei, and J. E. Repine, *J. Appl. Physiol.* **63,** 2159–2163 (1987).
9. J. S. Beckman and B. A. Freeman, *in* "Physiology of Oxygen Radicals" (A. Taylor and S. Matalon, eds.), pp. 39–53. Am. Physiol. Soc., 1986.
10. J. A. Royall, P. D. Gwin, D. A. Parks, and B. A. Freeman, *Arch. Biochem. Biophys.* **294,** 686–694 (1992).
11. R. Radi, J. F. Turrens, L. Y. Chang, K. M. Bush, J. D. Crapo, and B. A. Freeman, *J. Biol. Chem.* **266,** 22028–22034 (1991).

12. R. Radi, K. M. Bush, and B. A. Freeman, *Arch. Biochem. Biophys.* in press (1992).
13. P. Panus, R. Radi, P. Chumley, and B. A. Freeman, *Free Radical Biol. Med.* in press (1992).
14. H. A. Paler-Martinez, P. C. Panus, P. A. Chumley, and B. A. Freeman. *Free Radical Biol. Med.* submitted, (1992).
15. J. S. Beckman, D. A. Parks, J. Pearson, P. Marshall, and B. A. Freeman. *Free Radical Biol. Med.* **6,** 607–615 (1989).
16. E. D. Jarasch, G. C. Grund, and G. Bruder, *Cell (Cambridge, Mass.)* **25,** 67–82 (1981).
17. G. Bruder, H. W. Heid, E. D. Jarasch, and I. M. Mather, *Differentiation* **23,** 218–225 (1983).
18. E. D. Jarasch, G. Bruder, and H. W. Heid, *Acta Physiol. Scand. Suppl.* **548,** 39–46 (1986).
19. Y. Hattori, T. Hishino, C. Usami, K. Tsushima, and M. Ichikawa, *Adv. Exp. Med. Biol.* **253B,** 505–509 (1989).
20. D. A. Clare and J. G. Lecce, *Arch. Biochem. Biophys.* **233,** 233–237 (1991).
21. T. Nishino, T. Nishino, and K. Tsushima, *FEBS Lett.* **131,** 369–372 (1981).
22. P. C. Panus, B. Burgess, and B. A. Freeman, *Biochim. Biophys. Acta* **1091,** 303–309 (1991).
23. J. M. Thompson, J. S. Nickels, and J. R. Fisher, *Biochim. Biophys. Acta* **568,** 157–176 (1979).
24. N. Prajda, H. P. Morris, and G. Weber, *Cancer Res.* **36,** 4639–4646 (1976).
25. P. C. Panus, J. Shearer, and B. A. Freeman, *Exp. Lung Res.* **14** (Suppl.), 959–976 (1988).
26. C. M. Grum, R. A. Ragsdale, L. H. Ketai, and M. Shlafer, *Biochem. Biophys. Res. Commun.* **141,** 1104–1108 (1986).
27. R. M. Jackson, C. F. Veal, C. B. Alexander, A. L. Brannen, and J. D. Fulmer, *Am. Rev. Respir. Dis.* **137,** 1165–1171 (1988).
28. R. R. Baker, P. C. Panus, B. A. Holm, P. C. Engstrom, B. A. Freeman, and S. Matalon, *Am. J. Physiol.* **259,** L328–L334 (1990).
29. N. M. Hasan, R. B. Cundall, and G. E. Adams, *Free Radical Biol. Med.* **11,** 179–185 (1991).
30. T. Spector and R. Ferone, *J. Biol. Chem.* **259,** 10784–10786 (1984).
31. P. C. Lee, *Arch. Biochem. Biophys.* **157,** 322–323 (1973).
32. L. S. Terada, C. J. Beehler, A. Banerjee, J. M. Brown, M. A. Grosso, A. H. Harken, J. M. McCord, and J. E. Repine, *J. Appl. Physiol.* **65,** 2349–2353 (1988).
33. P. Gorog, J. D. Pearson, and V. V. Kakkar, *Atherosclerosis* **72,** 19–27 (1988).
34. U. P. Steinbrecher, *Biochim. Biophys. Acta* **959,** 20–30 (1988).
35. J. A. Royall, R. B. Berkow, J. S. Beckman, M. K. Cunningham, S. Matalon, and B. A. Freeman, *Am. J. Physiol. (Lung Cell Mol. Physiol.)* **257,** L499–L410 (1989).
36. K. L. Brigham, B. Meyrick, L. C. Berry, and J. E. Repine, *J. Appl. Physiol.* **63,** 840–850 (1987).
37. H. O. Friedl, G. O. Till, U. S. Ryan, and P. A. Ward, *FASEB J.* **3,** 2512–2518 (1989).
38. T. Oda, T. Akaike, T. Hamamoto, F. Suzuki, T. Hirano, and H. Maeda, *Science* **244,** 974–976 (1989).
39. T. Akaike, M. Ando, T. Oda, T. Doi, S. Ijiri, S. Araki, and H. Maeda, *J. Clin. Invest.* **85,** 739–745 (1990).
40. U. Yokoyama, J. S. Beckman, T. K. Beckman, J. K. Wheat, T. G. Cash, B. A. Freeman, and D. A. Parks, *Am. J. Physiol. (Gastrointest. Liver Physiol.* **21**) **258,** G564–G570 (1990).
41. C. M. Grum, R. A. Radsdale, L. H. Ketaie, and R. H. Simon, *J. Crit. Care* **2,** 223–226 (1987).
42. H. P. Friedl, G. O. Till, O. Trentz, and P. A. Ward, *Am. J. Pathol.* **135,** 203–217 (1989).
43. G. Bruder, E. Jarasch, and H. W. Heid, *J. Clin Invest.* **74,** 783–793 (1984).
44. C.-F. Cheng, G. M. Oosta, A. Bensadoun, and R. D. Rosenberg, *J. Biol. Chem.* **256,** 12893–12898 (1981).

45. L. Ghitescu, A. Fixman, M. Simionescu, and N. Simionescu, *J. Cell Biol.* **102,** 1304–1311 (1986).
46. J. E. Schnitzer, W. W. Carley, and G. E. Palade, *Am. J. Physiol.* **254,** H425–H437 (1988).
47. S. Tan, R. Radi, F. Gaudier, R. A. Evans, A. Rivera, and D. A. Parks, *Ped. Res.* submitted (1992).
48. R. Radi, H. Rubbo, and B. A. Freeman, *Arch. Biochem. Biophys.* submitted, (1992).
49. R. Radi, K. M. Bush, T. P. Cosgrove, and B. A. Freeman, *Arch. Biochem. Biophys.* **286,** 117–125 (1991).
50. R. Radi, S. Tan, E. Prodanov, R. A. Evans, and D. A. Parks, *Biochim. Biophys. Acta* in press (1992).
51. S. Moncada, R. M. J. Palmer, and E. A. Higgs, *Hypertension* **12,** 365–372 (1988).
52. M. A. Marletta, *Trends Biochem. Sci.* **14,** 488–492 (1989).
53. R. M. J. Palmer, D. S. Ashton, and S. Moncada, *Nature* (*London*) **333,** 664–666 (1988).
54. A. H. Ding, C. F. Nathan, and D. J. Stuehr, *J. Immunol.* **141,** 2407–2411 (1988).
55. C. Thiemermann and J. Vane, *Eur. J. Pharmacol.* **182,** 591–595 (1990).
56. J. S. Beckman, T. W. Beckman, J. Chen, P. A. Marshall, and B. A. Freeman, *Proc. Natl. Acad. Sci. U.S.A.* **87,** 1620–1624 (1990).
57. R. J. Gryglewski, R. M. J. Palmer, and S. Moncada, *Nature* (*London*) **320,** 454–456 (1986).
58. M. Saran, C. Michel, and W. Bors, *Free Radical Res. Commun.* **10,** 221–226 (1990).
59. R. Radi, J. S. Beckman, K. M. Bush, and B. A. Freeman, *Arch. Biochem. Biophys.* **288,** 481–487 (1991).
60. R. Radi, J. S. Beckman, K. M. Bush, and B. A. Freeman, *J. Biol. Chem.* **266,** 4244–4250 (1991).
61. B. Halliwell, *Free Radical Res. Commun.* **5,** 315–318 (1989).
62. G. Z. Matheis, G. D. Buckberg, D. Hayborn, M. Sherman, and L. Ignarro, *Am J. Physiol.* **262,** H616–H620 (1992).
63. M. Mulligan, J. Hevel, M. Marletta, and P. Ward, *Proc. Natl. Acad. Sci. U.S.A.* **88,** 6338–6342 (1991).
64. M. S. Mulligan, J. S. Warren, C. W. Smith, D. C. Anderson, C. G. Yeh, A. R. Rudolph, and P. A. Ward. *J. Immunol.* **148,** 3086–3092 (1992).
65. J. R. Lancaster, J. M. Langrehr, H. A. Bergonia, N. Murase, R. L. Simmons, and R. A. Hoffman. *J. Biol. Chem.* **267,** 10994–10998 (1992).

CHAPTER 5

Composition of NADPH Oxidase of Phagocytes and Other Cell Types: Role of Flavoprotein in Proton Translocation and Oxidase Activity

O. T. G. Jones
Department of Biochemistry
School of Medical Sciences
University of Bristol
Bristol BS8 ITD, England

A. R. Cross
Department of Molecular and Experimental Medicine
The Scripps Research Institute
La Jolla, California 92037

I. Flavin and Cytochrome *b* Interactions in NADPH Oxidase

The superoxide-generating activity of NADPH oxidase requires the transfer of electrons from an obligatory two-electron donor (NADPH) to oxygen acting as a one-electron acceptor, with the liberation of one H^+ for each $O_2^-\cdot$ formed:

$$NADPH + H^+ + 2O_2 \xrightarrow{\text{oxidase}} NADP^+ + 2O_2^-\bullet + 2H^+ \tag{1}$$

There is good evidence that FAD acts as a transducer in the reaction: it is reduced to $FADH_2$ by accepting two electrons from NADPH together with two protons. Because FAD can form a relatively stable one-electron reduced form (a flavin semiquinone), it can transfer electrons singly to cytochrome b_{-245}, liberating H^+ as shown in Fig. 1. In Fig. 1 two separate molecules of cytochrome b_{-245} are shown, each forming a separate molecule of superoxide. Studies using electron spin resonance (ESR) and resonance Raman spectroscopy (1) suggest that two hemes might be present in one molecule of cytochrome b_{-245}, sufficiently close to interact. If this interesting work is confirmed, then in the mechanism illustrated in Fig. 1 there may be only one molecule of cytochrome b_{-245} involved, with two different heme prosthetic groups.

A. Flavin Component of NADPH Oxidase

The activity of Triton X-100-solubilized NADPH oxidase is increased by the addition of FAD (2,3), and in plasma membranes from neutrophils there was a ratio of FAD to cytochrome b_{-245} close to 1 : 1 whereas the FMN content was low (4). In neutrophils from patients with the autosomal recessive form of chronic granulomatous disease (CGD) the FAD/

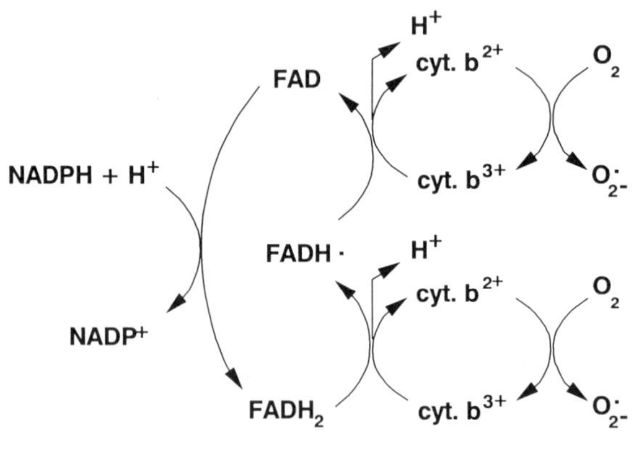

FIGURE 1

Possible arrangement of redox couples involved in NADPH oxidase. It is unclear whether one or two separate molecules of cytochrome *b* are involved.

cytochrome b_{-245} ratio was normal, but in membranes from patients with the X-linked form of CGD the cytochrome b_{-245} was absent, as expected, and the FAD content was diminished. This suggests that in normal neutrophils there is an association between an FAD-linked flavoprotein and cytochrome b_{-245}. This specific flavoprotein is apparently unstable or is synthesized at diminished rates in the absence of cytochrome b_{-245} synthesis.

Purification of NADPH oxidase in amounts sufficient for detailed analysis of its composition and kinetic properties has proved very difficult, and the published contents of cytochrome b_{-245} and FAD in these preparations are widely different, possibly because FAD and heme may be lost during purification. However, informative measurements can be made on isolated plasma membrane fractions from activated neutrophils and the detergent-soluble oxidase prepared from them. These show that in extracts of activated cells the major flavoprotein present is reduced by added NADPH (5,6). In membranes, or extracts, from resting cells FAD was present but was not reduced by NADPH. The extent of the reduction by FAD during enzyme turnover was proportional to the oxidase activity of the extract; partial inactivation of the oxidase by incubation at 25°C resulted in a diminished extent of reduction of FAD in the aerobic steady state. These experiments demonstrate the involvement of FAD in NADPH oxidase and show that electron transfer from cytosolic NADPH to the membrane flavoprotein is activation-dependent. From steady-state spectra, combined with measurements of the kinetics of oxidation of reduced cytochrome b_{-245}, it can be calculated (6) that every electron passing to oxygen to make $O_2^{-}\cdot$ passes through the cytochrome b_{-245} as shown in Fig. 1. It is thus very unlikely that FAD or its semiquinone reacts directly with O_2 to form $O_2^{-}\cdot$.

Despite its association with a protein, the FAD retains some fluorescence, with emission bands close to those of free FAD. Potentiometric titration of neutrophil membranes by ESR spectroscopy (7) detected a signal at $g = 2.004$, identified as a neutral semiquinone with a redox midpoint (Em_7) of −280 mV. This would be thermodynamically competent to transfer electrons from NADPH (Em_7 −320 mV) to cytochrome b_{-245} (Em_7 −245 mV). The relaxation properties of the semiquinone ESR signal suggested that it was near a transition metal (7), possibly the heme iron of cytochrome b_{-245}. The Em of the semiquinone, like that of the cytochrome b_{-245}, was unaltered by the transition from resting to active oxidase, but only the flavoprotein from unstimulated cells gave rise to a semiquinone ESR signal on the addition of NADPH.

The identification and isolation of the putative FAD protein has been difficult, in part because the FAD dissociates from detergent-solubilized proteins. Other experimental approaches have been adopted to label the flavoprotein, particularly using affinity labeling with NADPH dialdehyde. The reactivity of this affinity label with proteins in general has led to the identification of many different proteins as NADPH-binding proteins involved in the oxidase. There have been repeated reports that a cytosolic protein of 66–68 kDa (8) is predominantly labeled by the dialdehyde, although using the same approach a protein of 32 kDa has been identified as a specific NADH-binding protein (9). This protein was absent from the membranes of resting cells and from one CGD patient, and it was postulated to be an NADPH-binding protein which was transferred from cytosol to membrane on activation.

The purification of solubilized NADPH oxidase from neutrophil membranes using nondenaturing conditions has also yielded varied products. Kakinuma *et al.* (10) identified a protein of 67 kDa which catalyzed the oxidation of NADPH to yield $O_2^{-}\cdot$ under some conditions. This protein (p*I* 5.0) contained FAD but no cytochrome b_{-245}. Others [e.g., Glass *et al.* (11)] have suggested that purified oxidase contained FAD but not cytochrome b_{-245}. In a cell-free system NADPH oxidase can be reconstituted from a mixture of resting membranes, cytosol, and arachidonic acid (12). The transfer of an NADPH-binding protein from the cytosol fraction to the membrane as part of the activation process has sometimes been suggested [e.g., Smith *et al.* (13)]. Nisimoto and Otsuka-Murakami (14) have purified a soluble fraction from the cytosol containing major proteins of 45 and 40 kDa which catalyzes NADPH-dependent nitroblue tetrazolium (NBT) reduction and which activates NADPH oxidase in a cell-free system. A group of proteins of similar molecular mass was found to catalyze NBT reduction in extracts of active membrane (15), and it was proposed that a 45-kDa cytosolic NADPH–NBT reductase was translocated to the plasma membrane on activation.

An inhibitor, diphenylene iodonium (DPI), blocks the activity of the mitochondrial NADH dehydrogenase complex and covalently attaches to one subunit of this multisubunit flavoprotein complex (16). We have found that DPI (Fig. 2) is an even more potent inhibitor of NADPH oxidase (17) in whole neutrophils and in soluble membranes and extracts. Further, when labeled DPI was added to oxidase preparations, a 45-kDa protein was much the most labeled peptide. Spectroscopic studies showed that the addition of DPI to NADPH-reduced oxidase caused the disappearance of the absorption bands characteristic of reduced FAD and cytochrome b_{-245} (17) suggesting that DPI inhibited electron flow at, or before, the FAD level. The inhibitory effect of DPI on NADPH oxidase was manifest only when the oxidase was turning over. Nonactivated

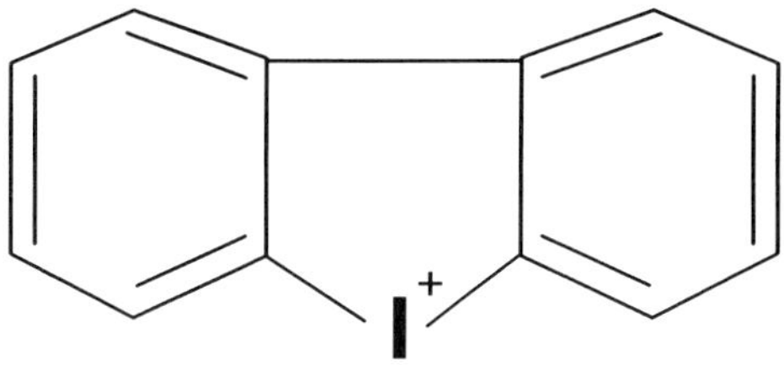

FIGURE 2

Structure of diphenylene iodonium.

neutrophils in 10 μM DPI, a concentration sufficient for complete inhibition of the active oxidase, can be transferred to fresh medium lacking DPI and the activity of the oxidase on phorbol addition found to be uninhibited. A likely explanation for these observations is that DPI is itself reduced by reduced electron transport components of the oxidase system to form the highly reactive DPI radical, DPI·. This radical would very rapidly attack adjacent flavins, hemes, or proteins causing inactivation of the oxidase. In model experiments we have shown that photoreduced FAD activates DPI and forms a stable addition complex with it (18). We have assumed that the 45-kDa protein labeled by DPI in neutrophil NADPH oxidase preparations is the flavoprotein, or is closely adjacent to it, and we have purified it using nucleotide affinity columns (19). A partial sequence of the protein established it as a novel protein which is induced during treatments of a monocyte–macrophage cell line with γ-interferon, a treatment which induces NADPH oxidase. The 45-kDa protein binds FAD, and polyclonal antibodies raised to it to inhibit soluble NADPH oxidase.

NADPH oxidase activity can be conferred on membranes from resting neutrophils when electrons are supplied from added flavoprotein NADPH–cytochrome *P*-450 reductase (20). This system has been exploited further by Isogai *et al.* (21) to show that *P*-450 reductase will reconstitute superoxide-generating capacity in a purified neutrophil cytochrome b_{-245}. Antibodies to *P*-450 reductase inhibited NADPH oxidase (19,22), perhaps because the homology of FAD and NADPH binding sites (23) means that many flavoproteins have common epitopes. Antibodies to *P*-450 reductase precipitated a 45-kDa protein from soluble extracts of NADPH oxidase (19) indicating that it, too, has epitopes in common with *P*-450 reductase and may be the flavoprotein reductase of NADPH oxidase.

In summary, the nature of the flavoprotein component of NADPH oxidase has yet to be decisively resolved. The absence of a clearly FAD-deficient CGD patient has delayed full clarification of this crucial part of the electron transport system, but this negative information is itself interesting. Analysis of sequence homologies suggests that cytochrome b_{-245} itself may have FAD and NADPH binding sites (56,57).

B. Proton Translocation Associated with NADPH Oxidase

NADPH oxidase is located in the plasma membrane of neutrophils and releases $O_2^-\cdot$ to the outer face (or into the interior of phagocyte vacuoles). Since NADPH is supplied at the cytoplasmic face of the membrane, the transfer of electrons is from inside to outside and must be electrogenic unless directly associated with movement of a compensating positive charge. There is evidence that activation of the oxidase in whole neutrophils is accompanied by changes in the plasma membrane potential; most frequently a depolarization has been recorded (24–29), although there have been reports of hyperpolarization.

Membrane potential changes are commonly measured by following the changes in fluorescence of cationic cyanine dyes [e.g., 3,3-dipropyloxadicarbocyanine (di-O-C_3), 3,3-dipentyloxadicarbocyanine (di-O-C_5)] or from absorbance changes of the anionic oxonols (e.g., Oxonol V). The granules of neutrophils are each enclosed in a membrane, and the marker dyes may distribute in the granule compartments as well as across the plasma membrane, leading to results which are difficult to interpret. This difficulty has been overcome by using neutrophil cytoplasts in place of whole neutrophils. The cytoplasts are plasma membrane-enclosed organelle-free vesicles of cytosol (30) which maintain the normal plasma membrane potential and respond to the stimuli which activate the oxidase. The lack of azurophil granules from the cytoplasts also overcomes the risk of peroxidative attack by myeloperoxidase on the membrane potential probe.

Using Oxonol V as a probe it was found that the plasma membrane depolarized by about 30 mV when cytoplasts were activated. The depolarization coincided with the onset of $O_2^-\cdot$ generation, but although $O_2^-\cdot$ release continued at an approximately linear rate over several minutes, the plasma membrane potential was stable after 1 min at a value about 30 mV more positive than the resting potential (31). When NADPH oxidase was inhibited by addition of DPI, superoxide production ceased and the membrane repolarized. These observations are best explained by assuming that NADPH oxidase is electrogenic and depolarizes the plasma membrane: in order to maintain a stable membrane potential and to allow continuing superoxide production, a channel opens and permits

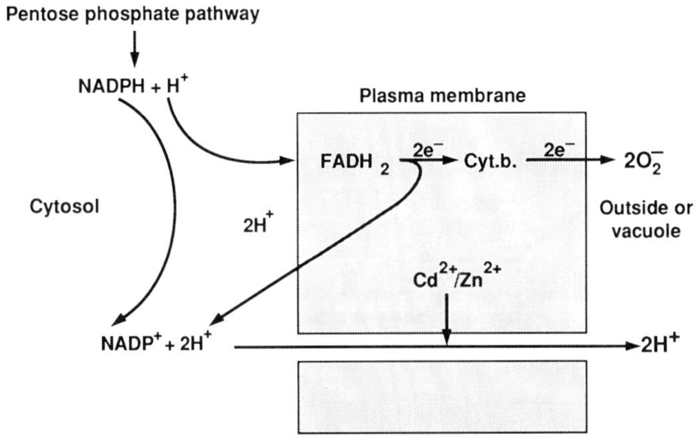

FIGURE 3

Suggested relationship of electron transfer by NADPH oxidase and transfer of H^+ via a channel.

the movement of a compensating ion (see Fig. 3). As discussed below, this ion is likely to be H^+. The early observation (26) that the membrane potential of neutrophils from CGD patients did not depolarize when they were stimulated with phorbol myristate acetate (PMA) or formylmethionylleucylphenylalanine (FMLP) accords with this suggestion. These CGD neutrophils responded to the stimuli normally with respect to degranulation and chemotaxis, showing that the receptor–response coupling was present but not making any contribution to membrane depolarization.

The oxidation of NADPH by an oxidase linked to O_2 must cause the release of H^+ [see Fig. 1 and Eq. (1)], and the oxidase might be arranged in the membrane so that this release of H^+ takes place either on the cytoplasmic face or exterior face of the plasma membrane. Internal pH of neutrophils or cytoplasts monitored using the fluorescence indicator 2′,7′-bis-2-carboxyethyl-5 (and -6) carboxyfluorescein (BCECF) showed that the internal pH became more acid when the NADPH oxidase was activated, and the changes were much more pronounced when the Na^+/H^+ exchanger was blocked by amiloride, or by suspending the cytoplasts in a K^+ medium (to remove Na^+ for exchange) (32). This increase in cytosolic acidity suggests that protons are released into the cytosol during NADPH oxidation. The coupling between internal pH and oxidase activity was shown by the addition of DPI to inhibit NADPH oxidase. This abolished the rise in cytosol $[H^+]$.

Outward proton movements through the plasma membrane of snail neurons are blocked by the addition of Zn^{2+} or Cd^{2+} ions (33). Treatment of neutrophil cytoplasts with Cd^{2+} caused increased acidification of the cytosol when NADPH oxidase was activated. Under optimum conditions for retention of H^+ within activated cytoplasts (Cd^{2+} present, together with valinomycin in an Na^+ medium to favor movement of K^+ from the cytosol as a charge compensator), the pH within the cytoplasts fell to around pH 6.7 and 0.8 H^+ was retained for every $O_2^-\cdot$ formed (32). This number is very close to that of 1 H^+ for each $O_2^-\cdot$ predicted by Eq. (1) and strongly supports a mechanism where reduced flavin transfers electrons to a cytochrome b_{-245} near the inner (cytosolic) face of the plasma membrane, with H^+ liberated into the cytosol for subsequent translocation through an H^+-conducting channel (Fig. 3).

The addition of Cd^{2+} to block the movement of a compensating H^+ for each electron transferred to O_2 on the outer face would be expected to increase depolarization of the plasma membrane when the oxidase is activated. This was indeed the effect found (31).

The plasma membrane potential of neutrophil cytoplasts becomes rapidly more positive when their NADPH oxidase is activated, but it then stabilizes as the H^+-translocating channel opens. The experiments of Henderson and Chappell (34) show that the channel is not voltage-regulated, but is activated by arachidonate. The addition of arachidonate made cytoplasts permeable to protons, but was without such effects on liposomes, showing that the arachidonate was not acting as a simple uncoupler. The involvement of arachidonate in activating the H^+ channel is particularly interesting since it is also an effective activator of NADPH oxidase in whole cells and *in vitro* reconstitutions.

II. Presence of "Phagocyte-Typic" NADPH Oxidase in Other Cell Types

A. Lymphocytes

The NADPH oxidase originally described in neutrophils (35) was first thought to be confined to the microbial phagocytic cells: polymorphonuclear leukocytes (PMN, neutrophils), monocytes, macrophages, and eosinophils. It is noteworthy that macrophage-derived cells are present in specialized forms in many tissues, frequently in large numbers (e.g., liver Kupffer cells, brain microglia). It is not yet clear to what extent and under what conditions these cells retain their capacity to produce superoxide. The function of the oxidase in these phagocytic cells is well understood; it is to produce toxic oxygen radicals to kill ingested microbes (by neutrophils, monocytes), invading parasites (by eosinophils), and virally infected or neoplastic cells (by macrophages). The severe, recurrent infections suffered by patients with chronic granulomatous disease in whom the NADPH oxidase is genetically dysfunctional is testimony to the importance of the role of oxygen radicals in host defense. It was therefore rather unexpected when it was first reported that Epstein-Barr virus (EBV)-transformed B-lymphocyte cell lines expressed low levels of the NADPH oxidase. Evidence that this superoxide-generating system was apparently identical to the "phagocyte" oxidase was provided by the demonstration that when patients with CGD were the donors of the lymphocytes, no NADPH oxidase was detected in the transformed cell lines (36). Subsequently it has been shown that the expression of the oxidase is not simply an abnormality created by the infection by EBV, but that normal B lymphocytes (but not T lymphocytes) express the superoxide-generating oxidase *in vivo*, as measured by superoxide dismutase (SOD)-inhibitable NBT reduction (37). The amount of superoxide produced by B lymphocytes is about 5% of that produced by a neutrophil on a cell/cell basis, when PMA is used as the stimulus (5 compared to 100 nmol/min/10^7 cells for neutrophils).

The superoxide-generating system in these transformed lymphocytes, like neutrophils, can be stimulated by a number of receptor-dependent and -independent stimuli and is inhibited by the same range of oxidase inhibitors. Included among the stimuli are the cytokines interleukin 1β (but not IL-1α unlike fibroblasts, Section II,C) and tumor necrosis factor α (TNF-α). These B cells also exhibit the phenomenon of priming, whereby preincubation of cells with a subthreshold concentration of one stimulus markedly potentiates the subsequent response to a second stimulus (38). One unexplained difference between the oxidase expressed in lymphocytes and the oxidase in normal neutrophils is the apparent variability in the K_m for NADPH among different cell lines, suggesting the oxidase may be incompletely assembled or activated in the membranes of the cells (39). The quantity of cytochrome b_{-245} in the B-cell lines is about 10% of that of a neutrophil (as determined by spectrophotometry at fixed redox potentials) (39,40), and the cells also contain the putative 45-kDa, DPI-binding oxidase flavoprotein (19) as detected by labeling with [^{125}I]DPI (40). Antibodies to one subunit of the cytochrome b_{-245} have been used to demonstrate that the cytochrome components of the oxidase are expressed at least at one developmental stage in the peripheral B lymphocytes, at the early B-cell stage, but the antigen is lost before the final differentiation into plasma cells (41). Antibodies have also been used to demonstrate that the cytochrome is present in tonsillar B cells (37). At the present time it is not known if B lymphocytes contain the 47- and 67-kDa cytosolic factors, p47-*phox* and p67-*phox*, which are an essential requirement for the activation of the neutrophil oxidase, although evidence has been presented that at least one of these factors is present in lymphoid cells (42). It is conceivable that superoxide generation by lymphocytes fulfills a signaling function related to proliferation or differentiation.

B. Endothelial Cells

Matsubara and Ziff (43) reported the increased production of superoxide by primary cultures of human endothelial cells after exposure to cytokines. The source of the superoxide has been attributed to the activity of xanthine oxidase (XO) in many preparations, and the conversion of xanthine dehydrogenase (which does not produce oxygen radicals) to XO (which produces superoxide and hydrogen peroxide) in response to inflammatory mediators has been reported (44). It is clear that the origin of at least part of the superoxide is a system apparently identical to that of the phagocyte. Endothelial cells from some sources do not contain XO, and in cases where XO is present, only part of the superoxide-generating activity is susceptible to XO inhibitors (45,46).

C. Fibroblasts

Superoxide production by a third nonphagocytic cell type has recently been described in which the "phagocyte" NADPH oxidase appears to be the origin of the radicals. Like the B-lymphocyte cell lines, primary cultures of human fibroblasts have been shown to contain both the low-potential cytochrome *b* (redox potential-243 ± 8 mV) and the 45-kDa flavoprotein (47). The rate of superoxide production was reported to be dose-dependent in response to IL-1α or TNF-α up to approximately 1 nmol/min/10^7 cells or about 1% of the capacity of a neutrophil. Unlike the neutrophil, however, the response of the fibroblasts continued in a linear fashion for at least 4 hr, and PMA was only a poor stimulus (48,49). There does appear to be a variability in the ability of cultured fibroblasts to release superoxide, which may be dependent on such factors as the cell cycle and composition of the culture medium (47,50,51).

Interestingly, superoxide release at similar concentrations to that reported by Murrell (51,52) stimulated fibroblast proliferation, whereas SOD and catalase inhibited proliferation, raising the possibility that superoxide could have a signaling role in wound healing and inflammation, leading to the increase in replicating fibroblasts found in certain fibrotic conditions (51,52). Oxygen-derived free radicals have similarly been reported to be released from osteoclasts and to stimulate their proliferation and bone resorption (53).

D. Glomerular Mesangial Cells

Kidney glomerular mesangial cells, which are believed to be mesenchymal in origin, resemble smooth muscle cells. Like fibroblasts and endothelial cells, human intrinsic mesangial cells respond poorly to PMA but exhibit a dose-dependent increase in the rate of superoxide production in response to the cytokine IL-1α (54). The most potent stimulus was the calcium ionophore A23187 which caused the release of 1.65 nmol/min/10^7 cells. The activity was unaffected by the XO inhibitor allopurinol or by inhibitors of mitochondrial respiration, but it was inhibited by the NADPH-oxidase inhibitor DPI (55). Membranes prepared from cultured human mesangial cells possessed a low potential (-250 mV) cytochrome *b* which had the spectral and carbon monoxide-binding characteristics of the neutrophil cytochrome b_{-245} (S. Jones and O. T. G. Jones, 1992, unpublished). Monoclonal antibodies were used to demonstrate the presence of both the α and β subunits of cytochrome b_{-245} (55), which was present at a concentration of 60 pmol/mg of crude membrane protein, approximately 30% of that found in an equivalent neutrophil preparation (S. Jones and O. T. G. Jones, 1992, unpublished). The cells have also been shown to contain the 45-kDa DPI-binding protein, but the presence of the 47-*phox* and 67-*phox* cytosolic activating factors has not yet been reported.

E. Function of Nonphagocytic NADPH Oxidase

The nonphagocytic "phagocyte oxidase"-containing cells seem to have the same molecular components of the NADPH oxidase found in neutrophils, but in lower concentration. They show a different type of response than the neutrophil, a relatively poor response to the potent neutrophil activator PMA, and a prolonged response to weak neutrophil stimuli such as cytokines. This is likely to be related to a distinct, nonmicrobicidal function in these other cell types, similar to the signaling role proposed for nitric oxide (endothelium-derived relaxation factor, EDRF). Nitric oxide, another short-lived radical, has a dual biological function. It is synthesized by an inducible system in macrophages at a concentration which is cytotoxic to target cells attacked by the macrophages but is also produced by a constitutive enzyme in a number of tissues (including macrophages and endothelial cells) where it appears to be identical with, or an immediate precursor of, endothelium-derived relaxation factor.

The capacity of these other types of cells to produce superoxide is likely to contribute to the tissue damage seen in a number of pathological conditions described elsewhere in this volume.

References

1. J. K. Hurst, T. M. Loehr, J. T. Curnutte, and H. Rosen, *J. Biol. Chem.* **266,** 1627–1634 (1991).
2. B. M. Babior and R. S. Kipnes, *Blood* **50,** 517–524 (1977).
3. T. G. Gabig and B. M. Babior, *J. Biol. Chem.* **263,** 9070–9074 (1979).
4. A. R. Cross, O. T. G. Jones, R. Garcia, and A. W. Segal, *Biochem. J.* **208,** 765–768 (1982).
5. A. R. Cross, J. F. Parkinson, and O. T. G. Jones, *Biochem. J.* **223,** 337–344 (1984).
6. A. R. Cross, J. F. Parkinson, and O. T. G. Jones, *Biochem. J.* **226,** 881–884 (1985).
7. K. Kakinuma, M. Kaneda, T. Chiba, and T. Ohnishi, *J. Biol. Chem.* **261,** 9426–9432 (1986).
8. S. Takasugi, K. Ishida, K. Takeshige, and S. Minakami, *J. Biochem. (Tokyo)* **105,** 155–157 (1989).
9. T. Umei, B. M. Babior, J. T. Curnutte, and R. M. Smith, *J. Biol. Chem.* **266,** 6019–6022 (1991).
10. K. Kakinuma, Y. Fukuhara, and M. Kaneda, *J. Biol. Chem.* **262,** 12316–12322 (1987).
11. G. A. Glass, D. M. DeLisle, P. DeTogni, B. E. Magee, M. Markert, and B. M. Babior, *J. Biol. Chem.* **261,** 13247–13251 (1986).
12. Y. Bromberg and E. Pick, *J. Biol. Chem.* **260,** 13539–13545 (1985).
13. R. M. Smith, J. T. Curnutte, and B. M. Babior, *J. Biol. Chem.* **264,** 1958–1962 (1989).
14. Y. Nisimoto and H. Otsuka-Murakami, *J. Biochem. (Tokyo)* **108,** 792–797 (1990).
15. Y. Nisimoto and H. Otsuka-Murakami, *Biochim. Biophys. Acta* **1040,** 260–266 (1990).
16. C. I. Ragan and D. P. Bloxham, *Biochem. J.* **163,** 605–615 (1977).
17. A. R. Cross and O. T. G. Jones, *Biochem. J.* **237,** 111–116 (1986).
18. V. B. O'Donnell, D. G. Tew, and O. T. G. Jones, *Eur. J. Clin. Invest.* **21**(2), 209 (Abstr.) (1991).
19. C. M. Yea, A. R. Cross, and O. T. G. Jones, *Biochem. J.* **265,** 95–100 (1990).
20. F. Sakane, H. Kojima, K. Takahashi, and J. Koyama, *Biochem. Biophys. Res. Commun.* **147,** 71–77 (1987).
21. Y. Isogai, A. Nasuda-Kouyama, and T. Iizuka, *J. Biol. Chem.* **266,** 13481–13484 (1991).
22. H. Takayama, S. Iwaki, K. Tamoto, and J. Koyama, *Biochim. Biophys. Acta* **799,** 151–157 (1984).
23. D. S. Bredt, P. M. Hwang, C. E. Glatt, C. Lowenstein, R. R. Reed, and S. H. Snyder, *Nature (London)* **351,** 714–718 (1991).
24. P. Naccache, H. J. Showell, E. L. Becker, and R. I. Sha'afi, *J. Cell Biol.* **75,** 635–649 (1977).
25. K. G. Lazzari, P. J. Proto, and E. R. Simons, *J. Biol. Chem.* **261,** 9710–9713 (1986).
26. B. E. Seligmann and J. I. Gallin, *J. Clin. Invest.* **66,** 493–503 (1980).
27. A. I. Tauber and E. R. Simons, *FEBS Lett.* **156,** 161–164 (1985).

28. A. R. Cameron, J. Nelson, and H. J. Forman, *Proc. Natl. Acad. Sci. U.S.A.* **80,** 3726–3728 (1983).
29. J. C. Whitin, C. E. Chapman, E. R. Simons, M. E. Chovaniec, and H. J. Cohen, *J. Biol. Chem.* **255,** 1874–1878 (1980).
30. D. Roos, A. A. Voetman, and L. J. Meerhof, *J. Cell Biol.* **97,** 368–377 (1983).
31. L. M. Henderson, J. B. Chappell, and O. T. G. Jones, *Biochem. J.* **246,** 325–329 (1987).
32. L. M. Henderson, J. B. Chappell, and O. T. G. Jones, *Biochem. J.* **255,** 285–290 (1988).
33. R. C. Thomas and R. W. Meech, *Nature (London)* **299,** 826–828 (1982).
34. L. M. Henderson and J. B. Chappell, *Biochem. J.* **283,** 171–175 (1992).
35. B. M. Babior, R. S. Kipnes, and J. T. Curnutte, *J. Clin. Invest.* **52,** 267–271 (1973).
36. D. J. Volkman, E. S. Buescher, J. I. Gallin, and A. S. Fauchi, *J. Immunol.* **133,** 3006–3009 (1984).
37. F.-E. Maly, M. Nakamura, J.-F. Gauchat, A. Urwyler, C. Walker, C. A. Dahinden, A. R. Cross, and O. T. G. Jones, *J. Immunol.* **142,** 1260–1267 (1989).
38. J. T. Hancock, L. M. Henderson, and O. T. G. Jones, *Immunology* **71,** 213–217 (1990).
39. J. T. Hancock, F.-E. Maly, and O. T. G. Jones, *Biochem. J.* **262,** 373–375 (1989).
40. F.-E. Maly, A. R. Cross, O. T. G. Jones, G. Wolf-Vorbeck, C. Walker, C. A. Dahinden, and A. L. de Weck, *J. Immunol.* **140,** 2334–2339 (1988).
41. S. Kobayashi, S. Imajoh-Ohmi, M. Nakamura, and S. Kanegasaki, *Blood* **75,** 458–461, (1990).
42. E. Pick, T. Kroizman, and A. Abo, *J. Immunol.* **143,** 4180–4187 (1989).
43. T. Matsubara and M. Ziff, *J. Immunol.* **137,** 3295–3298 (1986).
44. H. P. Friedl, G. O. Till, U. S. Ryan, and P. A. Ward, *FASEB J.* **3,** 2512–2518 (1989).
45. H. A. Kontos, *Chem.-Biol. Interact.* **72,** 229–255 (1989).
46. L. S. Terada, I. R. Willingham, M. E. Rosandich, J. A. Leff, G. W. Kindt, and J. E. Repine, *J. Cell. Physiol.* **148,** 191–196 (1991).
47. B. Meier, A. R. Cross, J. T. Hancock, F. J. Kaup, and O. T. G. Jones, *Biochem. J.* **275,** 241–245 (1991).
48. B. Meier, H. H. Radeke, S. Selle, M. Younes, H. Sies, K. Resch, and G. G. Habermehl, *Biochem. J.* **263,** 539–545 (1989).
49. B. Meier, H. H. Radeke, S. Selle, G. G. Habermehl, K. Resch, and H. Sies, *Biol. Chem. Hoppe-Seyler* **371,** 1021–1025 (1990).
50. G. A. C. Murrell, M. J. O. Francis, and L. Bromley, *Biochem. Soc. Trans.* **17,** 483–484 (1989).
51. G. A. C. Murrell, M. J. O. Francis, and L. Bromley, *Biochem. Soc. Trans.* **17,** 484 (1989).
52. G. A. C. Murrell, M. J. O. Francis, and L. Bromley, *Biochem. J.* **265,** 659–665 (1990).
53. I. R. Garrett, B. F. Boyce, R. O. C. Oreffo, L. Bonewald, J. Poser, and G. R. Mundy, *J. Clin. Invest.* **85,** 632–639 (1990).
54. H. H. Radeke, B. Meier, T. Topley, J. Flöge, G. G. Habermehl, and K. Resch, *Kidney Int.* **37,** 767–775 (1990).
55. H. H. Radeke, A. R. Cross, J. T. Hancock, O. T. G. Jones, M. Nakamura, V. Kaever, and K. Resch, *J. Biol. Chem.* **266,** 21026–21029 (1991).
56. A. W. Segal, I. West, F. Wientjes, J. H. A. Nugent, A. J. Chavan, B. Daley, R. C. Garcia, H. Rosen, G. Scrace, *Biochem. J.* **284,** 781–788 (1992).
57. D. Rotrosen, C. L. Yeung, T. L. Leto, H. L. Malech, C. H. Kwong, *Science* **256,** 1459–1462.

CHAPTER 6

Calcium-Modulated Cellular Effects of Oxidants

George E. N. Kass, Pierluigi Nicotera, and Sten Orrenius

Department of Toxicology
Karolinska Institute
S-104 01 Stockholm, Sweden

I. Introduction

It has become clear, over the past decade, that oxidative cell injury generated by chemicals, during reoxygenation of hypoxic tissue, or as a result of acute or chronic inflammatory processes is associated with a perturbation of intracellular calcium homeostasis. This perturbation can be a consequence of the impairment of the plasma membrane Ca^{2+}-translocating system(s), stimulation of Ca^{2+} channels, and inhibition of Ca^{2+} sequestration by the endoplasmic reticulum and mitochondria, all resulting in the inability of the cell to maintain its cytosolic free Ca^{2+} concentration ($[Ca^{2+}]_i$) within the physiological range ($\sim 0.1\ \mu M$). A sustained elevation of $[Ca^{2+}]_i$ has been causally linked to cell killing by a wide variety of unrelated compounds which display different chemical structures such as the heavy metals mercury and lead, organotin compounds, the hepatotoxins acetaminophen, carbon tetrachloride, and di-

Cellular and Molecular Mechanisms of Inflammation, Volume 4

quat, reactive oxygen metabolites, excitatory amino acids, quinones, and cyanide (see Refs. 1 and 2 for recent reviews). Ca^{2+} has also been implicated in the mechanism of immune cell killing by glucocorticoids and the environmental contaminant 2,3,7,8-tetrachlorodibenzo-*p*-dioxin (TCDD), and in the killing of target cells by neutrophils, macrophages, and natural killer cells. These findings led us and others to propose the Ca^{2+} hypothesis of cell injury which suggests that the disruption of intracellular Ca^{2+} homeostasis is a common step in cell killing by many toxic agents.

As discussed in the following sections, a number of mechanisms involving Ca^{2+}-dependent proteases, phospholipases, and endonucleases have been implicated in, and partially demonstrated to modulate, Ca^{2+}-mediated cell killing. In addition to this proposed mechanism of acute lethal injury by these catabolic processes, recent evidence has also been accumulating to implicate signal transduction processes as an important target for oxidant injury.

II. Cellular Calcium Sequestration Processes

In higher organisms most of the calcium is deposited in the bones and teeth as hydroxyapatite. The remaining calcium (~1%) is localized in the extracellular and intracellular fluids. Within the extracellular compartment the total concentration of calcium is dictated by the movements of Ca^{2+} in and out of the bone and teeth deposits and amounts to approximately 3 m*M* (of which about half is ionized). Although inside cells the total concentration of calcium varies from 20 μM in erythrocytes to 4 m*M* in cardiomyocytes, recent studies using cell-permeant indicators that are selective for calcium ions have shown that the free Ca^{2+} concentration in the cytosol is maintained between 0.1 and 0.2 μM (3,4). Thus, there is a concentration difference of approximately four orders of magnitude between the extracellular Ca^{2+} level (~1.3 m*M*) and the cytosolic free Ca^{2+} concentration; this results in a large electrochemical driving force in favor of net Ca^{2+} accumulation by the cells. This tendency to take up Ca^{2+} is balanced primarily by active Ca^{2+} extrusion systems located at the plasma membrane and by the coordinated activities of Ca^{2+}-sequestering systems located in the endoplasmic reticular, mitochondrial, and nuclear membranes (Fig. 1).

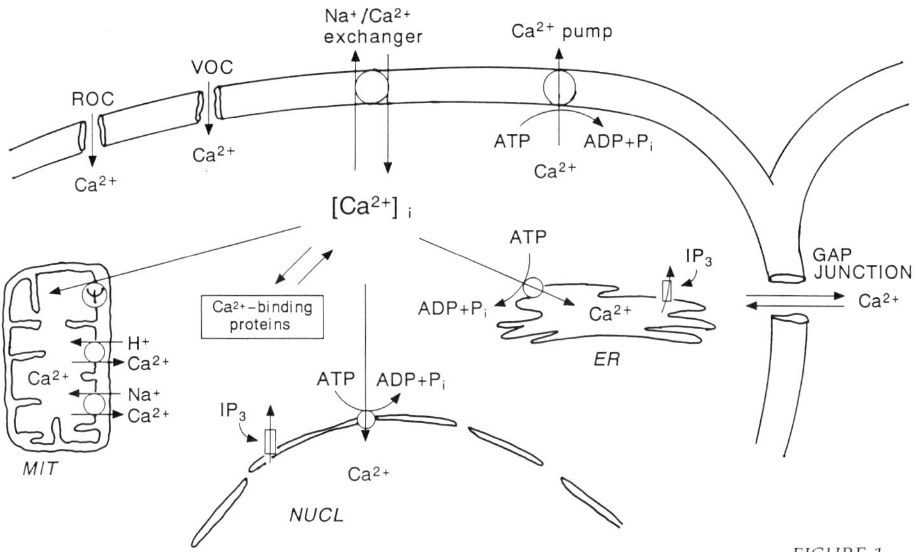

FIGURE 1
Intracellular Ca^{2+} transport processes.

A. Calcium Transport by the Plasma Membrane

1. *Calcium Entry*

Ca^{2+} enters the cell mainly through specific Ca^{2+} channels. One important group of Ca^{2+} channels comprises those activated by depolarization; these channels are commonly referred to as voltage-operated Ca^{2+} channels (VOC) (5). At least four types of voltage-operated Ca^{2+} channels with different pharmacological and electrophysiological properties have been identified in most excitable cells and in many nonexcitable cells. Recent studies in our and other laboratories have shown that, in nonexcitable cells, Ca^{2+} entry is also stimulated following the interaction of Ca^{2+}-mobilizing hormones and growth factors with their respective receptors. The mechanism by which Ca^{2+} influx through these receptor-operated channels (ROC) is regulated is still unclear; there is some evidence that G proteins or inositol phosphate turnover and the content of an intracellular pool identified as being part of the agonist-sensitive Ca^{2+} store may be involved (see Section IV). A third physiological route for Ca^{2+} entry involves an antiporter exchanging three Na^+ per Ca^{2+} ion translocated (see below). Additionally, it appears that Ca^{2+} enters through nonselective plasma membrane leak channels.

2. *Calcium Extrusion*

The two transport systems that can extrude Ca^{2+} against its concentration gradient to balance the basal as well as the hormone-stimulated influx of Ca^{2+} are the Ca^{2+}-ATPase and the Na^+/Ca^{2+} exchanger. The plasma membrane Ca^{2+}-ATPase, of which the enzyme found in erythrocytes is best characterized, utilizes the free energy liberated by the hydrolysis of ATP to electroneutrally expel Ca^{2+} in exchange for protons (6). The general kinetic properties of the Ca^{2+}-ATPase include a high affinity for Ca^{2+} but a low capacity for transport; however, these parameters may be modulated by calmodulin- and protein kinase C-dependent phosphorylation to favor Ca^{2+} extrusion.

In liver cells, the Ca^{2+}-ATPase is the predominant Ca^{2+} extrusion system. It has a molecular mass of around 140 kDa and a very high affinity for Ca^{2+} ($K_{0.5}$ 14 nM). In contrast to its erythrocyte counterpart, the liver plasma membrane enzyme does not appear to be stimulated by calmodulin. Recent evidence from our laboratory, however, suggests that the rate of Ca^{2+} efflux can be markedly increased by a currently unidentified second messenger generated by Ca^{2+}-mobilizing hormones (7).

The Na^+/Ca^{2+} exchanger is most active in heart and brain cells, and it catalyzes the electrogenic exchange of three Na^+ per Ca^{2+}. Consequently, the direction of the exchange depends on the transmembrane potential; with depolarization, Ca^{2+} influx occurs, whereas in the presence of a resting membrane potential Ca^{2+} is extruded from the cell.

B. Calcium Sequestration by the Endoplasmic and Sarcoplasmic Reticulum

Both the endoplasmic reticulum (ER) and the sarcoplasmic reticulum (SR) sequester Ca^{2+} through a Ca^{2+}-ATPase. Because of its high abundance in muscle tissue, the SR enzyme is the best characterized. The ATPase of the SR has high Ca^{2+} affinity and transport capacity, translocating 2 mol Ca^{2+} per mol ATP that is hydrolyzed. The SR and ER enzymes are very similar in many aspects, for example, molecular weight, reaction mechanism, and kinetic parameters. The liver ER Ca^{2+}-ATPase has recently been purified by the group of Kraus-Friedmann (8). This enzyme of 107 kDa has a high affinty for Ca^{2+} ($K_{0.5}$ 0.2–1 μM) and catalyzes the sequestration of 10–20 nmol Ca^{2+}/mg microsomal vesicle protein.

The regulation of Ca^{2+} sequestration by the hepatic endoplasmic reticulum is still poorly understood. Although the involvement of calmodulin in this process has been suggested, convincing evidence for this assumption is still missing. More recently, a role for glucose-6-phosphatase in the regulation of Ca^{2+} sequestration by the hepatic endoplasmic reticulum has been proposed in an attempt to couple the hydrolysis of glucose 6-phosphate to the termination of the $[Ca^{2+}]_i$ transient by enhancing Ca^{2+} sequestration through the intraluminal accumulation of inorganic phosphate (9).

C. Calcium Sequestration by Mitochondria

Ca^{2+} uptake and release by mitochondria occur via different routes (4,10). The Ca^{2+} uptake process is purely electrogenic, driven by the electrical component (membrane potential) of the total protonmotive force. Ca^{2+} is transported via a uniporter that has a relatively low affinity for Ca^{2+}, the reported $K_{0.5}$ values ranging from 5 to 30 μM, depending on the tissue of origin of the mitochondria and the composition of the medium. Spermine and inorganic phosphate stimulate the rate and extent of Ca^{2+} uptake, whereas ruthenium red (a hexavalent ammonium complex of Ru), lanthanides, and Mg^{2+} inhibit it.

Ca^{2+} release from isolated mitochondria occurs in exchange for Na^+ or H^+. For instance, Ca^{2+} release from heart and brain mitochondria can be stimulated by Na^+. The sodium-induced Ca^{2+} release is probably electroneutral and occurs at a high transmembrane potential. In liver mitochondria the Na^+/Ca^{2+} exchange is quantitatively not important, and the existence of a separate release pathway involving an electroneutral Ca^{2+}/H^+ antiporter, also operating under high transmembrane potential conditions, is now generally accepted. Release of Ca^{2+} from isolated liver mitochondria is inhibited by ADP, spermine, and *m*-iodobenzylguanidine, whereas it is stimulated by oxidants. Whether the latter phenomenon occurs through activation of the Ca^{2+}/H^+ antiporter is presently unclear (see Section V).

Under conditions of high intramitochondrial Ca^{2+} content, the Ca^{2+} efflux pathway becomes saturated, and isolated mitochondria act as efficient buffers of extramitochondrial Ca^{2+}. When isolated mitochondria contain little Ca^{2+}, as they have been found to *in situ* (11), the activity of the efflux pathway increases with matrix $[Ca^{2+}]$; under these conditions the mitochondria will not act as Ca^{2+} buffers, but matrix $[Ca^{2+}]$ will reflect the extramitochondrial $[Ca^{2+}]$. This is probably the mechanism by which the mitochondrial Ca^{2+}-regulated enzymes such as pyruvate dehydrogenase are regulated by $[Ca^{2+}]_i$ in the cell (12).

D. Calcium Sequestration by Liver Nuclei

The existence of pores in the nuclear envelope has generally been taken as evidence for the free diffusion of ions and small molecules in and out of the nucleus. However, using a suspension of isolated liver nuclei, we have recently identified and partially characterized a Ca^{2+} pump which promotes Ca^{2+} uptake into the nuclei and an increase in the intranuclear free Ca^{2+} concentration (13). The Ca^{2+} uptake is coupled to ATP hydrolysis and appears to be regulated by calmodulin. Additional studies have shown that liver nuclei can sequester about 2 nmol of Ca^{2+}/mg protein and have suggested a potential role for the nucleus in the regulation of $[Ca^{2+}]_i$ concentration (14).

III. Control of Cellular Calcium Homeostasis

As described above, the low resting $[Ca^{2+}]_i$ of 0.1–0.2 μM is achieved by the concerted action of the plasma membrane Ca^{2+} pump and active Ca^{2+} sequestration by the mitochondria, endoplasmic reticulum, and nucleus (Fig. 1). Isolated mitochondria can accumulate large amounts of Ca^{2+}; however, the affinity of the uniport carrier for Ca^{2+} is low. Therefore, mitochondria have been suggested to play a minor role in buffering cytosolic Ca^{2+}. Electron probe X-ray microanalysis of rapidly frozen liver sections has also demonstrated that mitochondria contain little Ca^{2+} *in situ* (~1 nmol Ca^{2+}/mg protein), whereas the endoplasmic reticulum represents the major intracellular Ca^{2+} store (11). It should, however, be noted that estimates of the ability of mitochondria to lower $[Ca^{2+}]_i$ have mainly been derived from experiments performed in the absence of possible natural modulators of Ca^{2+} uptake and release. With this point in mind, Rottenberg and Marbach (15) have recently shown that mitochondria isolated from brain tissue can lower the Ca^{2+} concentration of the incubation medium to 0.1 μM when in the presence of physiological concentrations of spermine and ADP. However, it is generally believed that in most tissues the ER is the main regulator of $[Ca^{2+}]_i$. Our recent finding that the nucleus has a high Ca^{2+}-buffering capacity opens the possibility that this compartment may also be involved in the regulation of the cytosolic free Ca^{2+} concentration within cells.

IV. Modulation of Calcium Homeostasis during Cell Signaling

Stimulation of cells with Ca^{2+}-mobilizing hormones, such as vasopressin, angiotensin II, or phenylephrine, produces a transient elevation of $[Ca^{2+}]_i$

from 0.1 to 0.4–1 μM. These hormone-induced $[Ca^{2+}]_i$ transients in populations of cells appear to be comprised of two phases, an initial rapid increase in $[Ca^{2+}]_i$ followed by a slow return to basal, or near basal, levels. With the recent development of digital imaging techniques, it has become possible to study $[Ca^{2+}]_i$ transients in individual cells. This has led to the observation that at low, close to threshold concentrations of Ca^{2+}-mobilizing hormones, cells respond to these agents with oscillating $[Ca^{2+}]_i$ spikes (16).

The mechanisms by which Ca^{2+}-mobilizing hormones produce $[Ca^{2+}]_i$ transients have been extensively studied in recent years (17). The signal transduction pathway leading to the elevation of $[Ca^{2+}]_i$ can be summarized as follows (Fig. 2). Following the binding of hormone to its plasma membrane receptor, a specific phospholipase C becomes activated via stimulation of a G protein, resulting in the hydrolysis of phosphatidylinositol 4,5-bisphosphate to generate two second messengers, inositol 1,4,5-trisphosphate and diacylglycerol (17). Diacylglycerol is a potent activator of protein kinase C (18), and inositol 1,4,5-trisphosphate is the mediator for Ca^{2+} release from nonmitochondrial intracellular store(s); this release of Ca^{2+} is responsible for the initial rapid elevation of $[Ca^{2+}]_i$ (17). The exact intracellular localization of the inositol 1,4,5-trisphosphate-sensitive Ca^{2+} pool is still not known. Subcellular fractionation and immunocytochemical studies of the localization of the specific receptor for inositol 1,4,5-trisphosphate have suggested that at least part of this pool is located within the endoplasmic reticulum. In addition, recent work from our laboratory has produced evidence for the existence of a second,

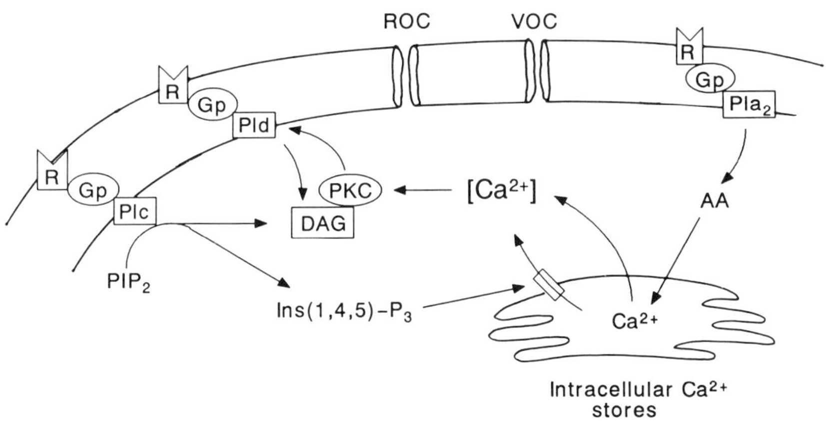

FIGURE 2

Ca^{2+}-utilizing signal transduction pathways.

inositol 1,4,5-trisphosphate-sensitive Ca^{2+} store located in the hepatocyte nucleus (14). However, the possible contribution of this pool to the agonist-induced elevation of cytosolic Ca^{2+} has yet to be elucidated.

In addition to mobilizing Ca^{2+} from intracellular stores, hormones promote Ca^{2+} influx from the extracellular compartment. Various mechanisms of agonist-stimulated Ca^{2+} entry have been described. In several cell types, receptor activation results in either a direct or a G protein-mediated opening of Ca^{2+} channels; these have termed receptor-operated Ca^{2+} channels (5). In other cases there is strong evidence that hormone-generated inositol polyphosphates are involved (second messenger-operated Ca^{2+} channels) (19). Additionally, a role for the depletion of the inositol 1,4,5-trisphosphate-sensitive Ca^{2+} store in activating Ca^{2+} entry has been proposed (the capacitative Ca^{2+} entry model) (20). Recent work from our laboratory has shown that liver cells possess at least two pathways for receptor-mediated Ca^{2+} entry (probably involving two types of Ca^{2+} channels) (21,22). The first of these two pathways is activated by the emptying of the agonist-sensitive intracellular Ca^{2+} store and does not require receptor activation (22). Emptying of this Ca^{2+} store in the absence of hormonal stimulation was experimentally achieved with inhibitors that are selective for the ER Ca^{2+}-ATPase, such as 2,5-di-(*tert*-butyl)-1,4-benzohydroquinone (tBuBHQ) (23) or thapsigargin (24). In contrast, the second pathway depends on receptor occupancy and requires a second messenger for activation (21,22). This pathway cannot exactly be defined as being of the capacitative type since emptying of the inositol 1,4,5-trisphosphate-sensitive Ca^{2+} pool with tBuBHQ or thapsigargin does not stimulate it. However, the prior emptying of this pool or pretreatment with cyclic AMP does reduce the latency period required for the activation of the second pathway and markedly increases the rate of ion flux through this Ca^{2+} channel (21).

V. Disruption of Intracellular Calcium Homeostasis by Toxic Agents

Cellular Ca^{2+} overload can result from either an enhanced influx of extracellular Ca^{2+} or an impairment of Ca^{2+} extrusion from the cell. In addition, interference with individual Ca^{2+} translocases can compromise the ability of the cell to buffer cytosolic Ca^{2+} changes and contribute to an increase in cytosolic Ca^{2+} level.

A. Calcium Sequestration by the Endoplasmic Reticulum and Its Role in Oxidant Injury

Over a decade ago, Moore and co-workers showed that Ca^{2+} sequestration by liver microsomes isolated from carbon tetrachloride-intoxicated rats was substantially inhibited (25). Since then a number of chemical toxins, including the oxidants *tert*-butyl hydroperoxide, diamide, and cystamine, have been found to impair Ca^{2+} sequestration by isolated microsomal fractions (26,27). The thiol-reducing agents dithiothreitol and glutathione (GSH) protected against the inhibition by the oxidants; therefore, the oxidation of essential sulfhydryl group(s) of the Ca^{2+}-ATPase molecule may be involved in the mechanism of oxidative inactivation of the ER Ca^{2+} translocase. However, recent work also suggests that the inhibitory effect on Ca^{2+} sequestration observed with low concentrations of oxidant may be due to the stimulation of a specific Ca^{2+} release pathway (28).

The findings by Moore and co-workers (25) also suggest that an impairment of Ca^{2+} sequestration may be the mechanism by which many chemical toxins cause liver cell death. However, recent work in our laboratory has shown that the selective inhibitor of the microsomal (ER) Ca^{2+}-ATPase, tBuBHQ, rapidly releases endoplasmic reticular Ca^{2+} (23) without correspondingly producing hepatotoxicity in isolated hepatocytes (G. E. N. Kass, 1988, unpublished observations) or in the isolated perfused rat liver (29). Hence, at least short-term interference with Ca^{2+} sequestration by the endoplasmic reticulum does not appear to play a major role in the development of acute hepatotoxicity (but see also Section VI,A).

B. Calcium Sequestration by Mitochondria and Its Role in Oxidant Injury

As discussed above, mitochondria contain little Ca^{2+} under physiological conditions, although they have the capacity to sequester large quantities of Ca^{2+} and could therefore act as efficient buffers of $[Ca^{2+}]_i$ under toxic conditions. However, this potentially important line of defense may not be operational under conditions of oxidative stress because many oxidants, such as *tert*-butyl hydroperoxide (30), menadione (31), and 3,5-dimethyl-*N*-acetyl-*p*-benzoquinone imine (3,5-Me_2-NAPQI) (32), have been found to stimulate the rapid release of Ca^{2+} from isolated liver mitochondria.

The mechanism by which oxidants cause mitochondrial Ca^{2+} efflux has been a matter of intense debate over the past 15 years (10). Several groups have suggested that oxidants, in the presence of Ca^{2+}, stimulate the reversible opening of a pore (33) which shows many of the characteristics of the adenine nucleotide carrier of the mitochondrial inner membrane (34,35). Other investigators have implicated nonselective damage to the inner membrane which results in the loss of the transmembrane potential and reversal of the uniport Ca^{2+} uptake route in the mechanism of oxidant-induced Ca^{2+} release (36). In apparent contrast, work from Richter's and our laboratories has demonstrated that (i) the initial Ca^{2+} release phase occurs from intact mitochondria under conditions of high transmembrane potential, and the observed loss of transmembrane potential is the result of the continuous reuptake of Ca^{2+} by the uniporter, and (ii) Ca^{2+} release following exposure to oxidants seems to be regulated by mitochondrial pyridine nucleotides. Addition of oxidants such as menadione, *tert*-butyl hydroperoxide, or 3,5-Me_2-NAPQI results in the rapid oxidation of NADH and NADPH followed by their hydrolysis to nicotinamide and ADP-ribose (Fig. 3). Pyridine nucleotide oxidation is necessary although not sufficient to cause Ca^{2+} release, and requires the further hydrolysis to nicotinamide and ADP-ribose.

Richter and co-workers have postulated that the oxidant-sensitive Ca^{2+} release mechanism involves the mono-ADP-ribosylation of a target protein (possibly the Ca^{2+}/H^+ antiporter) regulating Ca^{2+} efflux (10).

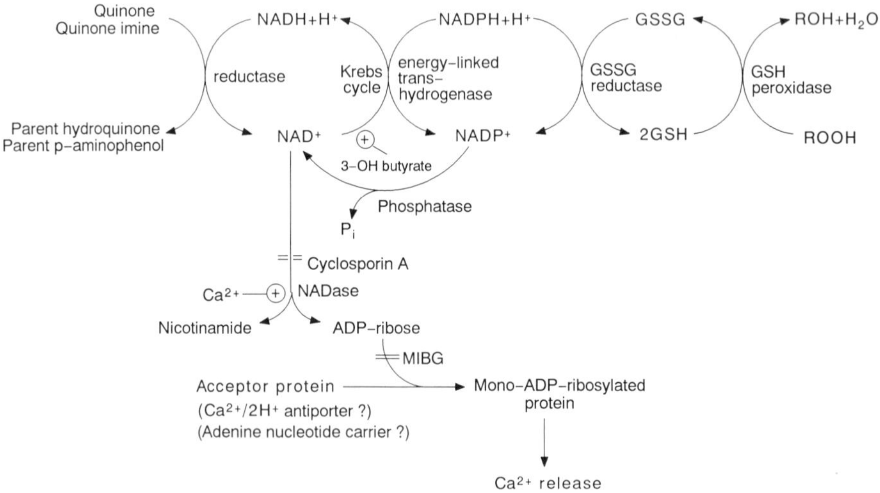

FIGURE 3

Proposed mechanism of oxidant-induced Ca^{2+} release from mitochondria.

Evidence in support of this mechanism is the prevention of oxidant-induced Ca^{2+} release by cyclosporin A, an inhibitor of mitochondrial pyridine nucleotide hydrolysis (37,38), and by *m*-iodobenzylguanidine, a competitive inhibitor of protein mono(ADP-ribose) formation (38,39). Furthermore, we have presented evidence that during oxidant-induced Ca^{2+} cycling (i.e., in the presence of Ca^{2+}) there is no release of ATP from the mitochondrial matrix. This demonstrates that, in liver mitochondria, the initial mechanism of oxidant-induced Ca^{2+} efflux does not involve the opening of a pore (33) or modification of the adenine nucleotide carrier into a nonselective channel (35,40).

The presence of separate routes for Ca^{2+} uptake and release, with the stimulation of the latter by oxidants, will result in Ca^{2+} cycling during oxidative stress. If excessive, this cycling has been suggested to lead to a loss of the transmembrane potential, inhibition of ATP synthesis, and damage to the mitochondria, thereby compromising cell survival. We have recently explored the role of mitochondrial Ca^{2+} release and cycling in the mechanism of oxidant-induced cell injury by using cyclosporin A as an inhibitor of mitochondrial Ca^{2+} release. Cyclosporin A protected hepatocytes from cell killing induced by *tert*-butyl hydroperoxide, cumene hydroperoxide, and 3,5-Me_2-NAPQI (41), and the mechanism of protection was confirmed to involve the inhibition of Ca^{2+} release from mitochondria *in situ* and subsequent cycling across the inner mitochondrial membrane. The oxidant-stimulated cycling of Ca^{2+} by mitochondria resulted in a rapid depletion of cellular ATP levels, which was blocked by cyclosporin A. Interestingly, there was only a narrow range of oxidant concentrations where cyclosporin A protected from cytotoxicity, and cyclosporin A failed to prevent cell killing by the redox-cycling quinone menadione or by the oxidants diamide and cystamine (M. J. Juedes and G. E. N. Kass, 1991, unpublished observations). These results clearly suggest that multiple, interacting pathways, possibly including plasma membrane damage and lipid peroxidation, are recruited during oxidant injury.

The oxidant stimulated a net decrease of NAD^+ levels in hepatocytes. A striking observation in that study was that the loss of this pyridine nucleotide could be accounted for by a converse increase in $NADP^+$ levels and therefore did not apparently result from the activation of poly(ADP-ribose) polymerase (41). The interconversion of NAD^+ to $NADP^+$ was probably catalyzed by NAD^+ kinase, an enzyme which is dependent on calmodulin for its activity (42,43) and which would have become activated by the increase in the cytosolic Ca^{2+} concentration that occurs after exposure of hepatocytes to oxidants (44,45). The significance of this prooxidant-mediated interconversion of NAD^+ to $NADP^+$ is at present not clear, but it may be important in providing additional cofactor for the pentose phosphate pathway, thereby supplying the cell with more NADPH for detoxification reactions (through the glutathione peroxidase–glutathione reductase system) and for the biosynthetic pathways involved in cellular repair mechanisms. Alternatively, diverting cellular NAD^+ to $NADP^+$ may represent an attempt by the cell to spare NAD^+ and avoid all the NAD^+ being consumed through poly(ADP-ribose) biosynthesis.

C. Calcium Fluxes across the Plasma Membrane

There is compelling evidence that many oxidants interfere with Ca^{2+} uptake and extrusion mechanisms at the level of the plasma membrane. Inhibition of Ca^{2+} efflux will result in the net accumulation of Ca^{2+} and in a pathological elevation of $[Ca^{2+}]_i$. In addition, it has become clear that chemical toxins can stimulate Ca^{2+} entry by interacting with existing Ca^{2+} channels or by increasing the plasma membrane permeability to Ca^{2+}. We have recently observed, for instance, that tributyltin, a highly immunotoxic environmental pollutant, stimulates Ca^{2+} influx in immature rat thymocytes in addition to inhibiting their plasma membrane Ca^{2+} translocase (46,47). Interestingly, tributyltin also releases intracellular Ca^{2+} stores including the tBuBHQ-sensitive pool located within the ER. The kinetic parameters for the tributyltin-induced Ca^{2+} influx across the plasma membrane are indistinguishable from those obtained with tBuBHQ. Hence, the stimulation of Ca^{2+} entry by tributyltin may involve a capacitative type of mechanism similar to that which applies to Ca^{2+}-mobilizing hormones and growth factors. It is clear from our previous work, however, that in most cases Ca^{2+} release from the ER pool and the subsequent capacitative Ca^{2+} entry is not sufficient to cause acute cytotoxicity (29) but additionally requires inhibition of the Ca^{2+} extrusion system.

VI. Mechanisms of Calcium-Mediated Cell Killing

The main evidence for the importance of Ca^{2+} overload in cell killing comes from experiments in which removal of extracellular Ca^{2+}, or loading of cells with intracellular Ca^{2+} chelators such as quin-2 or 1,2-bis (aminophenoxy) ethane-N,N,N′,N′-tetraacetic acid (BAPTA) prevented, or delayed, cell killing induced by various agents (1). In addition to Ca^{2+} chelators, Ca^{2+} channel blockers have also been used to prevent Ca^{2+} overload and cell death in several experimental systems.

Both the duration and the extent of the increase in $[Ca^{2+}]_i$ appear to be critical for the development of cytotoxicity. Even moderate increases in cytosolic Ca^{2+} can impair the ability of the cell to respond correctly to agonist stimulation and thereby inhibit cell control by hormones and growth factors. Another early effect of a sustained elevation of the cytosolic free Ca^{2+} concentration is the impairment of mitochondrial function. In addition, more prolonged and intense increases in cytosolic Ca^{2+} will result in the disruption of cytoskeletal organization and in the activation of a number of Ca^{2+}-stimulated catabolic processes, such as proteolysis, membrane degradation, and chromatin fragmentation. The involvement of these Ca^{2+}-dependent alterations in cell killing is briefly discussed in the following sections.

A. Alterations of Cell Signaling Processes by Oxidants

Calcium ions are required for many physiological functions, including the control of metabolic processes, cell differentiation and proliferation, and secretory functions (3). These Ca^{2+}-dependent processes are tightly controlled by hormones and growth factors. The loss of the ability of a cell to respond to such hormones and growth factors will not only deprive the cell of a trophic stimulus, but, as recent evidence (48) clearly indicates, it may also result in the activation of a suicide process that is characteristic of apoptotic cell death (see Section VI,C,3).

The inability of cells to respond to Ca^{2+}-mobilizing hormones can be the consequence of the selective depletion of the intracellular agonist-sensitive Ca^{2+} pool by compounds such as tBuBHQ (23) or bromotrichloromethane (49). Also, G_q, which is the transducing G protein for inositol 1,4,5-triphosphate-generating receptors, has been reported to be susceptible to inactivation by oxidants (50). Another possible target for toxicants are Ca^{2+} channels, as recently demonstrated with maitotoxin (51). This potent dinoflagellate toxin opens verapamil-sensitive Ca^{2+} channels in the myocyte plasma membrane and causes cell death by inducing a sustained elevation of $[Ca^{2+}]_i$ in these cells. Finally, prolonged increases in $[Ca^{2+}]_i$ may obliterate the Ca^{2+} transients normally evoked by physiological agonists, thereby resulting in an impairment of cell signaling.

In contrast to the above-mentioned examples where oxidants appear to block the cell signaling machinery at concentrations that are highly lethal to the cell, it has recently become clear that low levels of oxidants can have quite the opposite effect. For instance, it has been reported on several occasions (see, e.g., Ref. 52) that low levels of oxidants can stimulate cell proliferation. A similar observation has recently been made in our laboratory with the redox-cycling quinone 2,3-dimethoxy-1,4-naphthoquinone in RINm5F cells (J. Dypbukt and P. Nicotera, 1992, unpublished observations). Noncytotoxic levels of prooxidants can also lead to tumor promotion as evidenced by the work from the laboratory of Cerutti (53). Tumor promotional activity has been demonstrated for reactive oxygen species and organic peroxides such as benzoyl peroxide.

Because the Ca^{2+}-stimulated, phospholipid-dependent protein kinase (protein kinase C) plays a crucial role in cell proliferation and the activation of this enzyme by phorbol esters has been associated with tumor promotion, we investigated the effects of oxidants on protein kinase C. Exposure of rat hepatocytes to low levels of oxidants resulted in a rapid, 2- to 3-fold increase in the specific activity of protein kinase C (54). Only the cytosolic protein kinase C displayed the increase in specific activity, whereas the activity of the membrane-bound form remained unchanged. The increase in protein kinase C specific activity was not due to induction of protein kinase C. Rather, the oxidative modification of the protein kinase C enzyme itself, most likely through oxidative stress-induced modification of the thiol/disulfide balance of the enzyme, was responsible for the activation. The involvement of thiol residues in the activation phenomenon was confirmed when we found that partially purified protein kinase C from rat brain could be activated using low concentrations of GSSG in a glutathione redox buffer.

It has not yet been established whether the oxidative modification of protein kinase C results in the stimulation of substrate phosphorylation *in situ*. However, the oxidatively modified enzyme may overexpress responses to various physiological stimuli, and this represents a potential mechanism for oxidative stress-mediated tumor promotion (Fig. 4). Indeed, exposure of V79 cells to noncytotoxic concentrations of the oxidants menadione, diamide, *tert*-butyl hydroperoxide, or benzoyl peroxide was recently found to markedly decrease the requirement for 12-*O*-tetradecanoylphorbol 13-acetate (PMA) to inhibit cell-to-cell communication (S. K. Duddy, G. E. N. Kass, and L. Wärngård, unpublished observations). Inhibition of intercellular communication is thought to be involved in the process of tumor promotion. Also, the induction of the enzyme ornithine decarboxylase (which is controlled by protein kinase C) and skin tumor promotion by PMA has been reported to be enhanced by adriamycin, a redox-cycling anthracycline antibiotic (55). Thus, it seems that overamplified protein kinase C-dependent responses has a significant impact on the control of cellular growth and differentiation. This has recently been

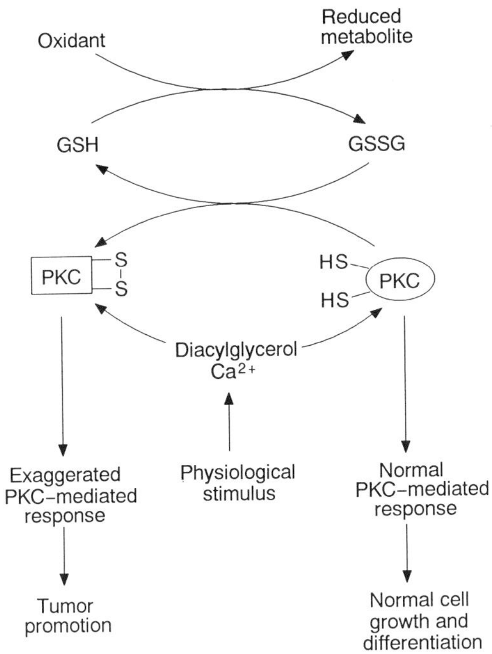

FIGURE 4

Proposed role of protein kinase C in tumor promotion by oxidants.

corroborated by Weinstein and colleagues (56) using cells that overexpressed a protein kinase C isoenzyme and displayed a number of characteristic features of transformed cells following exposure to PMA.

In addition to protein kinase C, other protein kinases have been shown to become activated under conditions of oxidative stress. Oxidants can, for instance, activate the rat liver insulin receptor tyrosine kinase (57,58). More recently, exposure of mouse epidermal cells to oxidants has been found to stimulate phosphorylation of the ribosomal protein S6 (59) through an aparently Ca^{2+}-dependent event. Analysis of the primary structure of a number of protein kinases (serine, threonine, and tyrosine kinases) has revealed a substantial sequence homology in the catalytic (kinase) domains (60). Thus, a common structural feature may predispose different protein kinases to activation through alteration(s) of their thiol/disulfide status. Consequently, modulation of kinase activities involved in signal transduction and cellular metabolism could constitute a mechanism by which a noncytotoxic state of oxidative stress is able to have profound implications on cell division and differentiation.

B. Cytoskeletal Alterations

One of the early signs of cell injury caused by a oxidants and a variety of other toxic agents is the appearance of multiple protrusions (blebs) on the cell surface (61). The events leading to bleb formation have not yet been fully elucidated, and several mechanisms may independently contribute to their formation. However, it is generally accepted that a perturbation of cytoskeletal organization and of the interaction between the cytoskeleton and the plasma membrane plays an important role. Evidence for this contention stems from the observation that agents which modify the cytoskeleton, such as cytochalasins, phalloidin, and microcystin LR, stimulate bleb formation and from the recent demonstration that the bundles of actin microfilaments present at the base of the bleb appear to be completely dissociated from the bleb-forming portion of the plasma membrane (62). The finding that Ca^{2+} ionophores induce similar blebbing, and that this is prevented by the omission of Ca^{2+} from the incubation medium, led to the proposal that Ca^{2+} is involved in the cytoskeletal alterations associated with the formation of surface blebs during cell injury (61).

The cytoskeleton is organized into a complex array of fibers which belong to three main classes: microfilaments, microtubules, and intermediate filaments (63). Microfilaments are mainly composed of actin and several actin-binding proteins. Many of the actin-binding proteins, such as caldesmon, gelsolin, and villin, require Ca^{2+} to be able to interact with other cytoskeletal constituents. Moreover, Ca^{2+} regulates the function of three other actin-binding proteins which are directly involved in the association of microfilaments with the plasma membrane. Among these proteins, α-actinin is involved in the normal organization of actin filaments into regular, parallel arrays. However, in the presence of micromolar Ca^{2+} concentrations, α-actinin dissociates from the actin filaments (64). The other two actin-binding proteins, vinculin and actin-binding protein, are substrates for Ca^{2+}-dependent proteases (65). Thus, an increase in the cytosolic free Ca^{2+} concentration to micromolar levels will result in the proteolysis of these two polypeptides.

Recent work has provided a great deal of evidence for the involvement of Ca^{2+} in the toxic alterations of actin microfilaments and actin-binding proteins. For example, the incubation of human platelets with the redox-active quinone menadione resulted in the dissociation of α-actinin from the whole cytoskeleton and in the proteolysis of actin-binding protein (66). These changes were largely prevented in cells preloaded with the intracellular Ca^{2+} chelator quin-2. Furthermore, immunocytochemical investigations revealed that dissociation of α-actinin from the actin filaments may be responsible for bleb formation during oxidant injury (67). Other studies on canine heart during the development of ischemia and reperfusion injury have revealed a progressive loss of vinculin staining along the lateral margin of myocytes (68). This loss was associated with the appearance of subsarcolemmal blebs and breaks in the plasma membrane. Since vinculin is a substrate for Ca^{2+}-dependent proteases and since the cytosolic Ca^{2+} concentration during ischemia and reperfusion rises well above the level necessary for protease activation, it appears that Ca^{2+}-activated proteases may be responsible for the loss of vinculin.

Microtubule structure and distribution are also controlled by Ca^{2+}. In addition, the turnover and distribution of microtubules are controlled by microtubule-associated proteins (MAPs), whose activities are modulated by Ca^{2+}- and calmodulin-dependent protein kinase (69). Other studies have demonstrated that microinjection of Ca^{2+}–calmodulin complexes in 3T3 fibroblasts results in the complete depolymerization of microtubules, which is spatially limited to the site of injection (70). Although the depolymerization of microtubules during oxidant injury has been reported (71), the possible involvement of Ca^{2+} in this process has not been clarified. Likewise, little is known about the role of Ca^{2+} in toxic modifications of intermediate filaments. In fact, our knowledge of the composition of intermediate filaments and of the role of these structures in cell physiology is still fragmentary. It has been shown that several intermediate filament proteins, including vimentin and cytokeratins, are substrates for a Ca^{2+}-activated protease. However, direct evidence is still missing for a physiological role of proteolysis in the control of intermediate filament function and for a possible contribution of cleavage of intermediate filaments to the cytoskeletal alterations occurring during cell injury.

C. Calcium-Dependent Degradative Enzymes

The catabolism of phospholipids, proteins, and nucleic acids involves enzymes most of which require Ca^{2+} for activity. Ca^{2+} overload can result in a sustained activation of these enzymes and in the degradation of cell constituents, which may ultimately lead to cell death (Fig. 5).

1. *Phospholipases*

Phospholipases catalyze the hydrolysis of membrane phospholipids. They are widely distributed in biological membranes and generally require Ca^{2+} for activation. A specific subset of phospholipases, collectively known as phospholipase A_2, has been proposed to participate in the detoxication of phospholipid hydroperoxides by releasing fatty acids

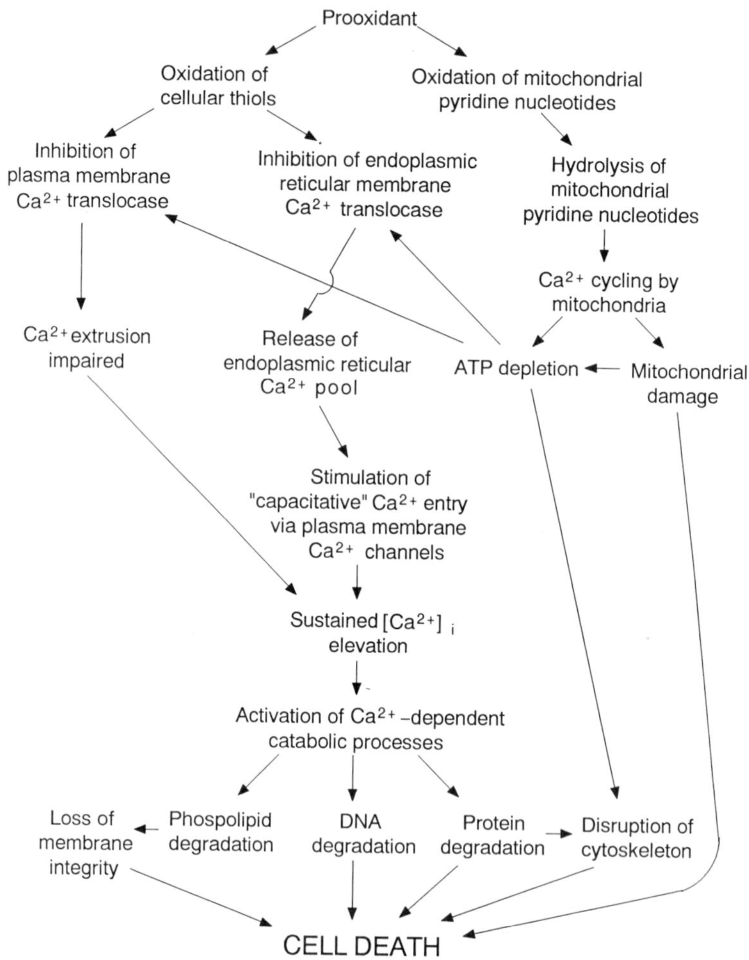

FIGURE 5

Ca^{2+}-dependent mechanisms involved in oxidant-induced cell killing.

from peroxidized membranes (72). However, phospholipase activation can also mediate pathophysiological reactions by stimulating membrane breakdown or by generating toxic metabolites. One of the best known examples for phospholipase-mediated toxicity is probably that caused by phospholipase-based snake and bee venoms. Therefore, phospholipase activation has been proposed as an important mechanism of cell killing. Phospholipase A_2 is Ca^{2+}- and calmodulin-dependent, and thus it is susceptible to activation following an increase in cytosolic Ca^{2+} concentration. Hence, it has been suggested that a sustained increase in cytosolic Ca^{2+} can result in enhanced breakdown of membrane phospholipids and, in turn, in mitochondrial and cell damage. Although a number of studies have indicated that accelerated phospholipid turnover occurs during anoxia or toxic cell injury (73), the importance of phospholipase activation in the development of cell damage by oxidants remains to be established.

2. *Proteases*

During the past 10 years the involvement of nonlysosomal proteolysis in several cell processes has become progressively clear. Proteases which have a neutral pH optimum include the ATP- and ubiquitin-dependent proteases and the calcium-dependent proteases, or calpains. Calpains are present in virtually all mammalian cells, and they appear to be largely associated with membranes in conjunction with a specific inhibitory protein (calpastatin). The extralysosomal localization of this proteolytic system allows the proteases to participate in several specialized cell functions, including cytoskeletal and cell membrane remodeling, receptor cleavage and turnover, enzyme activation, and modulation of cell mitosis.

Cellular targets for these enzymes include cytoskeletal elements and membrane integral proteins (66). Thus, the activation of Ca^{2+} proteases has been shown to cause modification of microfilaments in platelet and to be involved in cell degeneration during muscle dystrophy and in the development of ischemic injury in nervous tissue. Studies from our laboratory have suggested the involvement of Ca^{2+}-activated proteases in oxidant injury in liver (45,74). Although the substrates for protease activity during cell injury remain largely unidentified, it appears that cytoskeletal proteins may be a major target for Ca^{2+}-activated proteases during chemical toxicity.

3. *Endonucleases*

During physiological cell killing a suicide process is activated in affected cells which is known as "apoptosis" or programmed cell death. Several early morphological changes occur within apoptotic cells, including widespread plasma and nuclear membrane blebbing, compacting of organelles, and chromatin condensation (75). The most reliable and characteristic marker for this process is the activation of a Ca^{2+}-dependent endonuclease which results in the cleavage of cell chromatin into oligonucleosome-length fragments. Endonuclease activation has been implicated in the killing of target cells by cytotoxic T lymphocytes and natural killer cells, as well as in thymocytes exposed to glucocorticoid hormones.

The results of several recent studies have shown that Ca^{2+} overload can trigger endonuclease activation. The Ca^{2+} ionophore A23187 stimulates DNA fragmentation in thymocytes, and endonuclease activity in isolated nuclei is dependent on Ca^{2+} (76). In addition, Ca^{2+}-mediated endonuclease activation appear to be involved in the cytotoxicity of TCDD and tributyltin in thymocytes (46,77). Although Ca^{2+}-dependent endonuclease activation has been most extensively studied in thymocytes, it appears that this process may also be important in a variety of other tissues. For example, we have identified a constitutive endonuclease in liver nuclei that is activated by submicromolar Ca^{2+} concentrations in intact nuclei incubated in the presence of ATP to stimulate Ca^{2+} uptake (76). Endonuclease activation has also been implicated in damage to macrophages caused by oxidative stress (78). Although the responsible endonuclease requires Ca^{2+} for activity, its regulation appears more complex, however, and probably involves additional signals (79).

Ca^{2+} overload may also stimulate other enzymatic processes that result in DNA damage. Elevated Ca^{2+} levels can lock topoisomerase II in a form that cleaves, but does not religate, DNA, and topoisomerase II-mediated DNA fragmentation has been implicated in the cytotoxic action of some anticancer drugs (80). DNA single strand breaks in cells exposed to oxidative stress can also be generated through a Ca^{2+}-dependent mechanism (81). Thus, further work is required not only to identify other situations in which endogenous endonuclease activation can mediate Ca^{2+}-dependent cell killing, but also to identify additional Ca^{2+}-dependent catabolic processes which may generate DNA damage.

VII. Summary and Concluding Remarks

From the examples described in this chapter, it is clear that oxidant injury is a process with many facets. Whereas relatively low levels of oxidant do not kill the target cell but stimulate it to proliferate or differentiate, increasing the degree of oxidative stress will be cytotoxic to the cell (Fig. 6). Even then, the mode and mechanisms of cell killing may greatly vary depending on the target cell type as well as the nature of the oxidant. For instance, low levels of oxidant will produce a pattern of DNA fragmentation that is typical of that produced by agents which activate the

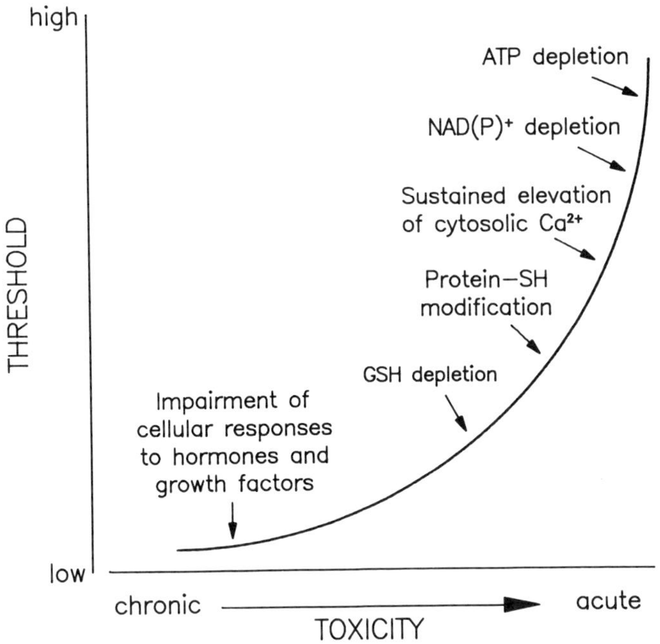

FIGURE 6

Overview of mechanisms involved in oxidant-mediated cell injury.

Ca^{2+}-dependent endonuclease(s), and therefore the mode of cell killing by the oxidant is characteristic of apoptosis. However, a further increase in oxidant level will promote cell necrosis rather than apoptosis, probably as a result of shifting from endonuclease activation to protease activation, phospholipase activation, and mitochondrial damage. Our work has also pointed to the variety of mechanisms and cellular targets recruited during necrotic cell killing depending on the type and dose of oxidant used. It is nevertheless reasonable to conclude that, in many types of oxidant injury, calcium ions do play an important role and in numerous cases may be considered as a common final link leading to cell death.

References

1. P. Nicotera, G. Bellomo, and S. Orrenius, *Chem. Res. Toxicol.* **3**, 484–494 (1990).
2. G. E. N. Kass, P. Nicotera, J. Llopis, and S. Orrenius, *in* "Regulation of Hepatic Function" (N. Grunnet and B. Quistorff, eds.), pp. 344–354. Munksgaard, Copenhagen, 1991.

3. A. K. Campbell, "Intracellular Calcium: Its Universal Role as Regulator," Wiley, New York, 1983.
4. E. Carafoli, *Annu. Rev. Biochem.* **56,** 395–433 (1989).
5. R. W. Tsien and R. Y. Tsien, *Annu. Rev. Cell Biol.* **6,** 715–760 (1990).
6. E. Carafoli, *Physiol. Rev.* **71,** 129–153 (1991).
7. S. K. Duddy, G. E. N. Kass, and S. Orrenius, *J. Biol. Chem.* **264,** 20863–20866 (1989).
8. N. Kraus-Friedmann, *Cell Calcium* **11,** 625–640 (1990).
9. A. Benedetti, R. Fulceri, M. Ferro, and M. Comporti, *Trends Biochem. Sci.* **11,** 284–285 (1986).
10. C. Richter and G. E. N. Kass, *Chem.–Biol. Interact.* **77,** 1–23 (1991).
11. A. P. Somlyo, M. Bond, and A. V. Somlyo, *Nature (London)* **314,** 622–625 (1985).
12. R. M. Denton and J. G. McCormack, *Annu. Rev. Physiol.* **52,** 451–466 (1990).
13. P. Nicotera, D. J. McConkey, D. P. Jones, and S. Orrenius, *Proc. Natl. Acad. Sci. U.S.A.* **86,** 453–457, 1989.
14. P. Nicotera, S. Orrenius, T. Nilsson, and P.-O. Berggren, *Proc. Natl. Acad. Sci. U.S.A.* **87,** 6858–6862.
15. H. Rottenberg and M. Marbach, *Biochim. Biophys. Acta* **1016,** 77–86 (1990).
16. M. J. Berridge and R. F. Irvine, *Nature (London)* **341,** 197–205 (1989).
17. M. J. Berridge, *Annu. Rev. Biochem.* **56,** 159–193 (1987).
18. Y. Nishizuka, *Nature (London)* **308,** 683–698 (1984).
19. R. F. Irvine, *FEBS Lett.* **263,** 5–9 (1990).
20. J. W. Putney, *Cell Calcium* **11,** 611–624 (1990).
21. G. E. N. Kass, J. Llopis, S. C. Chow, S. K. Duddy, and S. Orrenius, *J. Biol. Chem.* **265,** 17486–17492 (1990).
22. J. Llopis, G. E. N. Kass, A. Gahm, and S. Orrenius, *Biochem. J.* **284,** 243–247 (1992).
23. G. E. N. Kass, S. K. Duddy, G. A. Moore, and S. Orrenius, *J. Biol. Chem.* **264,** 15192–15198 (1989).
24. J. Llopis, S. C. Chow, G. E. N. Kass, A. Gahm, and S. Orrenius, *Biochem. J.* **277,** 553–556 (1991).
25. L. Moore, G. R. Davenport, and E. J. Landon, *J. Biol. Chem.* **251,** 1197–1201 (1976).
26. D. P. Jones, H. Thor, M. T. Smith, S. A. Jewell, and S. Orrenius, *J. Biol. Chem.* **258,** 6390–6393 (1983).
27. H. Thor, P. Hartzell, S.-Å, Svensson, S. Orrenius, F. Mirabelli, V. Marinorni, and G. Bellomo, *Biochem. Pharmacol.* **34,** 3717–3723 (1985).
28. L. Missiaen, C. W. Taylor, and M. J. Berridge, *Nature (London)* **352,** 241–244 (1991).
29. G. C. Farrell, S. K. Duddy, G. E. N. Kass, J. Llopis, A. Gahm, and S. Orrenius, *J. Clin. Invest.* **85,** 1255–1259 (1990).
30. G. Bellomo, A. Martino, P. Richelmi, G. A. Moore, S. A. Jewell, and S. Orrenius, *Eur. J. Biochem.* **140,** 1–6 (1984).
31. G. A. Moore, P. J. O'Brien, and S. Orrenius, *Xenobiotica* **16,** 873–882 (1986).
32. M. Weis, G. A. Moore, I. A. Cotgreave, S. D. Nelson, and P. Moldéus, *Chem.–Biol. Interact.* **76,** 227–240 (1990).
33. M. Crompton, A. Costi, and L. Hayat, *Biochem. J.* **245,** 915–918 (1987).
34. K. Lê Quôc and D. Lê Quôc, *Arch. Biochem. Biophys.* **265,** 249–257 (1988).
35. A. P. Halestrap and A. M. Davidson, *Biochem. J.* **268,** 153–160 (1990).
36. M. C. Beatrice, J. W. Palmer, and D. R. Pfeiffer, *J. Biol. Chem.* **255,** 8663–8671 (1980).
37. C. Richter, M. Theus, and J. Schlegel, *Biochem. Pharmacol.* **40,** 779–782 (1990).
38. M. Weis, G. E. N. Kass, S. Orrenius, and P. Moldéus, *J. Biol. Chem.* **267,** 804–809 (1992).
39. C. Richter, *Free Radical Res. Commun.* **8,** 329–334 (1990).
40. T. Dierks, A. Salentin, C. Heberger, and R. Krämer, *Biochim. Biophys. Acta* **1028,** 268–280 (1990).

41. G. E. N. Kass, M. J. Juedes, and S. Orrenius, *Biochem. Pharmacol.* submitted for publication.
42. J. M. Anderson and M. J. Cormier, *Biochem. Biophys. Res. Commun.* **84,** 595–602 (1978).
43. G. Epel, G. Patton, R. W. Wallace, and W. Y. Cheung, *Cell (Cambridge, Mass.)* **23,** 543–549 (1981).
44. P. Nicotera, D. McConkey, S.-Å. Svensson, G. Bellomo, and S. Orrenius, *Toxicology* **52,** 55–63 (1988).
45. P. Nicotera, M. Rundgren, D. J. Porubek, I. Cotgreave, P. Moldéus, S. Orrenius, and S. D. Nelson, *Chem. Res. Toxicol.* **2,** 46–50 (1989).
46. T. Y. Aw, P. Nicotera, L. Manzo, and S. Orrenius, *Arch. Biochem. Biophys.* **283,** 46–50 (1990).
47. S. C. Chow, G. E. N. Kass, M. J. McCabe, and S. Orrenius, *Arch. Biochem. Biophys.* **298,** in press.
48. D. M. Barnes, *Science* **242,** 1510–1511 (1988).
49. A. Benedetti, P. Graf, R. Fulceri, A. Romani, and H. Sies, *Biochem. Pharmacol.* **38,** 1799–1805 (1989).
50. G. Bellomo, H. Thor, and S. Orrenius, *J. Biol. Chem.* **262,** 1530–1534 (1987).
51. R. K. Kutty, Y. Singh, G. Santostasi, and G. Krishna, *Toxicol. Appl. Pharmacol.* **101,** 1–10 (1989).
52. R. H. Burdon and C. Rice-Evans, *Free Radical Res. Commun.* **6,** 345–358 (1989).
53. P. A. Cerutti, *Science* **227,** 375–381 (1985).
54. G. E. N. Kass, S. K. Duddy, and S. Orrenius, *Biochem. J.* **260,** 499–507 (1989).
55. J. P. Perchellet, G. S. Kishore, and E. M. Perchellet, *Cancer Lett.* **29,** 127–137 (1985).
56. G. M. Housey, M. D. Johnson, W.-L. Hisao, C. A. O'Brian, J. P. Murphy, P. Kirschmeier, and I. B. Weinstein, *Cell (Cambridge, Mass.)* **52,** 343–354 (1988).
57. T. M. Chan, E. Chen, A. Tatoyau, N. S. Shargill, M. Pleta, and P. Hochstein, *Biochem. Biophys. Res. Commun.* **139,** 439–445 (1986).
58. G. R. Hayes and D. H. Lockwood, *Proc. Natl. Acad. Sci. U.S.A.* **84,** 8115–8119 (1987).
59. R. Larsson and P. Cerutti, *J. Biol. Chem.* **263,** 17452–17458 (1988).
60. P. J. Parker, L. Coussens, N. Totty, L. Rhee, S. Young, E. Chen, S. Stabel, M. D. Waterfield, and A. Ullrich, *Science* **233,** 853–859 (1986).
61. S. A. Jewell, G. Bellomo, H. Thor, S. Orrenius, and M. T. Smith, *Science* **217,** 1257–1259 (1982).
62. J. E. Eriksson, G. I. L. Paatero, J. A. O. Meriluota, G. A. Codd, G. E. N. Kass, P. Nicotera, and S. Orrenius, *Exp. Cell Res.* **185,** 86–100 (1989).
63. A. D. Berdshadski and J. M. Vasiliev, "Cytoskeleton," Plenum, New York, 1988.
64. S. Rosenberg, A. Stracher, and R. C. Lucas, *J. Cell Biol.* **91,** 201–211 (1991).
65. W. R. Dayton, J. Shollmayer, R. A. Lepley, and L. R. Cortes, *Biochim. Biophys. Acta* **659,** 48–61 (1991).
66. F. Mirabelli, A. Salis, M. Vairetti, G. Bellomo, H. Thor, and S. Orrenius, *Arch. Biochem. Biophys.* **270,** 478–488 (1989).
67. G. Bellomo, F. Mirabelli, P. Richelmi, W. Malorni, F. Iosi, and S. Orrenius, *Free Radical Res. Commun.* **8,** 391–399 (1990).
68. C. Steenbergern, M. L. Hill, and R. B. Jennings, *Circ. Res.* **60,** 478–486 (1987).
69. J. B. Olmsted, *Annu. Rev. Cell Biol.* **2,** 421–457 (1986).
70. M. L. Shelanski, *Ann. N.Y. Acad. Sci.* **568,** 121–124 (1990).
71. G. Bellomo, F. Mirabelli, M. Vairetti, F. Iosi, and W. Malorni, *J. Cell. Physiol.* **143,** 118–128 (1990).
72. F. J. G. M. Van Kuijk, A. Sevanian, G. J. Handleman, and E. A. Dratz, *Trends Biochem. Sci.* **12,** 31–34 (1987).

73. K. R. Chien, R. G. Pfau, and J. L. Farber, *Am. J. Pathol.* **97,** 505–530 (1979).
74. P. Nicotera, P. Hartzell, C. Baldi, S.-Å. Svensson, G. Bellomo, and S. Orrenius, *J. Biol. Chem.* **261,** 14628–14635 (1986).
75. M. J. Arends, R. G. Morris, and A. H. Wyllie, *Am. J. Pathol.* **136,** 593–608 (1990).
76. D. P. Jones, D. J. McConkey, P. Nicotera, and S. Orrenius, *J. Biol. Chem.* **264,** 6398–6403 (1989).
77. D. J. McConkey, P. Hartzell, S. K. Duddy, H. Håkansson, and S. Orrenius, *Science* **242,** 256–259 (1988).
78. P. Warings, R. D. Eichner, A. Müllbacher, and A. Sjaarda, *Science* **246,** 1165–1168 (1988).
79. B. Brüne, P. Hartzell, P. Nicotera, and S. Orrenius, *Exp. Cell Res.* **195,** 323–329 (1991).
80. A. Udvardy, P. Schedl, M. Sander, and T. Hsieh, *J. Mol. Biol.* **191,** 231–246 (1986).
81. J. M Dypbukt, H. Thor, and P. Nicotera, *Free Radical Res. Commun.* **8,** 347–354 (1990).

CHAPTER 7

Mechanisms of Inflammatory Oxidant Damage in Tissues

Michael S. Mulligan, Kent J. Johnson, and Peter A. Ward

Department of Pathology
The Univeristy of Michigan Medical School
Ann Arbor, Michigan 48109

I. Introduction

There is abundant evidence that the generation of toxic oxygen products by activated neutrophils results in the damage or killing of endothelial cells both *in vitro* and *in vivo* (1–4). Macrophages also produce significant amounts of O_2^-, H_2O_2, as well as the nitrogen-centered radical nitric oxide (·NO) and contribute to oxidant mediated injury *in vitro* and *in vivo* (5–7). Neutrophils and mononuclear cells are recruited to sites of acute inflammation through a complex series of events that has recently been shown to require the participation of leukocyte adhesion molecules (8–13). Once circulating leukocytes have slowed, begun to roll, and adhere to the endothelium, transmigration occurs and the cells migrate to sites of inflammation in response to various chemoattractants. Many of these chemoattractants are also

Cellular and Molecular Mechanisms of Inflammation, Volume 4

capable of activating neutrophils, resulting in enhanced generation of toxic oxygen products in a manner known as "priming" (14,15). The extent of neutrophil recruitment often closely correlates with the degree of inflammatory tissue damage.

Once recruited to an extravascular site, neutrophils undergo additional stimulation which results in the release of products that are toxic to tissues and cells. In addition to the injurious effects of neutrophil-derived oxygen products, these cells also release proteases which have been shown to act synergistically with oxy radicals to damage endothelial cells (16). Neutrophils, macrophages, and endothelial cells also generate an array of mediators that amplify the inflammatory response. In addition to the generation of toxic oxygen products, cytokines such as tumor necrosis factor (TNF-α) and interleukin-1 (IL-1) [each of which can induce production of the other (17–19)] may be released and fed into the network of mediators that bring about tissue injury. Activated endothelial cells and macrophages can also generate neutrophil chemotactic factor (NCF, IL-8) and platelet-activating factor (PAF) (20–23). Other cells such as fibroblasts can also be induced to generate cytokines (17). Thus, a multitude of mediators derived from several sources are capable of directly or indirectly influencing inflammatory cell recruitment and enhancing production of tissue damaging oxy radicals by neutrophils and macrophages (24).

This chapter will focus on several animal models of acute inflammatory lung injury mediated by leukocyte-derived oxygen and nitrogen activated radicals as well as other mediators such as cytokines which have been demonstrated to play important roles in the events leading to lung injury, *In vitro* evidence supporting the conclusions from animal model studies will also be presented. Three models are lung injury have been selected. Lung injury following intravascular activation of complement is a relatively straightforward type of injury in which intravascular activation of neutrophils occurs, leading to oxygen radical injury of endothelial cells. Products of macrophages do not appear to be involved in the process leading to injury. In the model of immunoglobulin G (IgG) immune complex-induced injury, the events leading to cell injury can be ascribed to products of both neutrophils and macrophages, whereas in the model of IgA immune complex-induced injury, products exclusively generated by macrophages appear to be responsible for lung injury. In each model, details of the pathophysiological events will be presented. Finally, we will discuss information regarding the mechanisms by which neutrophils kill endothelial cells.

II. Acute Lung Injury Developing after Systemic Activation of Complement

Intravascular activation of complement is associated with intrapulmonary sequestration of neutrophils (25–29). This phenomenon is observed in patients undergoing leukopheresis, hemodialysis, and cardiopulmonary bypass. Contact of human plasma with dialysis membranes appears to lead to complement activation by the alternative pathway (30). These ideas are supported by the clinical findings of increased C3a and C5a in plasma from patients undergoing cardiopulmonary bypass and increased C5a in plasma from patients with adult respiratory distress syndrome (31,32). Intravascular activation of complement presumably leads to the stimulation of neutrophils and their subsequent sequestration in capillaries.

Experimentally, *in vitro,* activation of neutrophils by C5a can lead to cytotoxic injury of endothelial cells related to the generation by neutrophils of O_2^-, H_2O_2, and HO· (33,34). *In vivo,* complement-mediated lung injury is initiated by the bolus intravenous injection of 80 μg (20 units) of chromatographically purified cobra (*Naja naja*) venom. This results in complete abolition of CH_{50} hemolytic activity* within 3 min (4). Lung vascular permeability, as assessed by extravasation of ^{125}I-labeled bovine serum albumin (^{125}I-BSA), increases at least 3-fold above negative control values over the ensuing 30 min. Histologically (Fig. 1), intravascular aggregates of neutrophils are present in the pulmonary capillary beds, and, when aggregates are in direct contact with endothelial cells, necrosis of endothelial cells is evident. Neutrophil depletion by selective antibodies has been shown to attenuate the increase in lung vascular permeability by 68% (4). Treatment with catalase and superoxide dismutase has also been shown to limit increases in permeability by 66% and 53%, respectively (4). These findings demonstrate that lung injury developing after systemic activation of complement is neutrophil dependent and likely mediated by polymorphonuclear leukocyte (PMN) production of H_2O_2 and O_2^-. There is also strong evidence that HO·, a product of the interaction of H_2O_2 and O_2^-, is an important mediator of cobra venom factor (CVF)-induced lung injury, since pretreatment with the powerful HO· scavengers dimethyl sulfoxide (DMSO) or dimethylthiourea (DMTU) is protective, as is pretreatment with the iron chelator deferoxa-

* CH_{50}, the amount of serum required to cause complement-mediated 50% hemolysis of sensitized red cells.

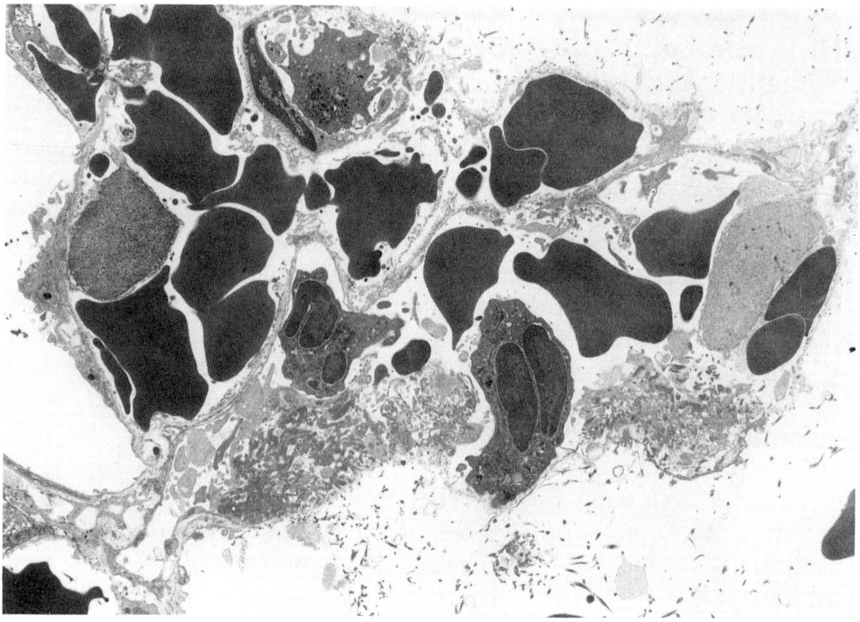

FIGURE 1

Histological alterations seen in the CVF model of lung injury. CVF-induced complement activation is associated with the rapid sequestration (within minutes) of neutrophils into the pulmonary capillary bed. The activation of neutrophil oxidant pathways induces endothelial cell necrosis, disruption of alveolar septae, and intraalveolar hemorrhage and fibrin deposition. (Transmission electron microscopy, X5600.)

mine. This supports the idea that HO· may be generated from O_2^- and H_2O_2 by the iron-dependent Fenton reaction (35). HO· may then act as the important final toxin in the development of CVF-induced lung injury (3).

Most recently, additional studies with this model have been conducted examining the roles of the $\beta 2$ leukocyte integrins. Infusion of monoclonal antibodies to CD18 or CD11b resulted in reductions in lung vascular permeability by 69 and 50%, respectively, and reductions in lung hemorrhage by 91 and 72%, respectively (36). Studies examining the involvement of CD11a and CD11c await the availability of appropriate monoclonal antibodies, but the results to date support a role for the $\beta 2$ integrin family of adhesion molecules in this model of injury. It seems likely that complement activation products such as C5a upregulate $\beta 2$ integrins of PMNs and that this family of leukocyte adhesion molecules is important for the full expression of PMN-induced injury. TNF-α and IL-1 have been shown to play no role in this model of lung injury. The roles of ICAM-1 and the selectin family of molecules remains to be examined.

III. Acute Lung Injury Following Deposition of Immunoglobulin G Immune Complexes

Following the intratracheal instillation of IgG antibody to bovine serum albumin and intravenous injection of BSA, immune complexes form at the alveolar–capillary interface (37). Over the next 4 hr acute alveolitis develops, characterized by a pronounced neutrophilic infiltrate, which is associated with increases in pulmonary vascular permeability and intraalveolar hemorrhage. A representative section of an IgG immune complex-injured lung is shown in Fig. 2. Quantitation of permeability and hemorrhage is accomplished by accumulation of ^{125}I-BSA or ^{51}Cr-labeled erythrocytes (RBC) in lung parenchyma (13,38). H_2O_2 and O_2^- are important mediators of injury in this model, as supported by the protective effects of treatment of animals with catalase and, to a lesser extent, superoxide dismutase (SOD) (3). While catalase provides protection in a dose-dependent fashion, it does not alter the extent of neutrophil influx; in contrast, pretreatment with SOD is associated with inhibition of the PMN influx (3). This finding may be related to the ability of oxygen metabolites (perhaps HO·) to generate a chemotactic lipid for neutrophils in that the addition of oxidants to human plasma generates a lipid-related chemotactic activity that is apparently dependent on generation of HO· (39).

The role of oxidants as mediators of IgG immune complex-induced injury is also supported by the fact that intratracheal instillation of glucose and glucose oxidase generating H_2O_2 produces a similar type of alveolitis (40). In the presence of myeloperoxidase or lactoperoxidase, but not horseradish peroxidase, interstitial pulmonary fibrosis also ensues, suggesting a role for products such hypochlorous acid (HOCl) (40). The oxygen radical scavengers DMTU and DMSO also signficantly attenuate IgG immune complex-induced lung injury, suggesting that HO· may be an important mediator of injury (3). In support of this concept, treatment with deferoxamine markedly reduces injury as measured by ^{125}I-BSA extravasation into lung parenchyma (3). It is therefore likely that H_2O_2 and O_2^- participate in the iron-dependent Fenton reaction resulting in

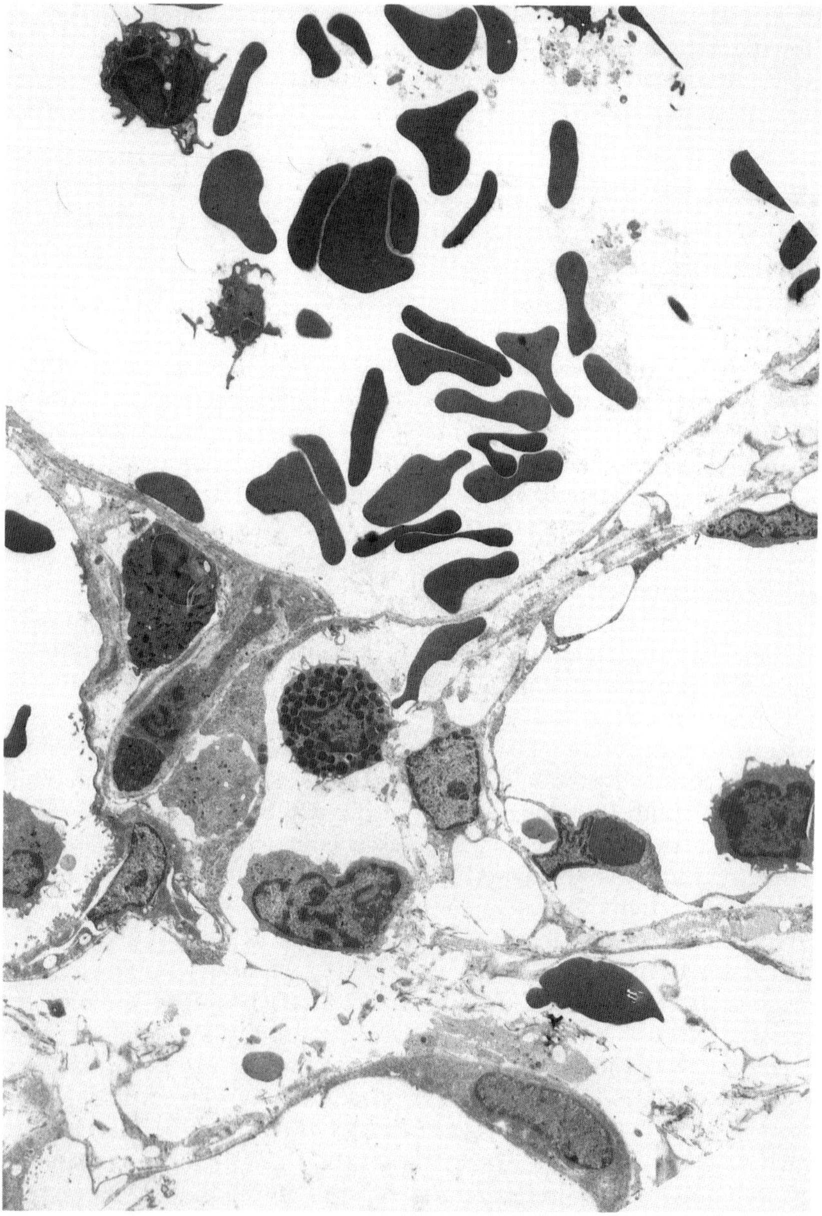

FIGURE 2

IgG immune complex-induced lung injury. In this model, the formation of IgG immune complexes in the lung induces acute injury which peaks at 4 hr and is characterized histologically by neutrophilic infiltrates, extensive injury to the pulmonary vascular bed, and intraalveolar hemorrhage. (Transmission electron microscopy, X2650.)

the generation of tissue toxic ·OH, which is the most toxic of the oxygen products of activated PMN (35).

The source of toxic oxygen products in the IgG immune complex model of lung injury appears to be the neutrophil. As expected, neutrophil depletion substantially blocks the development of IgG immune complex alveolitis (41). Immune complex deposition leads to complement activation with the generation of the C5a anaphylotoxin, which appears to be necessary for the accumulation in tissues of neutrophils and is also known to enhance oxy radical production by these cells. As expected, therefore, complement depletion prior to anti-BSA instillation markedly attenuates the development of injury (41). To what extent lung macrophages also contribute to the oxygen radical burden in this experimental model is not known, although it is known that IgG immune complexes are quite powerful stimulants of the respiratory burst in rat alveolar macrophages (24).

In these models, stimulated neutrophils generate oxidants and also release proteolytic enzymes into the surrounding tissues. Neutrophil elastase, which has been isolated in lung tissue from patients with acute respiratory distress syndrome (42–44), induces acute pulmonary injury and the development of pulmonary emphysema when instilled into the airways of lungs (38). It seems likely that lung injury induced by products of activated neutrophils is the result of the effects of both oxidants as well as proteases.

In addition to the tissue-damaging effects of O_2^-, ·OH, and H_2O_2, the nitrogen-centered radical nitric oxide (NO·) has also been implicated in the pathogenesis of IgG immune complex alveolitis and dermal vasculitis. Intratracheal instillation or intradermal injection of the L-arginine analog N^G-monomethyl-L-arginine acetate (NMA) together with the anti-BSA markedly attenuates the increases in vascular permeability and hemorrhage following tissue deposition of IgG immune complexes (45). Protection is correlated with diminished appearance of the degradation products of ·NO, namely, NO_2 and NO_3^-, in the bronchoalveolar (BAL) fluids of injured animals that have been pretreated with NMA. NMA competitively inhibits ·NO synthetase, and when L-arginine is coinstilled with NMA the protective effects of NMA are lost (45). It is known that ·NO interferes with the adherence of neutrophils to endothelial cells and that O_2^-, by interacting with ·NO to form $ONOO^-$ (peroxynitrite anion), "scavenges" ·NO in a manner that should enhance adhesive interactions between leukocytes and endothelial cells. However, recent data from our laboratory describing the protective effects of NMA IgG immune complex-induced pulmonary injury are not associated with diminished recruitment of neutrophils (45). More likely, NMA presents formation of toxic derivatives of ·NO, namely, $ONOO^-$ and HO· (46). While the source of the ·NO in these lung inflammatory reactions is not known, macrophages appear to be the likely source, and ·NO or its derivatives appear to be important purveyors of inflammatory injury.

The roles of platelet-activating factor and the cytokines TNF-α and IL-1 have also been explored in IgG immune complex-induced tissue injury models involving disorders. Platelet-activating factor is known to enhance immune complex-induced production *in vitro* of O_2^- by neutrophils (47). Treatment with a PAF receptor antagonist has been shown to attenuate IgG immune complex-induced vasculitis involving the lung or dermis of rats (47). In addition, TNF-α is also required for the development of IgG immune complex alveolitis (48). Treatment of rats with anti-TNF-α is highly protective, which can be correlated with blocking of the influx of neutrophils. The most likely explanation for this finding is that activated pulmonary macrophages release TNF-α (and IL-1), which then causes up-regulation of leukocyte adhesion molecules on pulmonary vascular endothelial cells.

Alveolar macrophages produce significant amounts of TNF-α and IL-1 following immune complex stimulation *in vitro* and *in vivo.* A similar requirement for IL-1 has been demonstrated in the immune complex-induced alveolitis model where high levels of IL-1 are also found in the BAL following IgG immune complex deposition (49). TNF-α *in vitro* can activate endothelium to cause up-regulation of adhesion molecules (50). *In vivo,* TNF-α is known to be able to induce endothelial leukocyte adhesion molecule (ELAM-1) expression in the pulmonary microvasculature (Fig. 3). As stated above, this appears to have a key parallel in IgG immune complex deposition in lung, in which TNF-α prevents elaboration that is associated with expression of ELAM-1 and neutrophil influx. Blocking of TNF-α prevents ELAM-1 expression and, correspondingly, influx of neutrophils. Also, blocking of ELAM-1 interferes with neutrophil influx. Somewhat surprisingly, TNF-α does not appear to be required for the development of reverse passive dermal Arthus reaction, whereas a requirement for IL-1 has been established in this model. Indeed, treatment with anti-IL-1, IL-1 receptor antagonist, or anti-ELAM-1 is associated with protection against injury and diminution of tissue neutrophil influx in both the lung and dermis following deposition of IgG immune complexes (13,51).

The $\beta2$ leukocyte intregrins have also been recently shown to play a role in the pathogenesis of IgG immune complex-induced alveolitis. Treatment with a monoclonal antibody to CD18 results in a reduction in neutrophil accumulation and an attenuation of vascular permeability and hemorrhage at sites of immune complex deposition in lung or skin (36).

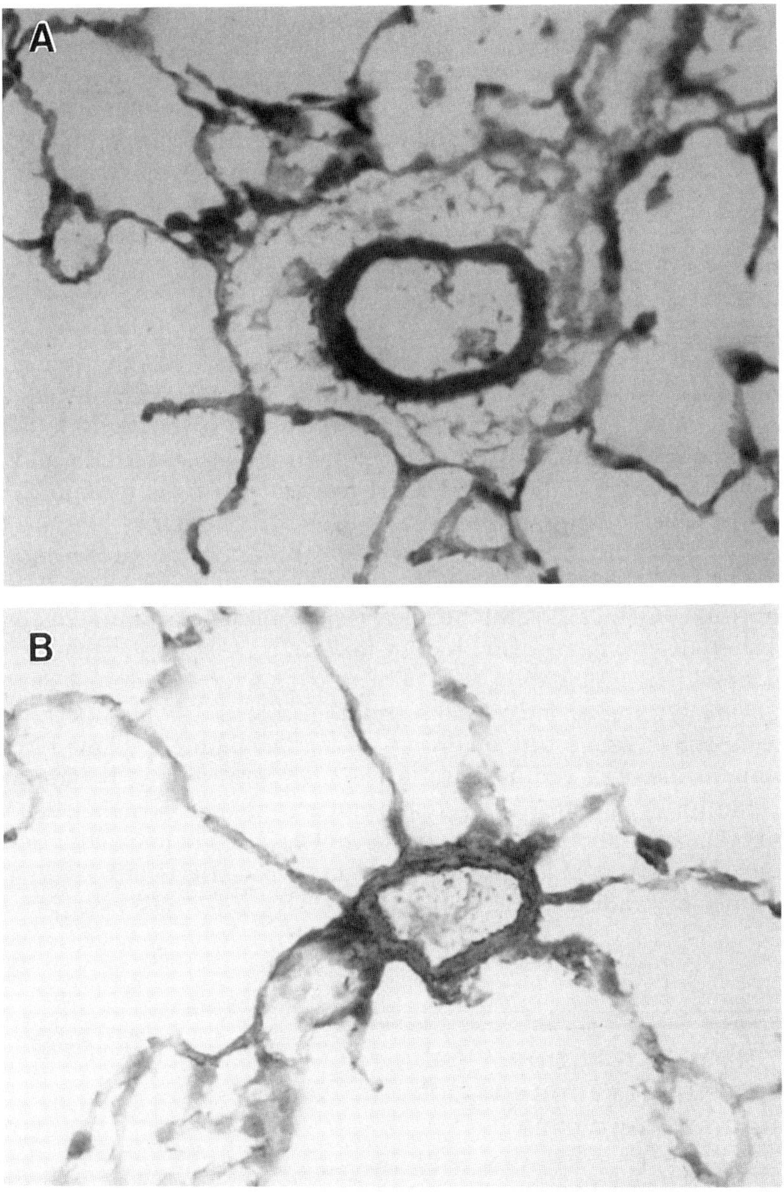

FIGURE 3

TNF-induced ELAM-1 expression in the lung vasculature. Normal lungs do not show up-regulation of endothelial cell adhesion molecules (A). However, after TNF infusion (B) or the induction of acute inflammation by immune complexes, there is an up-regulation of adhesion molecules including ELAM-1. (Immunohistochemistry, X400.)

Similarly, treatment with an antibody to CD11b results in less pronounced but nonetheless significant attenuation of alveolar injury developing after intrapulmonary IgG immune complex deposition (36). This attenuation correlates directly with reduced tissue accumulation of neutrophils. The roles of CD11a and CD11c and other adhesion molecules have yet to be investigated, pending the availability of appropriate monoclonal antibodies.

A likely sequence of events related to development of IgG immune complex-induced lung injury is depicted in Fig. 4. Tissue deposition of IgG immune complexes activates alveolar macrophages, resulting in the generation of oxidants (·NO, O_2^-, H_2O_2), cytokines (TNF-α and IL-1), and PAF. The cytokines up-regulate expression of ELAM-1 and other adhesion molecules on adjacent interstitial vascular endothelial cells, resulting in the initial adhesive interactions with circulating PMNs. Following this, neutrophils under the influence of CB11b/CD18 and endothelial cells associated with ICAM respond to C5a and migrate into the interstitial and intraalveolar compartments where they become activated by immune complexes, complement activation products, and macrophage-derived PAF. This results in neutrophil production of oxidants (O_2^-, ·OH, H_2O_2) and the release of proteases. As indicated above, activated macrophages also produce toxic oxygen- and nitrogen-derived products. The combination of all of these events causes cytolytic damage of alveolar epithelial and vascular endothelial cells as well as proteolysis of connective tissue (involving basement membrane and matrix), resulting in the observed increase in vascular permeability, hemorrhage, and fibrin deposition. The precise cellular source of ·NO (neutrophils, macrophages, or endothelial cells) has not yet been delineated, but ·NO (or its derivatives) is likely to exert its cytotoxic effects in concert with the other oxy radicals.

IV. Acute Lung Injury Following Deposition of Immunoglobulin A Immune Complexes

Intrapulmonary deposition of IgA immune complexes also leads to the development of acute lung injury. These animal studies may have clinical relevance since IgA immune complex deposition has been implicated in the pathogenesis of several diseases (Berger's nephropathy, Henoch–Schonlein purpura and renal lesions associated with systemic lupus ery-

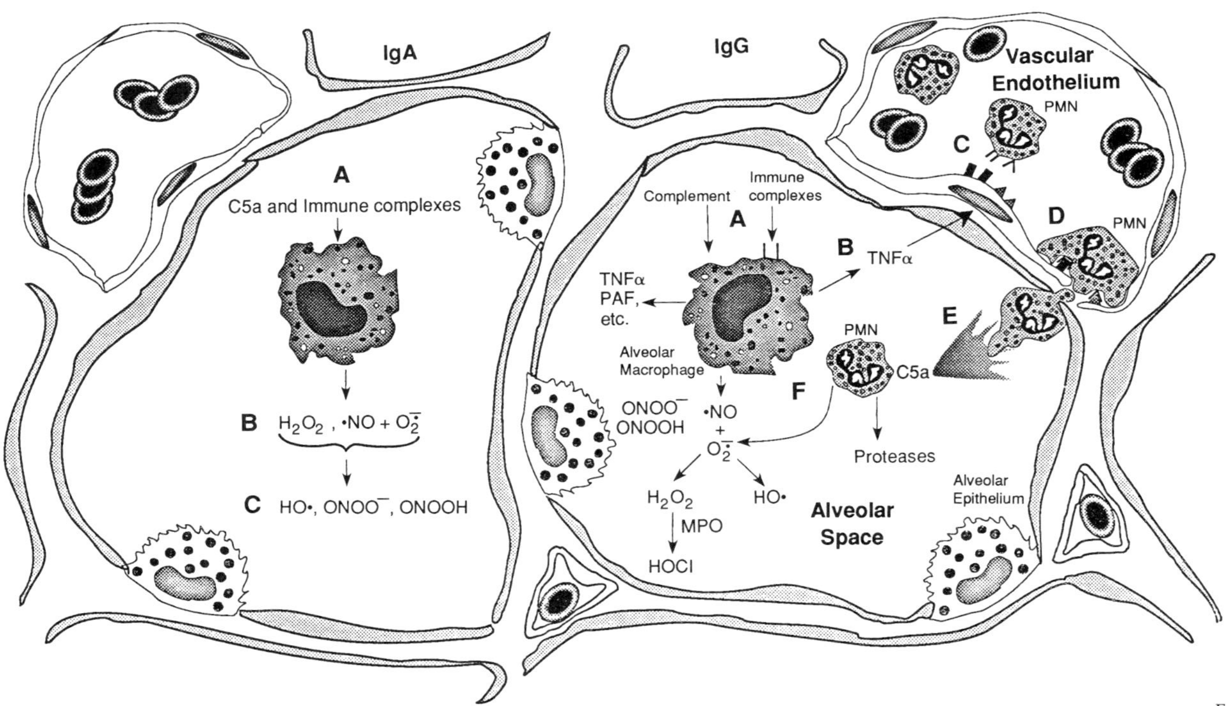

FIGURE 4

Postulated sequence of events in IgA- and IgG-induced lung injury. Left portion of figure, IgA: A, stimulation of MØ by IgA immune complexes and complement and engagement of MØ CD18; B, Oxidant production by macrophages; C, Formation of HO· and nitrogen centered radicals, and lung damage. Right portion of figure, IgG: A, Simulation of MØ by IgG immune complexes and complement; B, Release of TNFα from MØ; C, Upregulation of leukocyte adhesion molecules (including ELAM-1) on endothelial cells; D, Adherence of PMN to altered vascular endothelial cells; engagement of neutrophil CD18; E, Chemotaxis of PMN in response to C5a, PAF, and other mediators; F, Release of toxic oxygen products and proteases from PMN and MØ.

thematosus, and hepatic cirrhosis). The lung model of injury is similar to that found in IgG immune complex-induced alveolitis except for the fact that the antibody is an IgA directed against dinitrophenol (DNP), with DNP being conjugated to BSA (52). As is the case with IgG immune complex-induced injury, complement depletion is protective, but neutrophil depletion is not associated with attenuation of lung injury (52). This is not surprising, given the *in vitro* findings that IgA immune complexes stimulate alveolar macrophages (but not neutrophils) to produce O_2^-. In the *in vivo* model of IgA immune complex induced lung injury, there is a marked mononuclear cell infiltrate with very few neutrophils (52).

Oxygen radicals have also been implicated in the pathogenesis of IgA immune complex-induced alveolitis. Pretreatment of animals with superoxide dismutase, catalase, the iron chelator deferoxamine, or the hydroxyl radical scavenger DMSO suppresses the development of lung injury (5), in contrast to untreated positive control animals in which the lungs are characterized by the presence of increased numbers of alveolar macrophages, with interstitial edema and hemorrhage (Fig. 5). Futhermore, in this model of lung injury the L-arginine analog NMA is also highly protective, as demonstrated by greatly reduced vascular permeability and hemorrhage and reduced of injury of vascular endothelial and alveolar epithelial cells (53). These findings suggest that the macrophage is the source of damaging ·NO, O_2^-, H_2O_2 and ·OH. The protective interventions also suggest that ·OH may be the ultimate effector of the injury.

The possible roles of cytokines and adhesion molecules have also been investigated in this model of lung injury. Blocking of TNF-α and ELAM-1 in animals with IgA immune complexes is without effect, in striking contrast to the absolute requirements of TNF-α and ELAM-1 in neutrophil recruitment and lung injury following deposition of IgG immune complexes. In recent studies, the use of monoclonal antibodies to CD18 was associated with attenuation of lung vascular permeability and hemorrhage following intrapulmonary deposition of IgA immune complexes (53). The roles of VCAM-1, ICAM-1, CD18, and other selectins remains to be investigated.

A summary of the pathogenesis of IgA immune complex-induced injury is shown in Fig. 4. Following IgA immune complex deposition and complement activation, pulmonary macrophages are activated, perhaps through some interaction with CD18 of macrophages. Ultimately, the production of ·NO, ·OH, H_2O_2, and O_2^- results in alveolar epithelial and vascular endothelial cell damage, increased vascular permeability, and intraalveolar hemorrhage.

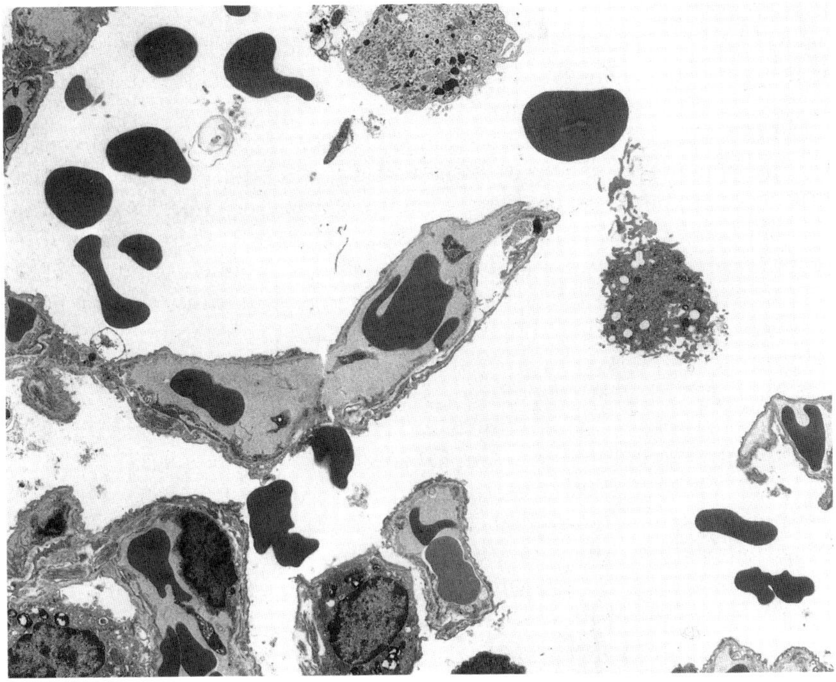

FIGURE 5

IgA immune complex-induced lung injury. Unlike the case for IgG, IgA immune complex-induced injury is not caused by neutrophils but rather is associated with an influx of monocytes/macrophages with subsequent injury to the pulmonary vascular bed and intraalveolar hemorrhage. (Transmission electron microscopy, X3050.)

V. Mechanism of *in Vitro* Injury of Endothelial Cells

Pulmonary vascular endothelial cell culture techniques have allowed for dissection of the pathway of neutrophil-mediated cytotoxicity. Both human endothelial cells harvested from umbilical veins (HUVEC) and rat pulmonary artery endothelial cells (RPAEC) have been evaluated. HUVEC demonstrate variability with respect to sensitivity to injury by activated neutrophils. This is related to their passage number. The same can be said of RPAEC after 10 passages. These findings only begin to describe the differences in endothelial cell physiology between species and vascular beds within the same species. The most likely explanation for these differences related to cell passage number is the reduction in iron content in passaged cells.

Neutrophil-mediated endothelial cell lysis is blocked by the presence of catalase but not consistently by superoxide dismutase (54), implicating H_2O_2 as a mediator of endothelial cell cytotoxicity (54). These results were supported by the findings that endothelial cells were damaged by incubation with xanthine and xanthine oxidase (which produce H_2O_2 and O_2^-) that this cytotoxicity was prevented by the addition of catalase. Since SOD catalyzes the conversion of O_2^- to H_2O_2, its ability to prevent endothelial cell lysis in these systems is not entirely surprising. Therefore, although PMA-activated neutrophils generate H_2O_2 and O_{2-}, only the former appears to be critical for endothelial cell killing (55). The addition of myeloperoxidase (MPO) inhibitors (azide, cyanide), which block the conversion of H_2O_2 to HOCl, or the use of HOCl scavengers does not attenuate endothelial cell killing by activated neutrophils, indicating that MPO products of H_2O_2 are not involved directly in the killing of endothelial cells by activated neutrophils (55). However HOCl may play a role in neutrophil-mediated vascular injury by activating the neutrophil metalloproteases collagenase and gelatinase, the result of which would be the lifting off of endothelial cells from the underlying basement membrane (56). This, by itself, could lead to an increase in permeability of vessels so affected.

The hydroxyl radical appears to be the ultimate mediator of neutrophil-produced injury of endothelial cells (55). Endothelial cytotoxicity mediated by neutrophils activated with immune complexes, opsonized zymosan particles, or PMA is attenuated by the catalase as well as by the iron chelator deferoxamine and by DMSO (55). These findings suggest that, in addition to H_2O_2, the ·OH generated by an iron-dependent reaction may be required for endothelial cell injury. One likely role for O_2^- that has been generated within endothelial cells is the reduction of Fe^{3+} to Fe^{2+}, permitting the role of the latter in the Fenton reaction (see above).

Recent evidence also suggests that nitric oxide or its metabolites may be important mediators of cytotoxicity (reviewed in Ref. 57). O_2^- combines with ·NO to form the peroxynitrate radical ($ONOO^-$), which, in turn, can yield HO·. Neutrophils generate relatively small amounts of ·NO in contrast to endothelial cells or macrophages stimulated with endotoxin. ·NO has been well-characterized as the endothelial cell-derived relaxing factor, but its role in endothelial cell injury has yet to be carefully defined. Deferoxamine will also react with perxynitrite to block HO· formation (58). It may be that part of the protective effects of deferoxamine are explained by this mechanism. Further studies are warranted. It is possible that the role of ·NO in injury to endothelial cells is most closely linked to its generation by monocytes and macrophages.

The role of neutrophil proteases in endothelial cell-induced injury is controversial. Neutrophil elastase appears to be responsible for the conversion of xanthine dehydrogenase to xanthine oxidase in endothelial cells, resulting in increased generation of intracellular O_2^- and H_2O_2 (59–60). Endothelial cell xanthine oxidase activity has also been implicated in endothelial cell injury associated with events following ischemia and reperfusion (61,62). The heightened production of these oxidants may then allow for HO· generation via the Haber–Weiss reaction. Neutrophil elastase has also been implicated in endothelial cell detachment from monolayers following addition of opsonized zymosan particles (63). Furthermore, known stimulants of neutrophil oxidant production like C5a and PMA (54,64) also trigger the release from neutrophils of granule contents. The extent to which these enzymes might be involved in endothelial cell injury functioning independently or synergistically with oxygen radicals is not completely understood.

Differences between species and differences with respect to vascular beds from the same animals make endothelial cell injury studies from different laboratories difficult to interpret. Work with RPAEC has revealed that adhesive interactions between neutrophils and endothelial cells facilitate oxygen radical-mediated endothelial cytotoxicity. The $\beta 2$ integrins (CD18) of PMN and ELAM-1 of the LEC-CAM family of endothelial cell adhesion mediators are important in cytotoxic interactions between PMN and endothelial cells (13,36). Sialyated Lewis^x antigen (Sial Le^x) is an important neutrophil ligand for ELAM-1 (65). ICAM-1 molecules on endothelial cells are recognized by the CD11a/CD18 and CD11b/CD18 molecules of neutrophils (66). These findings support the possibility that there are at least two independent adhesive interactions linked to endothelial cell cytotoxicity. The role of adhesion molecules may also help to explain how cytokine stimulation enhances endothelial cytotoxicity since ELAM-1 and other adhesion molecules are known to be up-regulated by TNF-α and other cytokines (62,67,68).

VI. Summary

Injury of the lung following the triggering of an inflammatory response by intravascular complement activation or by intrapulmonary deposition of immune complexes results in acute lung injury involving pulmonary vascular endothelial cells as well as alveolar epithelial cells. Depending on the circumstances, the injury can be linked to products of neutrophils, products of macrophages, or a combination of the two. The most likely leukocyte toxic products are proteases and derivatives of oxygen (O_2^-, H_2O_2, HO·) and nitrogen (·NO and $ONOO^-$). In addition, in situations in which products of macrophages are involved in events leading to injury, cytokines (IL-1, TNF-α) and PAF contribute to the complex series of events causing injury. Adhesion molecules on endothelial cells (ELAM-1, ICAM-1,2) and on leukocytes (β2 integrins) are also involved in leukocyte localization leading to injury. The *in vitro* study of endothelial cells has provided additional insights into mechanisms of their injury by activated neutrophils. The most current data suggest that the injury process is iron-dependent and that H_2O_2 generated from the neutrophil and O_2^- produced by the endothelial cell are related ultimately to the intracellular generation of HO· within the endothelial cell, which is responsible for the cytotoxic events. The combined approaches employing both *in vitro* and *in vivo* models of lung injury will lead to a clearer understanding of the pathophysiological events.

References

1. R. L. Baehner, R. B. Johnston, Jr., and D. G. Nathan, *J. Reticuloendothel Soc.* **12,** 150–169 (1972).
2. T. Sachs, C. F. Moldow, P. R. Craddock, J. K. Bowers, and H. S. Jacob, *J. Clin. Invest.* **61,** 1161–1167 (1978).
3. K. J. Johnson, and P. A. Ward, *J. Immunol.* **126,** 2365–2369 (1981).
4. G. O. Till, K. J. Johnson, and P. A. Ward, *J. Clin. Invest.* **69,** 1126–1135 (1982).
5. K. J. Johnson, P. A. Ward, R. G. Kunkel, and B. S. Wilson, *Lab. Invest.* **54,** 449–506 (1986).
6. J. B. Hibbs, R. R. Taintor, and Z. Vavrin, *Science* **235,** 473–476 (1987).
7. R. Iyengar, D. J. Stuehr, and M. A. Marletta, *Proc. Natl. Acad. Sci. U.S.A.* **84,** 6369–6373 (1987).
8. D. R. Freyer, M. L. Morganroth, and R. F. Todd, III, *Inflammation* **13,** 495–505 (1989).
9. P. J. Simpson, R. F. Todd, III, J. C. Fantone, J. K. Mickelson, J. D. Griffin, and B. R. Lucchesi, *J. Clin. Invest.* **81,** 624–629 (1988).
10. S. Nourshargh, M. Rampart, P. G. Hellewell, P. J. Jose, J. M. Harlan, A. J. Edwards, and T. J. Williams, *J. Immunol.* **142,** 3193–3198 (1989).
11. C. M. Doerschuk, R. K. Winn, H. O. Coxson, and J. M. Harlan, *J. Immunol.* **144,** 2327–2333 (1990).
12. C. W. Smith, S. D. Marlin, R. Rothlein, C. Toman, and D. C. Anderson, *J. Clin. Invest.* **83,** 2008–2017 (1989).

13. M. S. Mulligan, J. Varani, M. K. Dame, C. L. Lane, C. W. Smith, D. L. Anderson, and P. A. Ward, *J. Clin. Invest* **88,** 1396–1406 (1991).
14. J. A. Badwey, and M. L. Karnovsky, *Annu. Rev. Biochem.* **49,** 695–726 (1980).
15. D. Ross, *in* "The Cell Biology of Inflammation, Handbook of Inflammation," (G. Weissman, ed.), Vol. 2, pp. 337–385. Elsevier/North-Holland, New York, 1979.
16. J. Varani, I. Ginsburg, L. Schuger, D. F. Gibbs, J. Bromberg, K. J. Johnson, U. S. Ryan, and P. A. Ward, *Am. J. Pathol.* **135,** 435–438 (1989).
17. B. Sherry and A. Cerami, *J. Cell Biol.* **107,** 1268–1277 (1988).
18. C. A. Dinarello, *FASEB J.* **2,** 108–115 (1988).
19. P. Bachwich, S. W. Chensue, J. W. Larrick, and S. W. Kunkel, *Biochem. Biophys. Res. Commun.* **136,** 94–101 (1986).
20. R. M. Strieter, S. L. Kunkel, H. Showell, D. F. Remick, S. H. Phan, P. A. Ward, and R. M. Marks, *Science* **243,** 1467–1469 (1989).
21. F. Bussolino, G. Camussi, and C. Baglioni, *J. Biol. Chem.* **263,** 11856–11861 (1988).
22. J. S. Warren, P. A. Barton, D. M. Mandel, and K. Matrosic, *Lab. Invest.* **63,** 746–754 (1990).
23. R. M. Strieter, S. L. Kunkel, H. J. Showell, and R. M. Marks, *Biochem. Biophys. Res. Commun.* **156,** 1340–1345 (1988).
24. J. S. Warren, S. L. Kunke., T. W. Cunningham, K. J. Johnson, and P. A. Ward, *Am. J. Pathol.* **130,** 489–495 (1988).
25. P. R. Craddock, J. Fehr, A. P. Dalmasso, K. L. Brigham, and H. S. Jacob, *J. Clin. Invest.* **59,** 879–888 (1977).
26. P. L. Haslam, P. J. Townsend, and M. A. Branthwaite, *Anaesthesia* **25,** 22–26 (1980).
27. J. Nusbacher, S. I. Rosenfeld, J. L. MacPherson, P. A. Theim, and J. P. Leddy, *Blood* **51,** 359–365 (1978).
28. J T. O'Flaherty, P. R. Craddock, and H. S. Jacob, *Blood* **51,** 731–739 (1978).
29. P. R. Craddock, D. E. Hammerschmidt, C. F. Moldow, O. Yamada, and H. S. Jacob, *Semin. Hematol.* **16,** 140–147 (1979).
30. P. R. Craddock, J. Fehr, K. L. Brigham, R. S. Kronenberg, and H. S. Jacob, *N. Engl. J. Med.* **269,** 769–774 (1977).
31. E. D. Chenoweth, S. W. Cooper, T. E. Hugli, R. W. Stewart, E. H. Blackstone, and J. Kirklin, *N. Engl. J. Med.* **304,** 497–503 (1981).
32. D. E. Hammerschmidt, L. J. Weaver, L. D. Hudson, P. R. Craddock, and H. S. Jacob, *Lancet* **1,** 947–949 (1980).
33. T. Sachs, C. F. Moldow, P. R. Craddock, T. K. Bowers, and H. S. Jacob, *J. Clin. Invest.* **61,** 1161–1167 (1978).
34. M. A. Reidy, and S. M. Schwartz, *Lab. Invest.* **44,** 301–308 (1981).
35. J. M. McCord, and E. D. Day, Jr., *FEBS Lett.* **86,** 139–142 (1978).
36. M. S. Mulligan, J. Varani, J. S. Warren, G. O. Till, C. W. Smith, D. C. Anderson, R. F. Todd, III, and P. A. Ward, *J. Immunol.* **148,** 1847–1857 (1992).
37. K. J. Johnson, and P. A. Ward, *J. Clin. Invest.* **54,** 349–357 (1974).
38. A. Janoff, B. Sloan, G. Weinbaum, V. Damiano, R. A. Sandhaus, J. Elias, and P. Kimbel, *Am. Rev. Respir. Dis.* **115,** 461–478 (1977).
39. W. F. Petrone, E. K. English, K. Wong, and J. M. McCord, *Proc. Natl. Acad. Sci. U.S.A.* **77,** 1159 (1980).
40. K. J. Johnson, J. C. Fantone, J. Kaplan, and P. A. Ward, *J. Clin. Invest.* **67,** 983 (1981).
41. K. J. Johnson, and P. A. Ward, *J. Clin. Invest.* **54,** 349–357 (1974).
42. W. W. McGuire, R. G. Spragg, A. B. Cohen, and C. G. Cochrane, *J. Clin. Invest.* **69,** 543–553 (1982).
43. T. A. Merritt, C. G. Cochrane, K. Holcomb, B. Bohl, M. Hallman, D. K. Edward, and L. Gluck, *J. Clin. Invest.* **72,** 656–666 (1983).

44. C. T. Lee, A. M. Fein, M. Lippmann, H. Holtzman, P. Kimbel, and G. Weinbaum, *N. Engl. J. Med.* **304,** 192–196 (1981).
45. M. S. Mulligan, J. M. Hevel, M. A. Marletta, and P. A. Ward, *Proc. Natl. Acad. Sci. U.S.A.* **88,** 6338–6342 (1991).
46. J. S. Beckman, T. W. Beckman, J. Chen, P. A. Marshall, and B. A. Freeman, *Proc. Natl. Acad. Sci. U.S.A.* **87,** 1620–1624 (1990).
47. J. S. Warren, D. M. Mandel, K. J. Johnson, and P. A. Ward, *J. Clin. Invest.* **83,** 669–678 (1988).
48. J. S. Warren, K. R. Yabroff, D. G. Remick, S. L. Kunkel, S. W. Chensue, R. G. Kunkel, K. J. Johnson, and P. A Ward, *J. Clin. Invest.* **84,** 1873–1882 (1989).
49. J. S. Warren, *Biochem. Biophys. Res. Commun.* **175,** 604–610 (1991).
50. J. S. Pober, *Am. J. Pathol.* **133,** 426–433 (1988).
51. M. S. Mulligan, and P. A. Ward, *J. Immunol.* **149,** 331–339 (1992).
52. K. J. Johnson, B. S. Wilson, G. O. Till, and P. A. Ward, *J. Clin. Invest.* **74,** 358–369 (1984).
53. M. S. Mulligan, J. S. Warren, C. W. Smith, D. C. Anderson, C. G. Yeh, A. R. Rudolph, and P. A. Ward, *J. Immunol.* **148,** 3086–3092 (1992).
54. T. Sacks, C. F. Moldow, P. R. Craddock, T. K. Bowers, and H. S. Jacob, *J. Clin. Invest.* **61,** 1161 (1978).
55. J. Varani, S. E. Fligiel, G. O. Till, R. G. Kunkel, and U. S. Ryan, *Lab. Invest.* **53,** 656–664 (1985).
56. S. J. Weiss, *N. Engl. J. Med.* **320,** 365–376 (1989).
57. M. A. Marletta, *Trends Biochem. Sci.* **14,** 488–492 (1989).
58. J. S. Beckman, T. W. Beckman, J. Chen, *et al., Natl. Acad. Sci. U.S.A.* **87,** 1620–1624 (1990).
59. S. H. Phan, D. E. Gannon, and P. A. Ward, *Amer. J. Resp. Cell Mol. Biol.* **6,** 270–278 (1992).
60. D. N. Granger, *Am. J. Physiol.* **255,** H1269–H1275 (1988).
61. E. D. Jarasch, G. Bruder, and H. W. Heid, *Acta Physiol. Scand. (Suppl.)* **548,** 39–46 (1986).
62. H. P. Friedl, D. J. Smith, G. O. Till, P. D. Thompson, D. S. Louis, and P. A. Ward *Am. J. Pathol.* **136,** 491–495 (1990).
63. J. M. Harlan, P. D. Killen, L. A. Harker, G. E. Striker, and D. G. Wright, *J. Clin. Invest.* **68,** 1394 (1981).
64. S. J. Weiss, J. Young, A. F. LoBuflio, A. Slivka, and N. F. Nimeh, *J. Clin. Invest.* **68,** 714 (1981).
65. M. L. Phillips, E. Nudelman, F. C. Gaeta, M. Perez, A. K. Singhal, S. Hakomori, and J. C. Paulson *Science* **250,** 1130–1132 (1990).
66. S. M. Albelda, and C. A. Buck, *FASEB J.* **4,** 2868–2880 (1990).
67. L. Osborn, *Cell (Cambridge, Mass.)* **62,** 3–6 (1990).
68. J. Varani, M. J. Bendelow, D. E. Sealey, S. L. Kunkel, D. E. Gannon, U. S. Ryan, and P. A. Ward *Lab. Invest.* **59,** 292–295 (1988).
69. M. D. Bevilaqua, J. S. Prober, D. L. Mendrick, R. S. Letran, M. A. Ginsburg, Jr., *Proc. Natl. Acad. Sci. U.S.A.* **84,** 9238–9242 (1987).

CHAPTER 8

Contributions of Oxidants and Granulocytes to Ischemia–Reperfusion Injury

Paul Kubes* and D. Neil Granger

Department of Physiology and Biophysics
Louisiana State University Medical Center
Shreveport, Louisiana 71130
and
Department of Medical Physiology*
University of Calgary
Health Sciences Centre
Calgary T2N 4N1, Alberta, Canada

I. Introduction

A decade ago, we first obtained evidence which suggested that reactive oxygen metabolites may play an important role in mediating the microvascular dysfunction associated with reperfusion of the ischemic small intestine (1). In the ensuing years we have devoted considerable effort to determining the source and identity of the reactive oxygen metabolites that contribute to reperfusion injury in the intestine. The results of our studies and published work from other laboratories are largely consistent with the hypothesis that xanthine oxidase is a major source of the superoxide and hydrogen peroxide produced in the postischemic intestine. Support for this view is provided by observations that free radical scavenging enzymes (superoxide dismutase and catalase) and inhibitors of xanthine oxidase (allopurinol, pterin aldehyde) are equally effective in attenuating the microvascular injury induced by ischemia–reperfusion. Similar protection is afforded by iron chelators (deferoxamine), iron-binding proteins (apotransferrin), and hydroxyl radical scavengers (dimethyl sulfoxide), indicating that hydroxyl radicals, formed by the reaction of iron with superoxide and hydrogen peroxide (Haber–Weiss reaction), also contribute to reperfusion injury and lipid peroxidation (2).

Based on all of the aforementioned observations, it was initially held that the oxygen free radicals produced by xanthine oxidase were directly responsible for the microvascular dysfunction induced by ischemia–reperfusion. However, more recent studies from our laboratory indicate that xanthine oxidase-derived oxidants may play a more important role in initiating the formation of substances that attract, activate, and promote the adherence of granulocytes to microvascular endothelium. In this revised concept of xanthine oxidase-related reperfusion injury (see Fig. 1), activated granulocytes are considered the primary mediators of tissue injury, with xanthine oxidase-derived oxidants contributing to the initiation of the inflammatory response (2). In this chapter, we summarize studies from our laboratory which address the issue of granulocyte- and oxygen radical-mediated injury in the small intestine. Particular emphasis is given to describing our work on mechanisms of reperfusion-induced leukocyte infiltration and tissue injury.

II. Ischemia–Reperfusion-Induced Granulocyte Infiltration: Role of Oxidants

Our first attempt to examine the possible role of granulocytes in ischemia–reperfusion injury focused on whether granulocytes accumulate in intestinal mucosa exposed to ischemia and reperfusion (3). To achieve this objective, we measured tissue-associated myeloperoxidase (MPO) activity in mucosal biopsies obtained from feline intestine exposed to 3 hr of ischemia (blood flow reduced to 20% of baseline) and 1 hr of

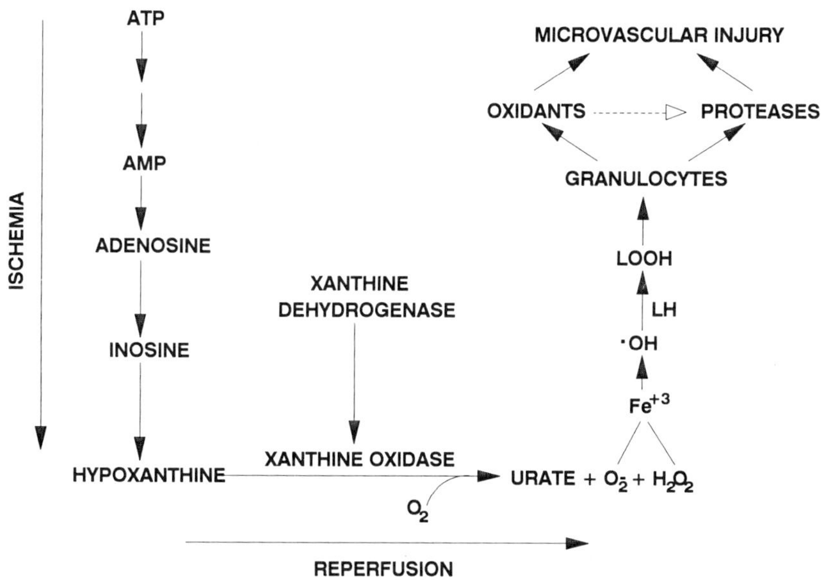

FIGURE 1

Mechanism proposed to explain the involvement of xanthine oxidase-derived oxidants and granulocytes in ischemia–reperfusion–induced microvascular injury. (From Ref. 2.)

reperfusion. The data from these experiments indicate that significant granulocyte accumulation occurs during the ischemic period, with a further, more dramatic increase observed following reperfusion. Since previous studies have demonstrated that feline eosinophils are devoid of peroxidase activity, it would appear that the ischemia–reperfusion (I/R)-induced increase in MPO activity largely reflects an accumulation of neutrophils. Based on the tissue MPO measurements and the number of circulating neutrophils per unit of MPO activity [10^6 polymorphonuclear leukocytes (PMNs) per unit MPO activity], we estimate that there are approximately 40 million neutrophils per gram of postischemic intestional mucosa.

To determine whether xanthine oxidase and superoxide play a role in I/R-induced neutrophil infiltration, cats were pretreated with either superoxide dismutase (SOD) or allopurinol (3). Both agents, when administered at concentrations which were previously shown to attenuate I/R injury in feline intestine, largely abolished the rise in tissue MPO normally observed in the postischemic intestine (see Fig. 2) (4). These observations were recently extended to include an analysis of the ef-

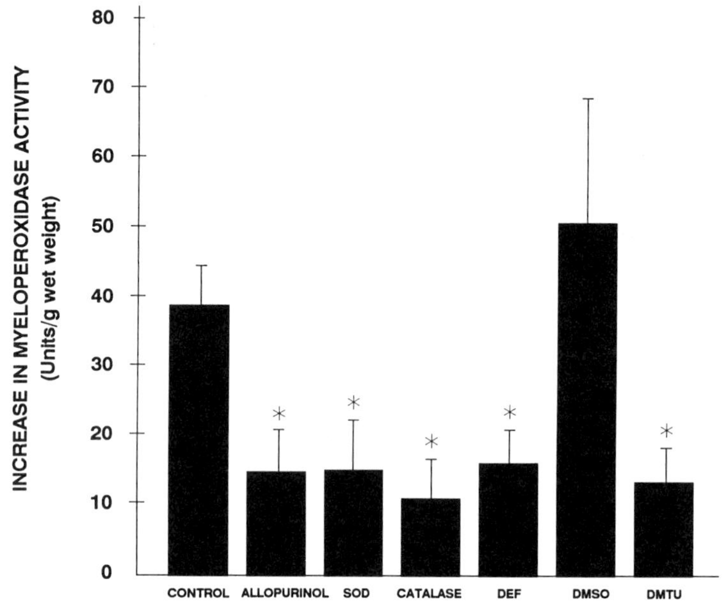

FIGURE 2

Effects of catalase, deferoxamine (DEF), dimethyl sulfoxide (DMSO), allopurinol, superoxide dismutase (SOD), and dimethylthiourea (DMTU) on increased myeloperoxidase (MPO) activity observed in intestine at 1 hr after reperfusion. *, significance from control. (From Ref. 4.)

fects of pretreatment with catalase, deferoxamine, dimethyl sulfoxide (DMSO), or dimethylthiourea (DMTU) on I/R-induced neutrophil infiltration (4). All of these agents, with the exception of DMSO, reduced the reperfusion-induced rise in tissue MPO in a manner similar to SOD and allopurinol (Fig. 2). Thus, the results obtained from the two studies (3,4) suggest that xanthine oxidase-derived oxygen radicals contribute significantly to the neutrophil recruitment elicited by I/R.

One possible explanation for the ability of SOD to reduce I/R-induced neutrophil infiltration is that superoxide formed following reperfusion diffuses out of endothelial and/or epithelial cells to interact with specific lipoproteins in extracellular fluid to yield the so called superoxide-dependent chemoattractant, which was previously described for human plasma (5). To test this possibility, we exposed feline plasma to different superoxide-generating systems (hypoxanthine–xanthine oxidase or potassium superoxide) and then tested the chemotactic potential of this plasma both *in vitro* and *in vivo* (4). The results of these experiments indicate that the direct interaction of superoxide with feline extracellular fluid does not lead to the production of a substance with significant chemotactic activity. However, the addition of H_2O_2 with either hemoglobin or ferrous iron to feline plasma caused significant chemotactic activity *in vitro*. These observations suggest that the H_2O_2 produced in postischemic tissues may interact with catalytically active iron (derived from either hemolysis or cellular release of low molecular weight iron) in extracellular fluid to form an inflammatory mediator such as platelet-activating factor (PAF), leukotriene B_4 (LTB_4), or C5a, which in turn promotes neutrophil infiltration.

The assumption that reperfusion causes granulocytes to adhere to microvascular endothelium and subsequently emigrate into the interstitial compartment is an important component of the hypothesis relating oxidant production to reperfusion-induced microvascular injury (2). Since the premise that reperfusion promotes leukocytes adherence to vascular endothelium was largely based on tissue MPO measurements, we directly addressed this issue by examining the influence of ischemia and reperfusion on leukocyte adherence and emigration in the postcapillary venules of the cat mesentery (6). For these studies, leukocyte adherence and emigration were monitored in venules exposed to 1 hr of ischemia followed by 1 hr of reperfusion.

Although there were a number of published reports dealing with leukocyte adherence in postcapillary venules, the experimental selection criteria for identification of an adherent leukocyte has not been standardized. Some investigators define an adherent leukocyte as a cell that is stationary for at least 1 sec, while others select either 30 sec or 1 min as the minimal stationary period for designation as adherence. We define an adherent leukocyte as one that is stationary for at least 30 sec based on the observation that the proportion (% of total) of leukocytes adherent for 1–30 sec decreases while those that are adherent for at least 30 sec increases in feline mesenteric venules exposed to either ischemia–reperfusion of PAF infusion (see Fig. 3). Furthermore, a relatively insignificant (<1%) proportion of leukocytes that are adherent in postcapillary venules for less than 30 sec will emigrate from the vessel, while approximately 20 and 60% of leukocytes adherent for at least 30 sec emigrate in response to ischemia–reperfusion and PAF infusion, respectively. Thus, it is our view that leukocytes which are adherent for at least 30 sec behave in a manner which is more consistent with an acute inflammatory response relative to leukocytes which adhere for shorter durations. Using these criteria, we observed that 1 hr of ischemia resulted in significant increases in leukocyte adherence and emigration, with reperfusion greatly enhancing these responses (Fig. 4).

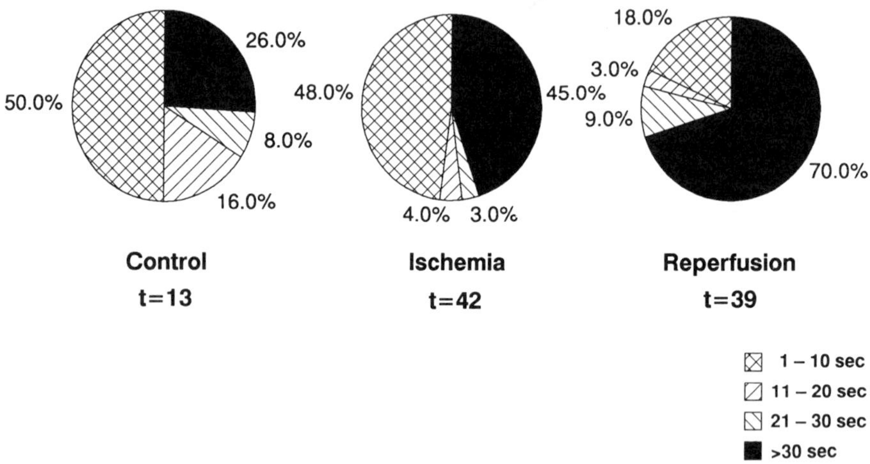

FIGURE 3

Duration of leukocyte adherence in mesenteric venules exposed to ischemia–reperfusion. t, total number of leukocytes.

To determine whether xanthine oxidase-derived oxidants play a role in the leukocyte–endothelial cell interactions initiated by ischemia–reperfusion, we examined the adherence and emigration responses to I/R in animals pretreated with either allopurinol or SOD (Fig. 4). Allopurinol treatment did not alter the responses to ischemia per se; however, it largely prevented the further increment in leukocyte adherence and emigration associated with reperfusion. SOD treatment attenuated the leukocyte adhesion responses elicited by both ischemia and reperfusion. The reductions in reperfusion-induced leukocyte emigration in SOD- and allopurinol-treated animals suggest that these treatments interfere either with the ability of leukocytes to adhere to endothelium or with their ability to move across the endothelial cell barrier, or both. However, we observed that the linear relationships between leukocyte emigration and adherence in allopurinol- and SOD-treated animals were not different from the relationships derived from untreated animals (6). This observation argues against the possibility that allopurinol and SOD interfere directly with the ability of leukocytes to emigrate from the vasculature.

In the aforementioned studies on I/R-induced, superoxide-mediated leukocyte adherence, SOD was administered prior to the induction of ischemia. To delineate whether superoxide simply initiates I/R-induced leukocyte adherence or if it contributes to the sustained leukocyte adhesion observed long after reperfusion, another series of adhesion experi-

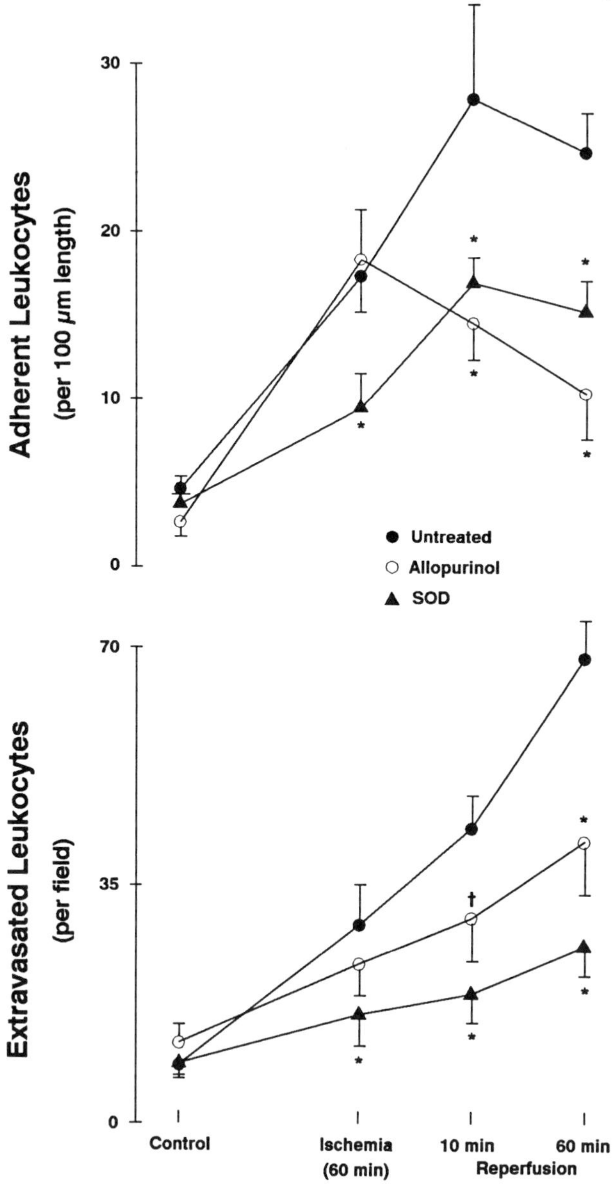

FIGURE 4

Effects of ischemia–reperfusion on adherence and emigration of leukocytes in cat mesenteric venules. *, significance from untreated group. (From Ref. 6.)

ments were performed in which SOD was administered at 1 hr after reperfusion (7). We observed that human recombinant CuZn-SOD (hSOD) reduced reperfusion-induced leukocyte adherence by 35–45% within 10 min after intravenous administration (Fig. 5). Human SOD also increases the ratio of leukocyte rolling velocity to erythrocyte velocity, indicating that the weaker adhesive interactions that mediate leukocyte rolling are also modulated by superoxide. Peroxide-inactivated hSOD did not affect either leukocyte adherence or rolling. Monoclonal antibody $1B_4$, which is directed against the common β subunit (CD18) of the leukocyte adhesion glycoprotein CD11/CD18, reduced reperfusion-induced leukocyte adherence by 75%, yet it did not alter leukocyte rolling velocity. These observations indicate that reperfusion-induced leukocyte adherence involves adhesive forces that are generated by both the interaction of superoxide with the endothelial cell and expression or activation of the leukocyte adhesion glycoprotein CD11/CD18, whereas leukocyte rolling is a superoxide-dependent, CD18-independent phenomenon.

The observation that SOD reduces leukocyte adherence in mesenteric venules raises the interesting possibility that other agents which have been used to either scavenge or prevent the production of oxygen radicals

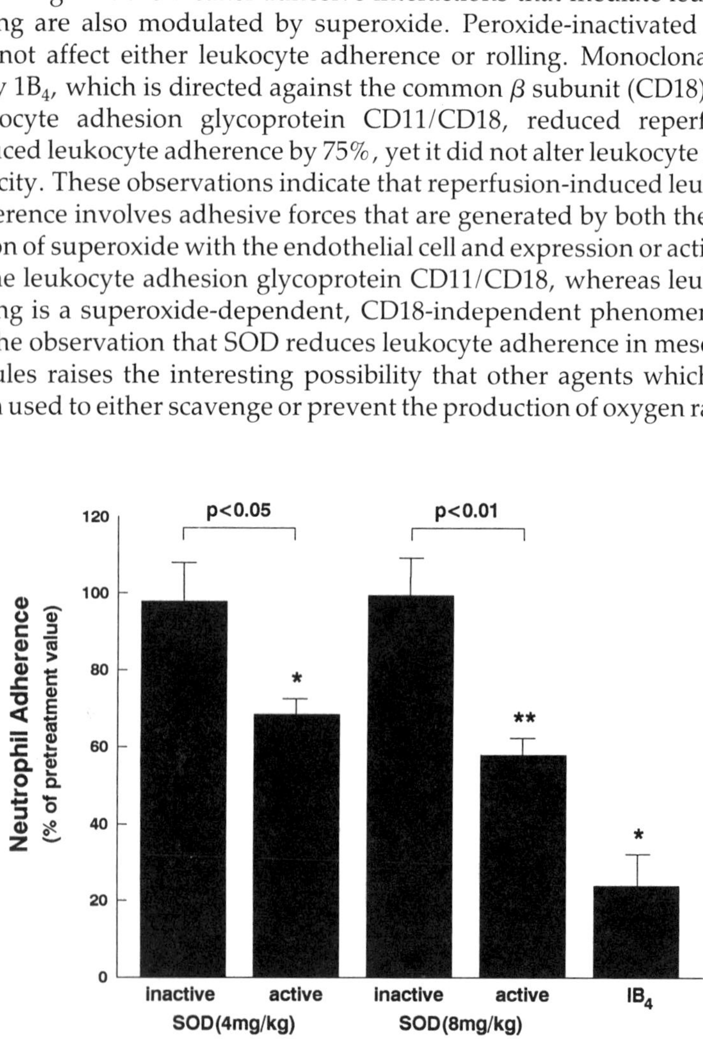

FIGURE 5

Effects of superoxide dismutase (SOD), peroxide-inactivated SOD, and anti-CD18 monoclonal antibody ($1B_4$) on reperfusion-induced neutrophil adherence to mesenteric venules. (From Ref. 7).

in postischemic tissues may also exert an influence on the adhesive interactions between leukocytes and venular endothelium. To address this possibility, we determined whether catalase, desferrioxamine, and oxypurinol alter leukocyte adhesion to microvascular endothelium when administered at concentrations that have been shown to protect against reperfusion injury (8). We observed that catalase and oxypurinol significantly attenuated leukocyte adhesion when administered 1 hr after reperfusion, while neither inactive catalase nor deferoxamine altered leukocyte adhesion (Fig. 6). These observations indicate that at least part of the protective effects previously observed with oxypurinol and catalase in models of I/R injury may be attributable to the antiadhesive actions of these drugs, while the beneficial effects of desferrioxamine cannot be ascribed to an influence on leukocyte adhesion. Our results also indicate that xanthine oxidase and H_2O_2 play an important role in mediating the leukocyte–endothelial cell adhesive interactions elicited by I/R.

Although CuZn-SOD is very efficient in catalyzing the dismutation of superoxide, the enzyme is known to exhibit low level, nonspecific peroxidase activity, a characteristic which is not shared by Mn-SOD (9).

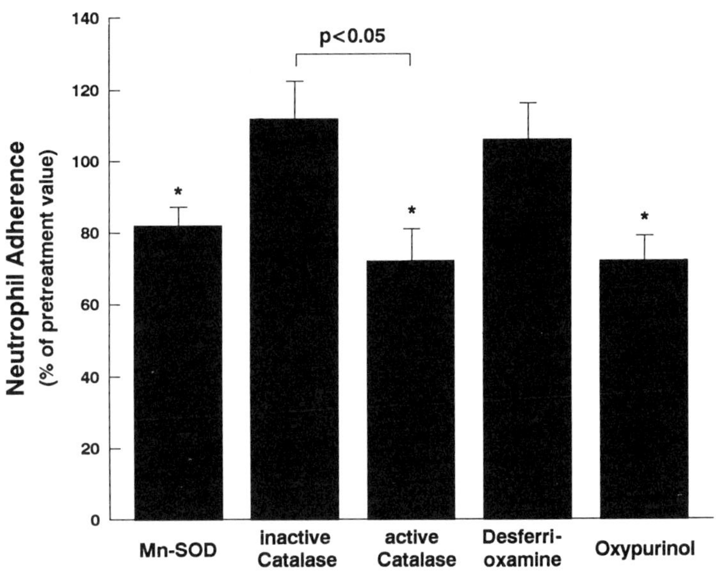

FIGURE 6

Effects of Mn-SOD, catalase, hypochlorous acid-inactivated catalase, desferrioxamine, and oxypurinol on reperfusion-induced neutrophil adherence in mesenteric venules (From Ref. 8.)

Thus, the similarity between the antiadhesive actions of CuZn-SOD and those of catalase raised the concern that CuZn-SOD attenuates leukocyte adherence as a result of its limited ability to decompose H_2O_2 rather than its ability to dismutate superoxide. To address this issue, we examined the influence of Mn-SOD on reperfusion-induced leukocyte adherence in a manner similar to that previously employed for CuZn-SOD (8). Our observation that Mn-SOD reduces leukocyte adhesion comparable to CuZn-SOD (Fig. 6) suggests that the antiadhesive actions of CuZn-SOD can be attributed to its ability to scavenge superoxide.

There are several possible explanations for the ability of SOD to reduce leukocyte adhesion in postcapillary venules. Superoxide dismutase may interfere with superoxide-induced (1) formation of inflammatory mediators, (2) expression of leukocyte and/or endothelial cell adhesion molecules, or (3) inactivation of an endothelial cell-derived antiadhesive substance. We have recently addressed the possibility that nitric oxide is an endogenous molecule that accounts for the antiadhesive actions of SOD (10). Nitric oxide (NO) is normally produced by microvascular endothelium and is rapidly inactivated by superoxide. Thus, if NO normally attenuates leukocyte adhesion to vascular endothelium, then conditions associated with enhanced formation of superoxide (e.g., ischemia–reperfusion) should lead to increased leukocyte adherence. To test this hypothesis, we examined the influence of inhibitors of nitric oxide production on leukocyte adherence in normal postcapillary venules. N^GNitro-L-arginine methyl ester (L-NAME) and N^G-monomethyl-L-arginine (L-NMMA), analogs of L-arginine that inhibit NO production, were superfused onto the surface of cat mesentery. Both inhibitors increased leukocyte adherence more than 15-fold (Fig. 7). Leukocyte emigration also increased, and the venular wall shear rate was reduced by nearly half. The CD18-specific antibody $1B_4$ abolished the leukocyte adherence induced by both analogs. Incubation of isolated feline neutrophils with L-NMMA and L-NAME did not lead to up-regulation of CD11/CD18 as assessed by flow cytometry. Only a minor component of the increased leukocyte adherence induced by NO inhibitors could be attributed to the reductions in venular shear rate. The L-NAME-induced leukocyte adherence was inhibited by L-arginine but not by D-arginine. Overall, these results indicate that NO may be an important endogenous inhibitor of leukocyte adherence in postcapillary venules and that inactivation of NO by superoxide may contribute to the increased leukocyte adherence observed in conditions associated with enhanced production of superoxide by endothelial cells and/or neutrophils.

A role for hydroxyl radicals in oxidant-mediated injury in tissues such as the intestine is often based on the observation that DMSO attenuates

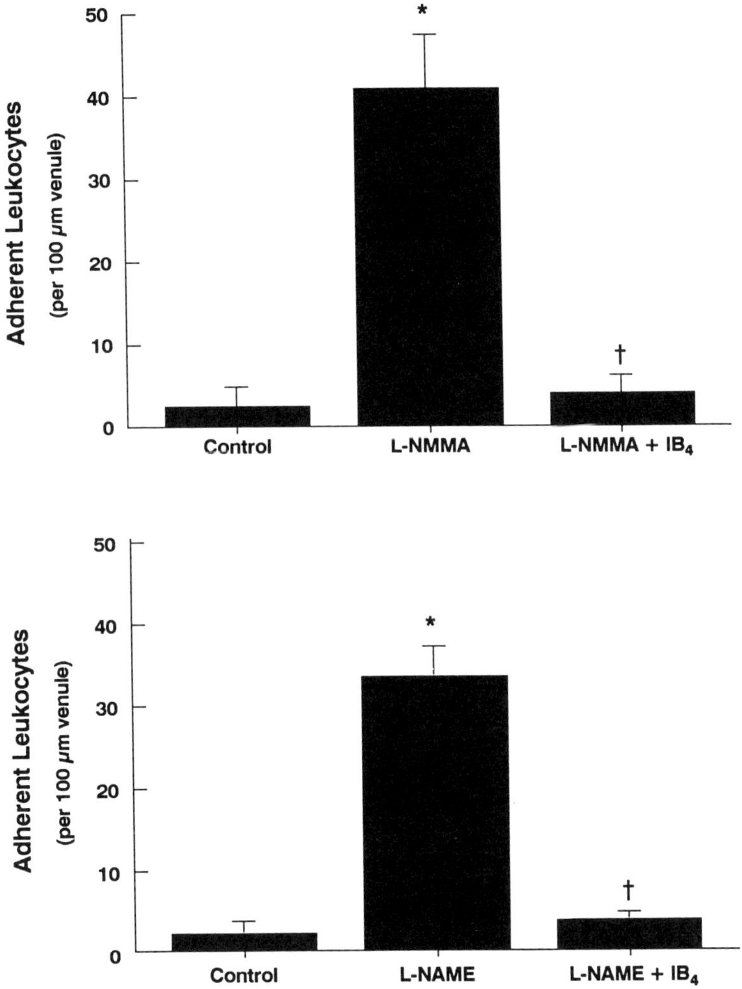

FIGURE 7

Effects of two inhibitors of nitric oxide synthesis (L-NMMA and L-NAME) on leukocyte adherence in mesenteric venules in the presence or absence of the CD18-specific monoclonal antibody ($1B_4$). *, significance from control; †, significance from L-NAME or L-NMMA alone. (From Ref. 10.)

this injury. We recently assessed whether DMSO, at concentrations used in previous studies for hydroxyl radical scavenging, prevents or attenuates leukocyte adherence to rat mesenteric venules (11). Leukocyte adherence was induced by superfusion of the mesentery with either *N*-

formylmethionylleucylphenylalanine (FMLP) or LTB_4 (both at 1 μM.) DMSO, at concentrations ranging between 2.5 and 140 mM, inhibited FMLP-induced adherence in a dose-related manner. The antiadhesive effect of DMSO was consistent with previously described reductions in neutrophil chemotaxis (Fig. 8). LTB_4-induced leukocyte adherence was also significantly attenuated by DMSO. Leukocyte rolling velocity and leukocyte flux were not affected by DMSO. These results indicate that DMSO dramatically reduces leukocyte adherence when employed at concentrations normally used for hydroxyl radical scavenging.

The antiadhesive action of catalase in mesenteric venules exposed to I/R raises the interesting possibility that neutrophil-derived hydrogen peroxide may promote adhesion either directly or indirectly via the formation of myeloperoxidase-derived oxidants such as hypochlorous acid (HOCl) and monochloramine (NH_2Cl). It has been estimated that most of the hydrogen peroxide produced by activated neutrophils is consumed by myeloperoxidase, which is released into extracellular fluid from azurophilic granules. MPO catalyzes the oxidation of chloride by hydrogen

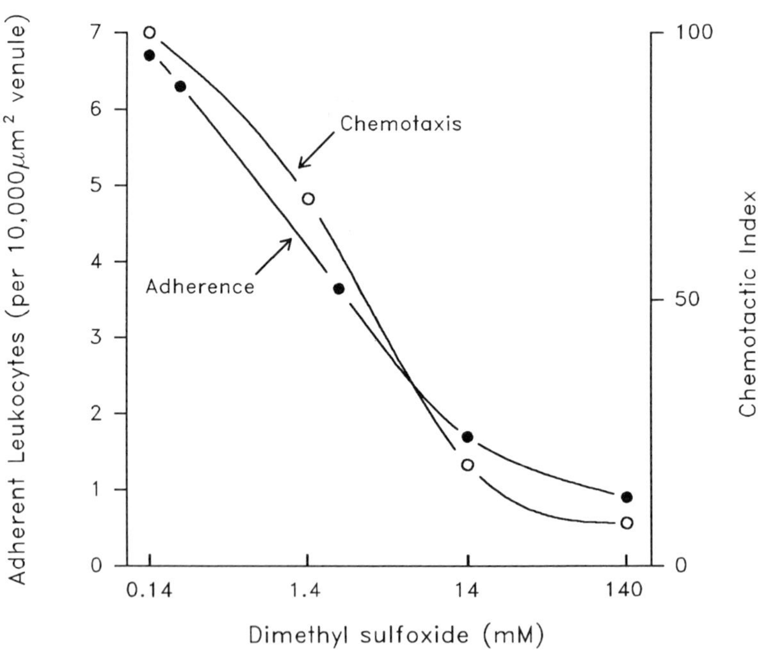

FIGURE 8

Dimethyl sulfoxide inhibits leukocyte adherence in colonic venules and zymosan-activated serum-induced neutrophil chemotaxis *in vitro*. (From Ref. 11.)

peroxide to yield HOCl, which in turn rapidly reacts with primary amines to yield *N*-chloramines, such as monochloramine and taurine monochloramine. HOCl and *N*-chloramines are highly reactive oxidants which may be more or less cytotoxic than hydrogen peroxide, depending on the lipophilicity of the compound.

To address the possible role of neutrophil-derived oxidants in modulating leukocyte adhesion we determined whether H_2O_2, HOCl, and NH_2Cl, at concentrations produced by activated neutrophils, promote leukocyte adherence to microvascular endothelium in postcapillary venules (12). The results derived from these experiments indicate that H_2O_2 and NH_2Cl, but not HOCl, promote leukocyte adhesion to venular endothelium. Incubation of isolated cat neutrophils with either NH_2Cl or H_2O_2 resulted in up-regulation of CD11/CD18, as assessed by flow cytometry. Although the leukocyte adhesion induced by both H_2O_2 and NH_2Cl was associated with a reduction in venular wall shear rate, corresponding decrements in shear rate induced by partial occlusion of the mesenteric artery did not lead to similar levels of leukocyte adherence. The leukocyte adherence induced by H_2O_2 and NH_2Cl were largely prevented by the CD18-specific monoclonal antibody $1B_4$ (Fig. 9), which indicates that both oxidants promote leukocyte adherence via up-regulation of CD11/CD18. The H_2O_2-induced leukocyte adherence was also attenuated by the PAF receptor antagonist WEB 2086. The latter observation supports the view that hydrogen peroxide stimulates the formation of PAF by vascular endothelial cells and subsequently promotes leukocyte adhesion via activation of CD11/CD18.

Although the results obtained from several of our studies implicated the leukocyte adhesion molecule CD11/CD18 in I/R-induced leukocyte adhesion in postcapillary venules, a systematic assessment of the influence of CD18-specific antibodies on I/R-induced leukocyte adhesion and emigration had not previously been undertaken. Thus, we performed an intravital microscopic and morphological assessment of the influence of pretreatment with monoclonal antibody $1B_4$ on leukocyte–endothelial cell adhesive interactions in mesenteric venules exposed to ischemia and reperfusion (13). In the same series of experiments, we also determined (1) whether neutrophils are the predominant leukocyte that adhere and emigrate in postischemic mesenteric venules and (2) whether leukocyte adherence and/or emigration is a prerequisite for reperfusion-induced increases in venular permeability. Horseradish peroxidase (HRP), administered intravenously, was used to assess vascular permeability by electron microscopy.

By light microscopy, the control (nonischemic) mesentery was sparsely populated by plasma cells, mast cells, and leukocytes; 30–50% of the resident population was neutrophils. Ischemia–reperfusion re-

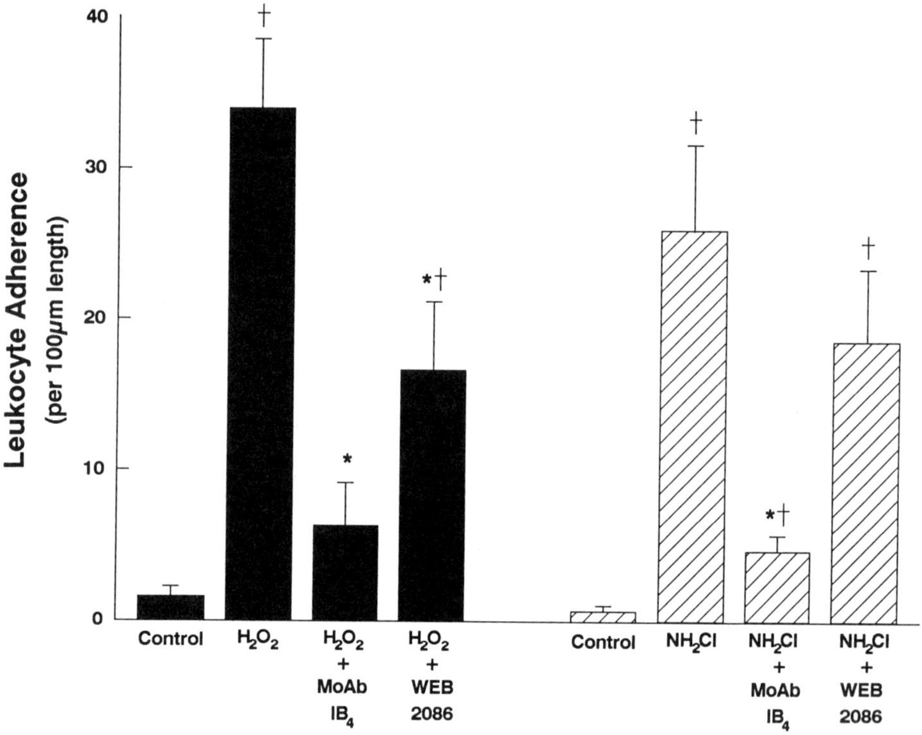

FIGURE 9

Effect of a CD18-specific antibody (MoAb $1B_4$) and a PAF-receptor antagonist on H_2O_2- and NH_2Cl-induced leukocyte adherence in mesenteric venules. Daggers denote significance relative to control; asterisks denote significance relative to oxidant alone. (From Ref. 12.)

sulted in a significant increase in the number of extravascular cells, with neutrophils accounting for over 80% of the total cell population. Control and ischemic venules demonstrated no leakage of HRP into the interstitium. However, venules exposed to ischemia and reperfusion demonstrated HRP leakage between endothelial cells and into the surrounding interstitium. In venules exposed to I/R, neutrophils were adherent to the luminal surface of the endothelium, were transmigrating the vessel wall, and were present in the surrounding interstitium. In animals pretreated with monoclonal antibody $1B_4$ the increases in leukocyte adherence and emigration normally observed (by intravital microscopy) during ischemia and reperfusion were largely abolished (Fig. 10). In addition, a lower

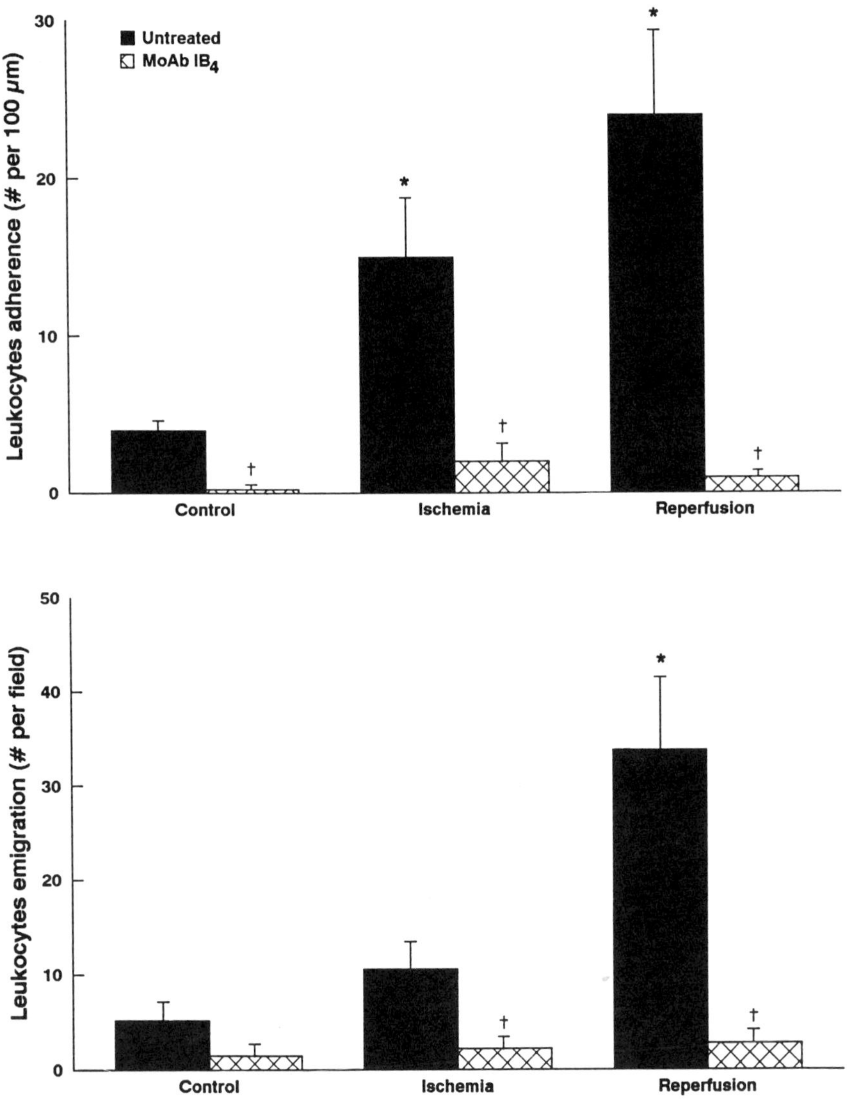

FIGURE 10

Intravital microscopic assessment of leukocyte adherence (top) and emigration (bottom) in mesenteric venules exposed to ischemia–reperfusion. *, significance from control (untreated); †, significance relative to corresponding value in untreated group. (From Ref. 13.)

level of HRP leakage was noted following reperfusion in venules treated with $1B_4$, when compared to control. The results of this study indicate that (1) neutrophils are the predominate leukocytes that adhere and emigrate in postischemic venules and (2) CD11/CD18 expression or activation is a requirement for I/R-induced neutrophil adherence and emigration.

Although allopurinol has been widely used to probe for the role of xanthine oxidase in various models of I/R-induced tissue injury, there are reports which suggest that the drug may act by directly scavenging free radicals rather than inhibiting xanthine oxidase. Thus, we undertook a series of experiments to determine whether the regimen of allopurinol administration used in most studies of I/R injury results in a significant modification of the free radical scavenging properties of extracellular fluid (14). Extracellular fluid (ECF) from allopurinol-treated animals contained approximately 10 μM each of allopurinol and oxypurinol. Although ECF from allopurinol-treated animals resulted in 80% inhibition of xanthine oxidase activity, it did not exhibit a greater potential to scavenge either HOCl or hemoprotein-derived oxidants. In view of the tremendous antioxidant potential of normal ECF, it seems unlikely that the presence of small quantities of either allopurinol or oxypurinol would enhance the free radical scavenging properties of plasma and lymph.

III. Endothelial Cell Monolayer Dysfunction Induced by Anoxia–Reoxygenation

Although the results of a number of *in vivo* studies indicate that microvascular endothelium is very vulnerable to ischemia–reperfusion injury, it is difficult to appreciate the exact nature of the endothelial cell alterations induced by I/R based on data derived from whole organ studies. Thus, we have developed an *in vitro* model to mimic I/R-induced microvascular injury in which cultured endothelial cells are exposed to anoxia followed by reoxygenation (15). In our initial study, cultured venular endothelial cells were grown to confluency, labeled with ^{51}Cr, and exposed to different durations of anoxia (0.5–4 hr). ^{51}Cr release and cell detachment were used to assess endothelial cell dysfunction at different times after reoxygenation (1–18 hr). In some experiments, human neutrophils were added to the endothelial cells on reoxygenation.

When endothelial cell monolayers were exposed to periods of anoxia of at least 2 hr, 70–80% ^{51}Cr release and 80–95% cell detachment were noted following reoxygenation, with the addition of neutrophils causing negligible enhancement of injury. Shorter periods of anoxia ($\leq$ 1 hr) resulted in 30–40% ^{51}Cr release and 50–60% cell detachment, and the addition of neutrophils greatly enhanced the anoxia–reoxygenation (A/R)-induced endothelial cell dysfunction. The activity of neutrophilic elastase in the medium bathing the endothelial cell monolayers was significantly elevated when neutrophils were added to monolayers exposed to A/R, as compared to normoxic monolayers. Using a 30-min period of anoxia, we demonstrated that either SOD or allopurinol significantly attenuated A/R-induced injury in the presence, but not in the absence, of neutrophils. The results of this study indicate that reoxygenation of anoxic endothelial cell monolayers results in cell injury, the degree of which is related to the duration of anoxia. The addition of neutrophils after reoxygenation exacerbates A/R-induced injury, indicating that neutrophils become activated by some factor(s) released by endothelial cells. The activated neutrophils then injure the monolayer via the release of proteases (elastase) and/or reactive oxygen metabolites.

The possibility that elastase may be responsible for A/R-induced, neutrophil-mediated injury to cultured microvascular endothelial cells was addressed in another study (16). In this series of experiments, four agents were used to inhibit neutrophilic elastase activity: Eglin C, methoxysuccinyl-Ala$_2$-Pro-Val-CH$_2$Cl (MAAPV), L658,758, and a monoclonal antibody against neutrophilic elastase. We observed that all of the elastase inhibitors attenuated the A/R-induced, neutrophil-mediated endothelial cell detachment but not ^{51}Cr release. When purified neutrophilic elastase was added to normal endothelial cell monolayers to mimic the levels released from neutrophils in our A/R model, no alteration in ^{51}Cr release and cell detachment were observed. However, addition of elastase to endothelial cell monolayers exposed to A/R (in the absence of neutrophils) produced a dose-dependent increase in cell detachment but did not affect ^{51}Cr release. These observations indicate that elastase is an important mediator of the nonlytic endothelial cell injury induced by neutrophils in our model of A/R. Furthermore, our results indicate that endothelial cell monolayers exposed to anoxia–reoxygenation are more susceptible to elastase-mediated cell detachment.

Because neutrophil adhesion is an important feature of our model of A/R-induced endothelial cell dysfunction, we have recently undertaken a series of experiments to determine the contributions of both neutrophil and endothelial cell adhesion molecules to the hyperadhesivity of neutrophils induced by A/R (17). Human umbilical vein endothelial cells (HUVEC) were subjected to 30 min of anoxia followed by 30 min of reoxygenation and then exposed to ^{51}Cr-labeled neutrophils. Anoxia–

TABLE I

Contribution of Adhesion Glycoproteins to Anoxia–Reoxygenation-Induced Neutrophil Adherence to Endothelial Cell Monolayers[a]

Condition	Adherence (%)
Normoxia	9.6 ± 1.0
Anoxia–reoxygenation	25.1 ± 0.9
Plus CD18 MAb	8.0 ± 0.7
Plus CD11a MAb	14.6 ± 1.2
Plus CD11b MAb	14.2 ± 1.2
Plus CD11a and CD11b MAbs	10.0 ± 1.0
Plus ICAM-1 MAb	13.9 ± 1.1
Plus ELAM-1 MAb	23.0 ± 2.7

[a] From Ref. 17.

reoxygenation resulted in a 2.7-fold increase in neutrophil adherence to HUVEC when compared to normoxic HUVEC (Table I). The A/R-induced increase in neutrophil adherence was significantly attenuated by monoclonal antibodies (MAb) directed against the leukocyte adhesion glycoproteins CD11a, CD11b, and CD18. The effects of the CD11a- and CD11b-specific antibodies were additive and equivalent to that observed with a CD18-specific antibody. Although immunoneutralization of ELAM-1 on HUVEC did not modify A/R-induced neutrophil adherence, ICAM-1-specific antibodies reduced adherence to a level observed with CD11a and CD11b antibodies. A/R did not elicit increased levels if ICAM-1 or ELAM-1 mRNA or surface protein. However, incubation of neutrophils in supernatants of A/R-conditioned HUVEC elicited increases in neutrophil adherence and surface expression of CD18. The neutrophil adherence elicited by A/R-conditioned medium was significantly reduced by treatment with either catalase or a PAF receptor antagonist, which, in turn, promotes CD11/CD18 activation/expression on neutrophils. The adhesive interactions between CD11a/CD18 and CD11b/CD18 on neutrophils with ICAM-1 on endothelial cells ultimately results in firm attachment of neutrophils to the monolayer.

Alterations in microvascular permeability have frequently been used to assess the endothelial cell dysfunction caused by reperfusion of ischemic tissues (1,2). To determine whether these observations can be mimicked using monolayers of cultured endothelial cells, we monitored albumin permeability across endothelialized filters exposed to successive periods (30 min) of normoxia ($pO_2$145 mmHg), hypoxia ($pO_2$20 mmHg),

TABLE II

Effect of Hypoxia–Reoxygenation on Endothelial Cell Monolayer Permeability to Albumin[a]

Condition	Albumin permeability (× control)
Hypoxia	1.5 ± 0.2
Reoxygenation	2.3 ± 0.5[b]
Reoxygenation plus superoxide dismutase	1.2 ± 0.1[c]
Reoxygenation plus allopurinol	1.3 ± 0.1[c]

[a] From Ref. 18.
[b] Relative to hypoxia.
[c] Relative to reoxygenation alone.

and reoxygenation ($pO_2$145 mmHg). When compared to the control normoxic period, albumin permeability was 1.5 times higher during hypoxia and 2.3 times higher during reoxygenation (Table II) (18). The increased monolayer permeability associated with reoxygenation, but not hypoxia, was largely prevented by pretreatment with either oxypurinol or superoxide dismutase (18). The results obtained from this *in vitro* model of reperfusion injury indicate that the altered endothelial barrier function induced by hypoxia–reoxygenation is mediated by xanthine oxidase-derived oxygen radicals.

IV. Inflammatory Mediators and Ischemia–Reperfusion

Since our work indicates that adherence and emigration of leukocytes in postcapillary venules increases dramatically following ischemia/reperfusion, we began to explore the possible mechanisms that lead to leukocyte activation and adhesion in postischemic microvessels. As previously discussed, pretreatment of animals with either allopurinol or superoxide dismutase significantly attenuated the leukocyte adherence and emigration that is observed at the time of reperfusion. Although these studies would implicate xanthine oxidase-derived oxidants in reperfusion-induced leukocyte recruitment, it appears unlikely that reactive oxygen metabolites directly mediate leukocyte infiltration and adherence. It is, however, conceivable that exposure of cells to oxidants can activate phospholipase A_2, an event known to cause significant alterations in arachidonic acid metabolism leading to the formation of potent leukocyte chemoattractants and activators including platelet-activating factor and leukotriene B_4. Indeed, we provide evidence above which indicates that hydrogen peroxide may stimulate the synthesis of PAF by cultured endothelial cells exposed to anoxia–reoxygenation and that PAF subsequently promotes neutrophil adherence to endothelial cell monolayers. Therefore, we initially focused our attention on the potential role of platelet-activating factor as a mediator of the leukocyte–endothelial cell interactions elicited by reperfusion of ischemic mesenteric venules.

Our first objective was to determine whether the production of platelet-activating factor was increased following ischemia–reperfusion. Using the platelet aggregation bioassay, an approximate 6-fold increase in PAF activity was observed following 1 hr of ischemia and 1 hr of reperfusion in feline intestinal mucosa (19). Intravital microscopic techniques were then used to determine whether the increased PAF activity was responsible for the elevated leukocyte adhesion observed in postischemic vessels. Leukocyte rolling velocity and the rates of leukocyte adhesion (R_{LA}) and emigration (R_{LE}) were monitored in untreated animals and in animals pretreated with a PAF receptor antagonist (WEB 2086). Figure 11 illustrates that the rate of leukocyte adhesion increased approximately 5-fold following reperfusion and that WEB 2086 reduced the rate of leukocyte adhesion by 35–40%. The rate of leukocyte emigration, which was undetectable under control conditions, increased to approximately one leukocyte leaving the circulation every 2 min following reperfusion. The PAF receptor antagonist reduced R_{LE} by almost 90% during reperfusion. The ratio R_{LE}/R_{LA}, which represents the proportion of adherent leukocytes that ultimately emigrate from the vasculature, was greatly reduced by WEB 2086, which indicates that PAF plays a more important role in promoting leukocyte emigration than adherence in postcapillary venules exposed to ischemia–reperfusion.

The signal that activates PAF production in the intestine following ischemia–reperfusion remains unclear. However, studies from our laboratory suggest that H_2O_2 is a likely candidate since this oxidant promotes leukocyte adhesion in postcapillary venules and H_2O_2-induced adhesion can be attenuated by the PAF receptor antagonist WEB 2086 (12). This possibility is further supported by *in vitro* studies which demonstrate that H_2O_2 can stimulate cultured endothelial cells to produce PAF and consequently promote an adhesive interaction between leukocytes and endothelial cell monolayers which is reduced by PAF receptor antagonists (20).

Another phospholipase A_2 metabolite that has been studied extensively in the postischemic intestine is leukotriene B_4. It is well known that the intestinal mucosa is adept at metabolizing arachidonic acid to a variety of lipoxygenase products including the potent chemoattractant LTB_4, which is frequently implicated as a mediator of reperfusion-induced neutrophil infiltration. Although it is conceivable that oxidants may promote LTB_4 synthesis and release thereby causing PMN adhesion in the vasculature, a direct link between oxidants and enhanced LTB_4 production following reperfusion of the ischemic bowel has not been demonstrated. Several groups including our own have demonstrated a significant increase in LTB_4 production in mucosa subjected to ischemia–reperfusion (21). However, the question remained whether LTB_4 accumulation in the intestinal mucosa was a cause or a consequence of reperfusion-induced granulocyte infiltration. In a recent study (22), we reported that animals pretreated with either a lipoxygenase inhibitor (L663,536) or an LTB_4 antagonist (SC-41930) exhibited an attenuation in the magnitude of reperfusion-induced granulocyte infiltration, providing the first direct evidence that LTB_4 is an important signal for granulocyte recruitment. Because myeloperoxidase activity was measured in this study rather than leukocyte adhesion and emigration, it remains unclear whether LTB_4 contributes to the process of leukocyte adhesion, emigration, or both.

Although both PAF and LTB_4 receptor antagonists prevent reperfusion-induced PMN accumulation in the small bowel, the role of each inflammatory mediator in this process remains unresolved. We have recently directed our research toward understanding the specific role of these mediators in inflamed vessels. Much evidence would suggest that LTB_4 is an important chemotactic agent both *in vitro* and *in vivo*. Superfusion of the rat mesentery with LTB_4 has been reported to produce PMN adhesion and emigration (23). Figure 12 demonstrates that local intraarterial infusion of LTB_4 into the small bowel causes leukocyte adhesion in postcapillary venules but does not promote leukocyte emigration (24). These data suggest that leukocytes emigrate out of the vasculature if the LTB_4 concentration is greater in interstitium than plasma. This view is supported by *in vitro* studies (25) which demonstrate that PMNs will cross a membrane only if the concentration of LTB_4 is greater on the opposing side. If no chemotactic gradient is present (i.e., similar amounts of LTB_4 are present on the two sides of the membrane), then neutrophils would not emigrate. Thus, if LTB_4 contributes to the leukocyte emigration observed in postischemic mesenteric venules, then the inflammatory mediator must be produced by cells situated outside of the vasculature.

Platelet-activating factor has been reported to be a poor chemotactic agent *in vivo*. This is consistent with our previously mentioned observation that PAF receptor antagonists have only a limited effect on isch-

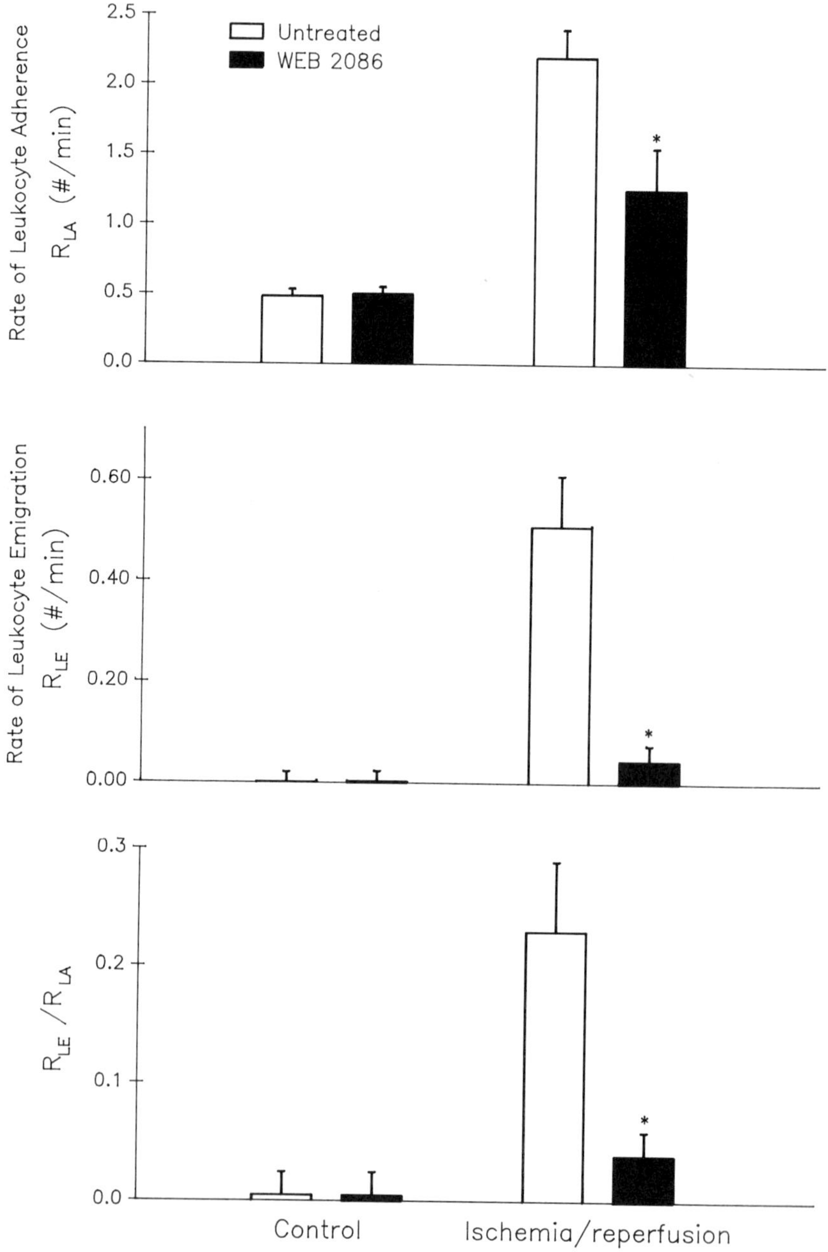
Untreated
WEB 2086
Rate of Leukocyte Adherence
R_{LA} (#/min)
2.5
2.0
1.5
1.0
0.5
0.0
*
Rate of Leukocyte Emigration
R_{LE} (#/min)
0.60
0.40
0.20
0.00
*
R_{LE} / R_{LA}
0.3
0.2
0.1
0.0
*
Control
Ischemia/reperfusion

emia–reperfusion-induced leukocyte adherence (30–40% reduction) to postischemic vessels. Nonetheless, the PAF receptor antagonist WEB 2086 exerts a profound effect on reperfusion-induced leukocyte emigration (90% attenuation). Unlike LTB_4, both superfusion (24) and local intraarterial infusion of PAF (Fig. 12) causes a large fraction (>60%) of adherent leukocytes to emigrate out of the vasculature (23,24). These data suggest that PAF may contribute more to reperfusion-induced leukocyte emigration than does LTB_4.

Another observation of interest is that intraarterial infusion of PAF, but not LTB_4, causes a large increase in microvascular protein and fluid leakage (Fig. 12). These data would suggest that leukocyte adhesion per se does not always result in microvascular dysfunction. Clearly, leukocyte adhesion may not be the most critical step in the microvascular dysfunction associated with acute inflammation. Indeed, microvascular dysfunction appeared to be more closely related to leukocyte emigration than leukocyte adherence. This contention is based on the observations that infusion of a proinflammatory agent which promotes leukocyte emigration (PAF) leads to microvascular dysfunction while infusion of an agent that only promotes leukocyte adhesion (LTB_4) does not. Further support for the view that leukocyte emigration and vascular protein leakage were closely correlated comes from the observations that superfusion of the mesentery with LTB_4 promotes both leukocyte emigration and microvascular dysfunction (22,26). Whether leukocyte emigration per se leads to enhanced microvascular protein and fluid leakage or whether a leaky vasculature is required for leukocyte emigration remains a source of controversy. Resolution of this issue will largely depend on the discovery of agents that specifically inhibit leukocyte emigration without altering leukocyte adhesion, superoxide production, and degranulation or endothelial cell function.

The mechanism by which leukocytes adhere to and emigrate from the vasculature and induce microvascular dysfunction under different inflammatory conditions remains unclear. Several *in vitro* studies indicate that adherent leukocytes are capable of degrading various structural

FIGURE 11

Average rate of leukocyte adherence (R_{LA}), rate of leukocyte emigration (R_{LE}), and the proportion of adherent leukocytes that ultimately emigrate (R_{LE}/R_{LA}) in mesenteric venules prior to and during the reperfusion period in untreated animals and animals that received the PAF receptor antagonist WEB 2086. Asterisks denote significance ($p < 0.05$) relative to corresponding untreated value. (From Ref. 19.)

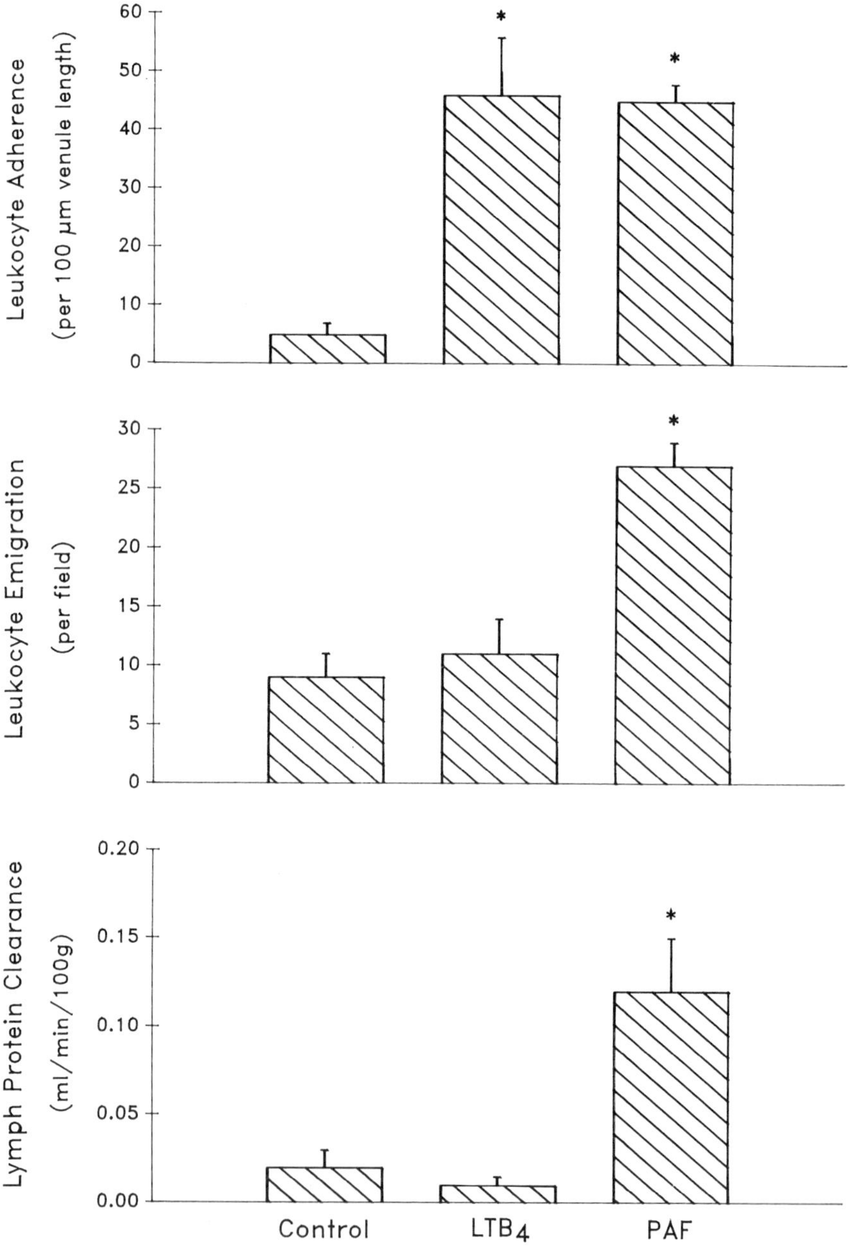

FIGURE 12

Leukocyte adherence, leukocyte emigration, and lymph protein clearance prior to and following either LTB_4 or PAF infusion. Asterisks denote significance ($p < 0.05$) relative to control value. (From Ref. 24).

components of the vascular basement membrane. It has also been demonstrated that neutrophil-mediated degradation of endothelial basement membrane can be prevented by inhibitors of neutrophilic elastase. These observations have led to the proposal that limited release of elastase is a prerequisite for the neutrophil emigration associated with acute and chronic forms of inflammation.

Recently, two structurally dissimilar elastase inhibitors, Eglin C and L658,758, were used to determine whether elastase plays a role in the leukocyte infiltration elicited by ischemia–reperfusion (27). The data suggest that the reperfusion-induced increase in mucosal myeloperoxidase activity is significantly attenuated in animals pretreated with either Eglin C (which inhibits both elastase and cathepsin G) or L658,758 (a specific elastase inhibitor). These results suggest that reperfusion-induced neutrophil infiltration into the intestinal mucosa is facilitated by limited release of elastase from activated phagocytes. Intravital microscopy was used to determine the rates of leukocyte adherence (R_{LA}) and leukocyte emigration (R_{LE}) in mesenteric venules exposed to ischemia–reperfusion. Figure 13 illustrates that L658,758 reduced by 90% the number of leukocytes that emigrated out of the vasculature. More importantly, this occurred independently of leukocyte adhesion inasmuch as the proportion of adherent leukocytes that eventually emigrated from postcapillary venules after reperfusion was reduced by approximately 75%. These data suggest that elastase is essential for activated leukocytes to migrate into the interstitium from microvessels exposed to ischemia–reperfusion.

While much emphasis has been given to the identification of inflammatory mediators (PAF, LTB_4) in I/R-induced PMN adhesion and emigration, there is some evidence to suggest that endogenous antiadhesion molecules (e.g., adenosine) may also accumulate during ischemia and following reperfusion. With this observation in mind, we set out to determine whether exogenous adenosine alters the granulocyte adherence and emigration in mesenteric venules exposed to I/R (28). Exogenous adenosine attenuated reperfusion-induced leukocyte adherence to venular endothelium by approximately 35%. Particularly impressive was the profound reduction (»70%) in leukocyte emigration induced by adenosine. This ability of adenosine to reduce leukocyte adhesion and emigration may explain why the purine is as effective as CD18-specific monoclonal antibodies or antineutrophil serum in protecting the intestinal vasculature from reperfusion injury. It remains to be established whether the effects of adenosine on PMN emigration results from cytoskeletal alterations in the PMN and/or endothelial cell or from an effect on neutrophil activation and degranulation. In support of the latter possibility is

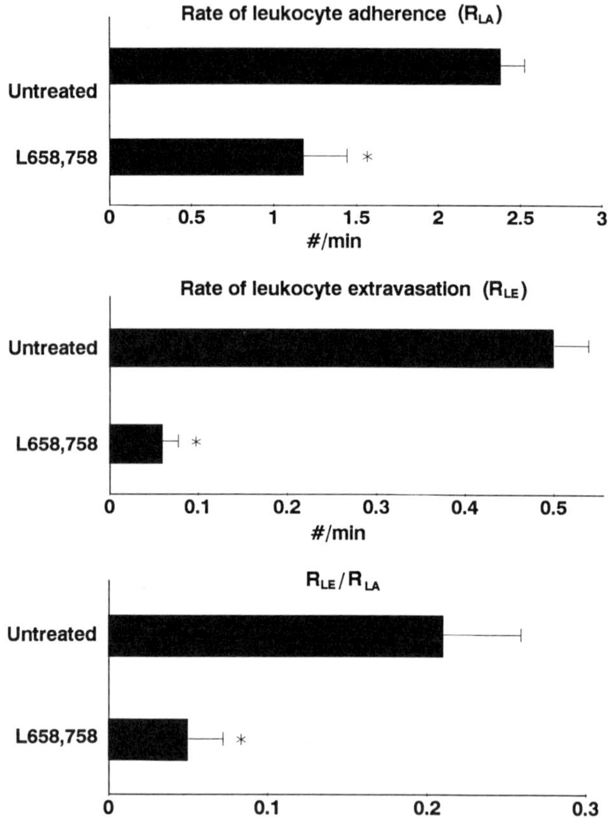

FIGURE 13

Average rate of leukocyte adherence (R_{LA}), rate of leukocyte emigration (R_{LE}) and the proportion of adherent leukocytes that ultimately emigrate (R_{LE}/R_{LA}) in mesenteric venules during the reperfusion period in untreated animals and animals that received the elastase inhibitor L658,758. Asterisks denote significance ($p < 0.05$) relative to corresponding untreated value. (From Ref. 27.)

the work by Cronstein and co-workers, who reported that adenosine and derivatives of adenosine inhibit production of superoxide and hydrogen peroxide by human granulocytes (29). Although adenosine does indeed accumulate in ischemic tissues, the increase in purine concentration is clearly insufficient to prevent the reperfusion-induced leukocyte adhesion and tissue injury. Nonetheless, agents which enhance the production of adenosine (e.g., methotrexate) may be beneficial in the treatment of PMN-mediated vascular injury.

V. Neutrophil-Mediated Injury

The neutrophil-mediated injury associated with ischemia–reperfusion of the small bowel is a major focal point of our research program. There is now a large body of evidence which suggests that leukocytes mediate the microvascular injury that occurs at the time of reperfusion of the small intestine. In 1986, we initially observed that myeloperoxidase-positive cells accumulate in the mucosa of postischemic intestine (3). An important question which arose from that study was whether neutrophils were a cause or an effect of I/R injury in the small bowel. Two approaches were used to test whether neutrophils mediate the I/R-induced microvascular dysfunction, namely, neutrophil depletion with polyclonal antiserum and prevention of neutrophil adherence with a monoclonal antibody (MAb 60.3) directed against a specific membrane-associated glycoprotein that modulates neutrophil adherence to endothelium (30). Intestinal microvascular permeability to plasma proteins was measured in control preparations, in preparations subjected to 1 hr ischemia and 1 hr reperfusion, and in two experimental groups that received either antineutrophil serum or MAb 60.3 (Table III). The data indicate that either depletion of circulating leukocytes or inhibition of PMN adherence to postcapillary venules significantly attenuates the increased microvascular permeability induced by I/R. These findings support the hypothesis that circulating neutrophils mediate the injury produced by reperfusion of the ischemic bowel. Moreover, the observation that neutrophil depletion and preven-

TABLE III

Role of Neutrophils in Ischemia–Reperfusion-Induced Increase in Microvascular Permeability[a]

Condition	Microvascular permeability
Control	0.08 ± 0.005
Ischemia	0.15 ± 0.03[b]
Ischemia–reperfusion	0.41 ± 0.02[b]
Plus antineutrophil serum	0.13 ± 0.01[c]
Plus monoclonal antibody 60.3	0.12 ± 0.01[c]
Plus monoclonal antibody $1B_4$	0.17 ± 0.04[c]

[a] From Refs. 2 and 30.
[b] $p < 0.05$ relative to control.
[c] $p < 0.05$ relative ischemia–reperfusion alone.

tion of neutrophil adherence are equally effective in attenuating the microvascular injury suggests that neutrophil adherence or a neutrophil adherence-dependent event (e.g., emigration) is a rate-limiting step in neutrophil-mediated microvascular injury.

In addition to the microvascular dysfunction that is observed in the intestine following reperfusion, it is likely that the mucosa and the mucosal barrier may be impaired following ischemia-reperfusion. Mucosal injury in the postischemic bowel has been assessed either morphologically or by measuring the permeability of the mucosal barrier to small solutes such as ^{51}Cr-labeled EDTA. Morphological studies have demonstrated that intestinal ischemia is typically associated with subepithelial edema after relatively short periods of ischemia, lifting of the epithelium from the villus basement membrane, and loss of villi as the duration and severity of the ischemic episode increase. We have shown that intestinal ischemia (3 hr, blood flow at 20% of control) followed by reperfusion results in a decrease in villus height and crypt depth as well as a reduction in mucosal thickness, with epithelial lifting down the sides of the villi and disruption of the lamina propria. These morphological alterations are accompanied by a dramatic increase in mucosal permeability to ^{51}Cr-EDTA following reperfusion of the ischemic intestine (31). Thus, it appears that the I/R-induced mucosal barrier dysfunction predicted by our ^{51}Cr-EDTA measurements is likely a result of damage to the epithelial barrier.

Associated with reperfusion-induced mucosal dysfunction is an increase in mucosal myeloperoxidase activity from 12 to 25 units/g wet weight, suggesting an influx of approximately 10–15 million myeloperoxidase-positive cells. To determine whether circulating leukocytes contribute to the mucosal dysfunction caused by 3 hr of ischemia followed by 1 hr of reperfusion, some animals received a monoclonal antibody (MAb 1B_4) directed against the common β subunit (CD18) of the leukocyte adhesion glycoprotein complex (CD11/CD18). This intervention did not prevent the increase in ^{51}Cr-EDTA clearance during ischemia or following reperfusion despite complete prevention of leukocyte infiltration into the postischemic mucosa, suggesting that the infiltrating leukocytes do not mediate the mucosal dysfunction associated with I/R. It should be noted that the baseline mucosal myeloperoxidase activity is approximately 10–15 units/g wet weight, which indicates that there is a significant resident population of myeloperoxidase cells within the mucosa. We have previously demonstrated that repeated injections of MAb 1B_4 over a 48-hr period reduces mucosal myeloperoxidase activity to less than 10% of baseline. This chronic regimen of MAb 1B_4 administration dramatically reduces the increased mucosal permeability induced by I/R. These observations indicate that the resident population of PMNs play a more important role in mediating reperfusion-induced increases in mucosal permeability than newly recruited leukocytes. Although an explanation for the different contributions of resident versus newly recruited granulocytes to I/R-induced mucosal dysfunction is not readily available, one possibility is that the resident population of granulocytes are situated in closer proximity to mucosal epithelium and thus are capable of inflicting greater damage to the mucosal barrier than newly recruited granulocytes.

Although the barrier function of the mucosa is clearly compromised in response to I/R, it remained unclear whether this was associated with a significant reduction in mucosal function. An important role of the small intestine is to absorb nutrients (e.g., monosaccharides, lipids) from the bowel lumen. Intestinal lipid absorption involves a number of complex processes, and so may be highly vulnerable to I/R. In a series of experiments, we examined the influence of I/R on the uptake and transport of lipids in rat intestine and then assessed the role of neutrophils in the functional impairment induced by I/R (32). In these studies a lipid test meal was infused into the bowel at either 24 or 48 hr following a 10-min occlusion of the superior mesenteric artery. Intestinal absorption and transport of lipid into lymph was markedly suppressed in response to I/R, but only at 24 hr (i.e., mucosal function returned to normal at 48 hr). This indicates that the small intestine is capable of fully recovering from the functional impairment caused by I/R within 48 hr. The impaired lipid absorption and transport into lymph at 24 hr was associated with significantly more fatty acid transported by portal blood of the animals exposed to 10 min of ischemia. Normally, fatty acids are incorporated into chylomicrons within epithelial cells and then transported into the bloodstream via the lymphatic system. In animals exposed to I/R, reesterification of absorbed monoglycerides and fatty acids to form triglycerides was unaffected, suggesting that the increased fatty acid concentration in portal blood might be a reflection of a leaky intestinal mucosa in response to I/R rather than an inability of the mucosa to produce chylomicrons. If indeed I/R creates a leaky mucosal barrier, then lipids might gain access to the interstitium and portal blood by circumventing the interior of epithelial cells. This conclusion is consistent with the increased mucosal permeability ^{51}Cr-EDTA during I/R previously described.

Another objective of the aforementioned study was to determine whether neutrophils play a role in the I/R-induced decrement in lipid absorption (32). Therefore, the same protocol was used as described above, but some animals were rendered neutropenic with antineutrophil serum (ANS). Rats were given repeated injections of antiserum over a 36-hr interval prior to the experiment. This regimen depleted circulating

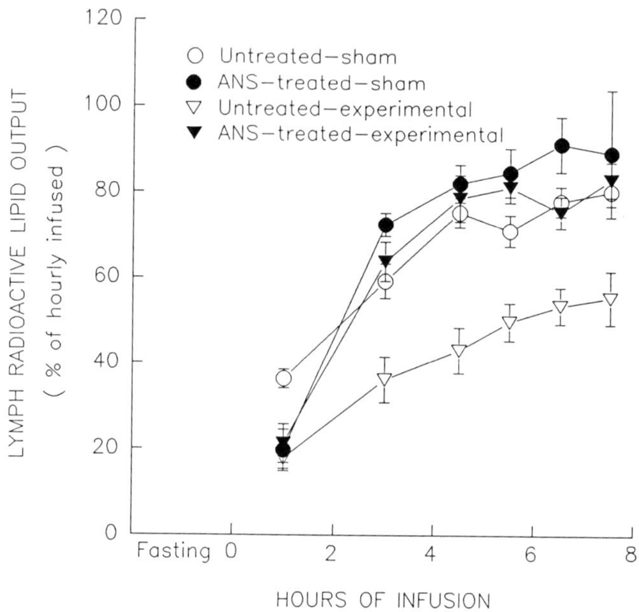

FIGURE 14

Effects of antineutrophil serum (ANS) on the decrement in intestinal lipid absorption induced by ischemia–reperfusion (From Ref. 32.)

as well as mucosal levels of leukocytes to less than 5% of control. Figure 14 demonstrates that the animals pretreated with ANS did not exhibit the reduction in lipid absorption and transport in lymph normally observed 24 hr after I/R. These results indicate that neutrophils mediate the impairment in lipid absorption and lymphatic lipid transport observed following I/R. Additionally, it was also observed that the increased portal blood transport of fatty acids following I/R was prevented in neutropenic animals. If the increased portal transport of lipids is due to compromised epithelial cell junctions as previously suggested, then one explanation for the ANS results is that depletion of neutrophils prevents the migration of these phagocytic cells through epithelial intercellular junctions and thereby prevents disruption of the mucosal barrier. Although the results of this study implicate neutrophils in the mucosal dysfunction induced by I/R, the mechanism by which PMNs impair the transport of lipid in intestinal lymph remains unclear. A likely possibility is that activation of leukocytes by proinflammatory agents released at the time of reperfusion cause the release of reactive oxygen metabolites and proteases which may injure the absorptive enterocyte and thereby limit the ability of the cell to produce and release chylomicrons.

VI. Other Models of Intestinal Inflammation

In recent years, we have used a number of models in addition to ischemia–reperfusion to assess the influence of acute inflammation on the integrity and function of the gastrointestinal mucosa. Platelet-activating factor has been implicated in the pathogenesis of intestinal injury associated with endotoxemia, inflammatory and immune reactions, and ischemia–reperfusion. Evidence supporting its role as a proinflammatory mediator is based on observations that PAF levels rise in affected tissues and that mucosal injury is attenuated by PAF receptor antagonists. It is therefore conceivable that intraarterial infusion of PAF into the superior mesenteric artery will induce intestinal dysfunction. We therefore examined the influence of local intraarterial infusions of PAF (4, 20, and 40 ng/min) on intestinal transcapillary, lymphatic, and transmucosal water and protein fluxes (33). PAF caused a significant rise in venous hematocrit without a corresponding increase in venous plasma protein concentration and a 14- to 37-fold increase in vascular protein flux. These data are consistent with a large increase in microvascular permeability to macromolecules. In addition, net secretory fluid flux into the lumen of the bowel was induced in a dose-dependent manner. The secreted fluid contained significant quantities of plasma proteins but no red blood cells. The results, coupled to previous reports that PAF leads to disruption of the mucosal membrane, suggest that filtration of interstitial fluid into the lumen (characterized by high lymph flow, protein in secreted fluid, and mucosal injury) is responsible for at least part of the PAF-induced fluid secretion.

There are several possible mechanisms by which PAF could lead to an increased rate of capillary fluid filtration, vascular protein leakage, and mucosal dysfunction. The hypotensive and splanchnic vasoconstrictor actions of PAF have led to speculations that the vascular and mucosal injury induced by PAF may reflect injury caused by ischemia or ischemia–reperfusion. However, the low dose of PAF infusion (4 ng/min) used in our study did not result in significant alterations in blood flow or vascular resistance, despite increased fluid and protein fluxes across the microvasculature and mucosa. This observation indicates that ischemia per se is not a prerequisite for the PAF-induced microvascular and mucosal dysfunction. Another well-known action of PAF is that it causes leukocyte activation and adhesion to postcapillary venules. Therefore, the phospholipid may cause tissue injury by promoting the activation of circulating and/or resident granulocytes. Pretreatment of animals with MAb $1B_4$ attenuated the PAF-induced increments in lymph flow and vascular protein flux but did not affect the augmented mucosal fluid and protein fluxes (Fig. 15) (34). These observations indicate that the PAF-induced, leukocyte-mediated intestinal injury is confined to the microvasculature.

It was also interesting that the beneficial effect of MAb $1B_4$ on vascular fluid and protein fluxes were not observed at the low PAF infusion rate (first 30 min), which initially led us to conclude that intravascular leukocytes are not responsible for the microvascular dysfunction produced by low levels of PAF and that higher levels are required to activate feline neutrophils. However, more recently we have observed that the initial rise (15–30 min) in vascular fluid and protein flux is independent of circulating leukocytes, and with prolonged PAF infusion the vascular fluid and protein leakage become more contingent on leukocyte adhesion. It is likely that PAF has an early, direct effect on microvascular integrity since *in vitro* studies indicate that PAF induces a direct and reversible change in endothelial cell shape due to rearrangement of the cytoskeleton.

From the aforementioned data, it is clear that simply preventing leukocyte adhesion to postcapillary venules during either infusion of PAF or ischemia–reperfusion does not prevent mucosal dysfunction. However, when the continuous influx of leukocytes into the mucosal interstitium was arrested by chronic administration of MAb $1B_4$ thereby reducing the resident population of myeloperoxidase-positive cells to less than 10%, the mucosal dysfunction in the reperfused intestine was prevented. In another series of experiments, PAF was infused at 30-min intervals in untreated animals and animals that received MAb $1B_4$ for 3 days. Figure 16 demonstrates that PAF induced a 4-, 25-, and 20-fold increase in ^{51}Cr-EDTA clearance at 4, 20, and 40 ng/min, respectively, and mucosal granulocyte depletion resulted in greatly reduced clearance of ^{51}Cr-EDTA, suggesting that resident granulocytes play an important role in mediating the mucosal dysfunction induced by PAF.

The mechanism by which resident granulocytes mediate the PAF-induced mucosal dysfunction remains unclear, but it may be dependent on the limited release of proteases and/or oxidants from the phagocytic cells. Therefore, in two other groups of animals, we assessed the mechanism by which leukocytes mediate the PAF-induced mucosal dysfunction

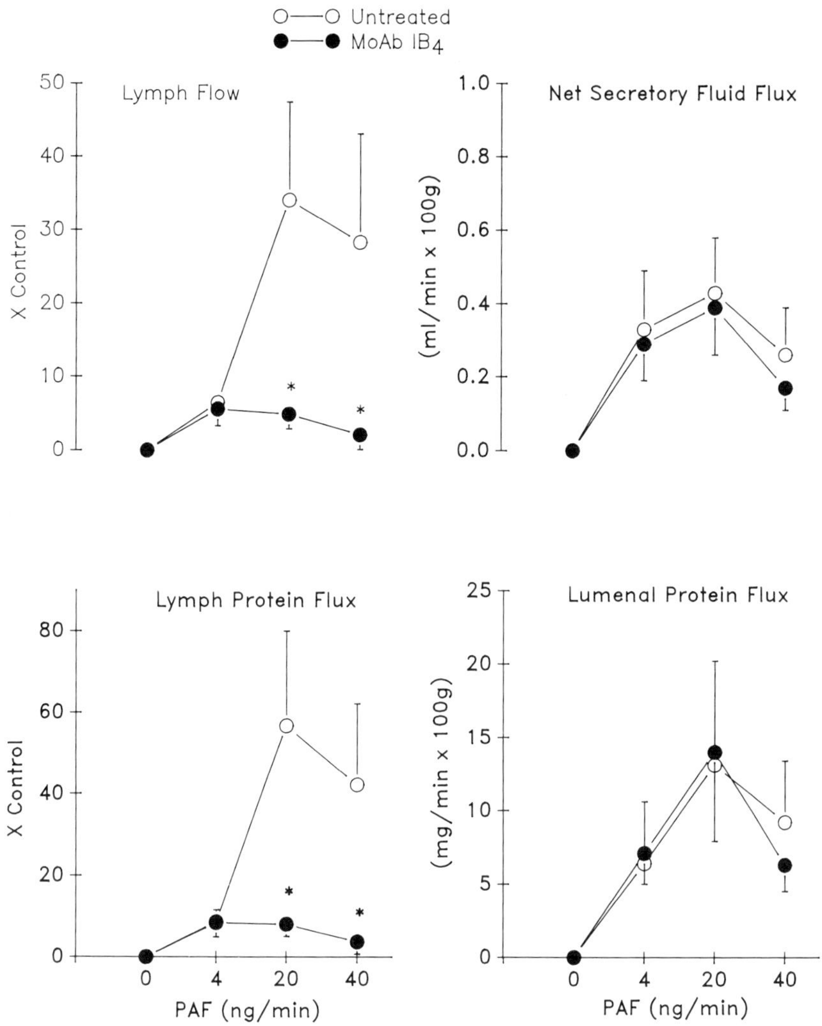

FIGURE 15

Alterations in lymph flow, lymph protein flux, net secretory (luminal) fluid flux, and luminal protein flux during PAF infusion in control animals and animals pretreated with antiadhesion antibody MAb $1B_4$. Asterisks denote significance ($p < 0.05$) relative to corresponding untreated value. (From Ref. 34.)

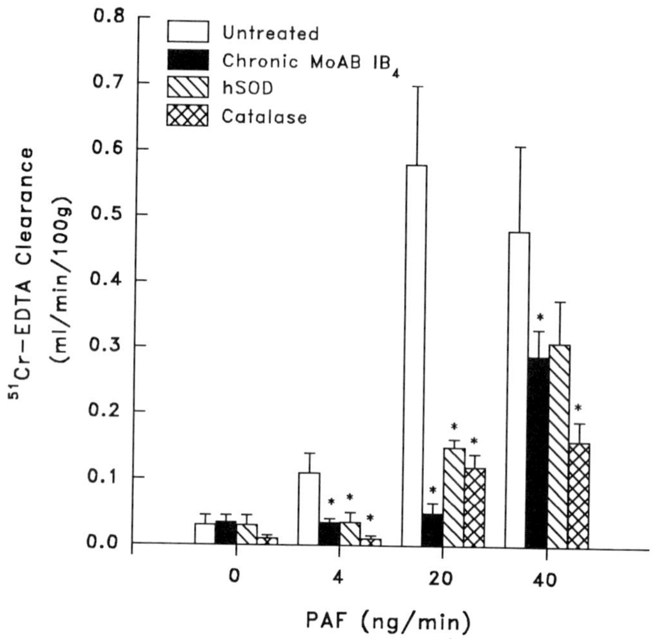

FIGURE 16

Clearance of ^{51}Cr-EDTA (index of mucosal permeability) during infusion of 4, 20, and 40 ng PAF/min in untreated animals and animals treated with MAb $1B_4$, superoxide dismutase or catalase. Asterisks denote significance ($p < 0.05$) relative to corresponding untreated value. (From Ref. 34.)

by pretreating with either superoxide dismutase or catalase. We observed that treatment with either antioxidant enzyme caused a dramatic reduction in ^{51}Cr-EDTA clearance, particularly at the two lower doses of PAF (Fig. 16). At the highest dose of PAF, ^{51}Cr-EDTA clearance was still markedly reduced in the catalase group but not in the hSOD group. These observations suggest that oxidants derived from phagocytic cells may be responsible for the PAF-induced mucosal dysfunction.

It is well established that *N*-formylmethionylleucylphenylalanine (FMLP), a peptide produced by resident ileal and colonic bacteria, attracts and activates leukocytes. To evaluate the sensitivity of the distal bowel and colon to FMLP, the bacterial peptide was perfused through the lumen of the rat colon and ileum and the integrity of the mucosal barrier assessed using blood-to-lumen clearance of ^{51}Cr-EDTA. In response to FMLP, mucosal permeability to ^{51}Cr-EDTA increased approximately 4-fold, yet the FMLP-induced mucosal dysfunction was not associated with an increased mucosal myeloperoxidase activity (35). Although FMLP did not induce recruitment of intravascular granulocytes into the mucosa, the increased mucosal permeability induced by FMLP was largely prevented by depletion of circulating granulocytes with antineutrophil serum (Table IV) (36,37).

The mechanism responsible for the neutrophil-mediated increase in mucosal permeability was addressed in additional studies (36,37). Neutrophils are known to cause tissue damage by both oxidative (reactive oxygen metabolites) and nonoxidative (proteases) mechanisms. *In vitro* data suggest that FMLP induces leukocyte chemotactic activity, leukocyte degranulation (release of proteases), and superoxide production at concentrations of FMLP that induce mucosal dysfunction *in vivo* (38). Of the various proteases produced and released by neutrophils, elastase has attracted most attention. Thus, we assessed whether neutrophil proteases, and in particular elastase, mediate the FMLP-induced increases in

TABLE IV

Effects of Various Antioxidants and Protease Inhibitors on Chemoattractant-Induced Injury to Ileal Mucosa[a]

Treatment	^{51}Cr-EDTA clearance (× control)
None	4.3 ± 1.2
Antineutrophil serum	0.88
Superoxide dismutase	3.4 ± 0.9
Catalase	3.2 ± 0.7
Deferoxamine	1.7 ± 0.2
Deferoxamine (iron-loaded)	4.6 ± 1.9
Deferoxamine (manganese-loaded)	1.5 ± 0.2
Dimethyl sulfoxide	1.5 ± 0.3
PZ-51	1.9 ± 1.0
Soybean trypsin inhibitor	1.8 ± 1.3
Eglin C	1.6 ± 0.5
MAAPV	1.7 ± 0.9
5-Aminosalicylic acid	1.8 ± 0.4
4-Aminosalicylic acid	1.7 ± 0.5
N-Acetyl-5-aminosalicylic acid	4.3 ± 0.8
Sulfapyridine	3.8 ± 1.2
Dapsone	1.7 ± 0.3

[a] Data from Refs. 35–37.

intestinal mucosal permeability. Table IV demonstrates that pretreatment with the nonspecific serine protease inhibitor, soybean trypsin inhibitor, significantly attenuated the clearance responses normally observed during luminal perfusion with FMLP. Additionally, the more specific elastase inhibitor MeOSuc-Ala-Ala-Pro-Val-CH_2Cl (MAAPV) and Eglin C (an inhibitor of elastase and cathepsin G) significantly reduced the FMLP-induced increases in ^{51}Cr-EDTA clearance. The results of this study indicate that neutrophilic proteases mediate at least part of the increased mucosal permeability induced by luminal exposure to FMLP.

Table IV also summarizes the effects of antioxidants on FMLP-induced mucosal dysfunction. The data suggest that superoxide dismutase and catalase do not provide significant protection but that dimethyl sulfoxide (hydroxyl radical scavenger) and deferoxamine (iron chelator) significantly attenuate the FMLP-induced increases in mucosal permeability. The effects of the latter two agents suggest that hydroxyl radicals formed by the iron-catalyzed Haber–Weiss reaction mediate the dysfunction associated with FMLP infusion into the lumen of the small bowel. An apparent contradiction to this interpretation is our inability to demonstrate a protective effect with either superoxide dismutase or catalase. These data suggest that neither superoxide nor H_2O_2 play a role in the FMLP-induced increases in mucosal permeability and that generation of the hydroxyl radical via the Haber–Weiss reaction is unlikely. One explanation that may reconcile the inconsistency between data obtained with the antioxidant enzymes and the other agents is that the former are excluded from sites of oxidant generation, whereas the smaller and more lipophilic molecules (desferrioxamine and dimethyl sulfoxide) have greater access to both extracellular and intracellular compartments. Data to support this view are provided by the observation that two low molecular weight antioxidants, namely, manganese-loaded desferrioxamine (SOD mimetic) and PZ 51 (H_2O_2 detoxifying agent), attenuate the FMLP-induced mucosal dysfunction. Therefore, the exclusion of SOD and catalase from a neutrophil-associated microenvironment may account for the inability of these enzymes to provide protection in models of FMLP-induced epithelial cell injury.

FMLP infusion into the bowel lumen also elicited an increased intestinal microvascular permeability, interstitial edema, and hyperemia (38). These findings suggest that luminal perfusion of FMLP affects the terminal ileum of the rat in a manner consistent with an inflammatory response. The data also demonstrate that peptides produced by microorganisms in the gut lumen can indeed increase microvascular permeability. To assess the importance of neutrophils in the microvascular dysfunction elicited by FMLP, antineutrophil serum was used. Treatment with antineutrophil serum reduced the circulating neutrophil count to 5% of control levels. The FMLP-induced increases in vascular protein flux were significantly attenuated by antineutrophil serum, indicating that neutrophils also mediate the FMLP-induced microvascular dysfunction.

The data from the PAF and FMLP models of inflammation as well as our ischemia–reperfusion model raise a new and complicating factor in the study of inflammation of the intestine. It appears that there are two distinct microscopic compartments, namely, the intravascular compartment and extravascular space, which are affected by PAF, FMLP, and ischemia–reperfusion. Based on the evidence presented in this chapter, it would appear likely that intravascular leukocytes mediate the microvascular dysfunction whereas the resident granulocyte population mediates the mucosal dysfunction associated with acute inflammation. There is a growing body of evidence that leukocyte-derived oxidants and proteases may play relatively different roles in mediating injury in each compartment. Thus, it is conceivable that therapeutic interventions that are effective in limiting the injury to one compartment may not be so effective in achieving a therapeutic effect in the other.

Acknowledgments

The work summarized in this chapter was funded by research grants from the National Institutes of Diabetes and Digestive and Kidney Diseases (DK33594, DK43785).

References

1. D. N. Granger, G. Rutili, and J. M. McCord, *Gastroenterology* **81,** 22–29 (1981).
2. D. N. Granger, *Am. J. Physiol.* **255,** H1269–H1275 (1988).
3. M. B. Grisham, L. A. Hernandez, and D. N. Granger, *Am. J. Physiol.* **251,** G567–G574 (1986).
4. B. J. Zimmerman, M. B. Grisham, and D. N. Granger, *Am. J. Physiol.* **258,** G185–G190 (1990).
5. W. F. Petrone, D. K. English, K. Wong, and J. M. McCord, *Proc. Natl. Acad. Sci. U.S.A.* **77,** 1159–1163 (1980).
6. D. N. Granger, J. N. Benoit, M. Suzuki, and M. B. Grisham, *Am. J. Physiol.* **257,** G683–G688 (1989).
7. M. Suzuki, W. Inauen, P. R. Kvietys, M. B. Grisham, C. Meininger, M. E. Schelling, H. J. Granger, and D. N. Granger, *Am. J. Physiol.* **257,** H1740–H1745 (1989).
8. M. Suzuki, M. B. Grisham, and D. N. Granger, *J. Leukocyte Biol.* **50,** 488–494 (1991).
9. E. K. Hodgson and I. Fridovich, *Biochemistry* **14,** 5299–5302 (1975).

10. P. Kubes, M. Suzuki, and D. N. Granger, *Proc. Natl. Acad. Sci. U.S.A.* **88,** 4651–4655 (1991).
11. E. Sekizuka, J. N. Benoit, M. B. Grisham, and D. N. Granger, *Am. J. Physiol.* **256,** H594–H597 (1989).
12. M. Suzuki, H. Asako, P. Kubes, S. Jennings, M. B. Grisham, and D. N. Granger, *Microvasc. Res.* **42,** 125–138 (1991).
13. M. G. Oliver, R. D. Specian, M. A. Perry, and D. N. Granger, *Inflammation* **15,** 331–346 (1991).
14. B. J. Zimmerman, D. A. Parks, M. B. Grisham, and D. N. Granger, *Am. J. Physiol.* **255,** H202–H206 (1988).
15. W. Inauen, D. N. Granger, C. J. Meininger, M. E. Schelling, H. J. Granger, and P. R. Kvietys, *Am. J. Physiol.* **259,** G134–G139 (1990).
16. W. Inauen, D. N. Granger, C. J. Meininger, M. E. Schelling, H. J. Granger, and P. R. Kvietys, *Am. J. Physiol.* **259,** H925–H931 (1990).
17. N. Yoshida, D. N. Granger, D. C. Anderson, R. Rothlein, C. Lane, and P. R. Kvietys, *Am. J. Physiol.* **262,** H1891–H1898 (1992).
18. W. Inauen, D. K. Payne, P. R. Kvietys, and D. N. Granger, *Free Radical Biol. Med.* **9,** 219–223 (1990).
19. P. Kubes, G. Ibbotson, J. Russell, J. L. Wallace, and D. N. Granger, *Am. J. Physiol.* **259,** G300–G305 (1990).
20. M. S. Lewis, R. E. Whatley, P. Chain, T. M. McIntyre, S. M. Prescott, and G. A. Zimmerman, *J. Clin. Invest.* **82,** 2045–2055 (1988).
21. M. J. Mangino, C. B. Anderson, M. K. Murphy, E. Brunt, and J. Turk, *Am. J. Physiol.* **257,** G299–G307 (1989).
22. B. J. Zimmerman, D. J. Guillory, M. B. Grisham, T. S. Gaginella, and D. N. Granger, *Gastroenterology* **99,** 1358–1363 (1990).
23. H. Asako, P. Kubes, B. A. Baethge, R. E. Wolfe, and D. N. Granger, *Inflammation* **16,** 45–56 (1992).
24. P. Kubes, M. G. Grisham, J. A. Barrowman, T. Gaginella, and D. N. Granger, *Am. J. Physiol.* **261,** H1872–H1879 (1991).
25. T. B. Casole and K. Abbas, *Am. J. Physiol.* **258,** C639–C647 (1990).
26. J. Bjork, P. Hedqvist, and K. E. Arfors, *Inflammation* **6,** 189–200 (1982).
27. B. J. Zimmerman and D. N. Granger, *Am. J. Physiol.* **259,** H390–H394 (1990).
28. M. B. Grisham, L. A. Hernandez, and D. N. Granger, *Am. J. Physiol.* **257,** H1334–H1339 (1989).
29. B. N. Cronstein, R. I. Levin, J. Belanoff, G. Weissman, and R. Hirschhorn, *J. Clin. Invest.* **78,** 760–770 (1986).
30. L. A. Hernandez, M. B. Grisham, B. Twohig, K. E. Arfors, J. M. Harlan, and D. N. Granger, *Am. J. Physiol.* **253,** H699–H703 (1987).
31. P. Kubes, J. Hunter, and D. N. Granger, *Gastroenterology* in press (1992).
32. H. Kurtel, K. Fujimoto, B. J. Zimmerman, D. N. Granger, and P. Tso, *Am. J. Physiol.* **261,** G490–G496 (1991).
33. P. Kubes, M. Suzuki, and D. N. Granger, *Am. J. Physiol.* **258,** G158–G163 (1990).
34. P. Kubes, K. E. Arfors, and D. N. Granger, *Am. J. Physiol.* **260,** G965–G971 (1991).
35. C. von Ritter, E. Sekizuka, M. B. Grisham, and D. N. Granger, *Gastroenterology* **95,** 651–656 (1988).
36. C. von Ritter, R. Be, and D. N. Granger, *Gastroenterology* **97,** 605–609 (1989).
37. C. von Ritter, M. B. Grisham, M. Hollwarth, W. Inauen, and D. N. Granger, *Gastroenterology* **97,** 778–780 (1989).
38. D. N. Granger, B. J. Zimmerman, E. Sekizuka, and M. B. Grisham, *Gastroenterology* **94,** 673–681 (1988).

CHAPTER 9

Macrophage-Derived Nitric Oxide: Generation and Consequences

Qiao-wen Xie and Carl Nathan

Beatrice and Samuel A. Seaver Laboratory
Division of Hematology–Oncology
Department of Medicine
Cornell University Medical College
New York, New York 10021

I. Introduction

Nitric oxide (NO), a short-lived radical gas, is generated by lightning from nitrogen and oxygen, and also accumulates in smog. Only in the last decade has the biochemically extraordinary finding emerged that mammalian macrophages can also generate this highly reactive inorganic molecule, along with its accumulating oxidation products, nitrite and nitrate. That mammalian cells can produce reactive nitrogen intermediates (RNI) recalled the equally surprising discovery decades earlier that phagocytes can produce another set of highly reactive inorganic species, the reactive oxygen intermediates (ROI). Thus, phagocytes make both bleach and smog.

Cellular and Molecular Mechanisms of Inflammation, Volume 4

Nitric oxide is of particular interest, not only as the newest and smallest known biosynthetically derived secretory product, but as one that is endowed with the potential both to destroy tumor cells and microbes and to regulate the cardiovascular, nervous, and immune systems. The diversity of the biological roles of NO derives from the wide variety of mammalian cells now known to generate it, differences in the circumstances of its production and quantities released, and the spectrum of enzyme prosthetic groups and side chains which are among its targets.

In this chapter we summarize current understanding of how macrophages accomplish the feat of synthesizing NO without lightning or the combustion of fossil fuels. We describe the striking dependence of macrophage NO synthase on immunological induction. Finally, we survey known and hypothesized functions of macrophage-derived NO and discuss the biochemical bases of these effects.

II. Discovery That Macrophages Release Reactive Nitrogen Intermediates, and Their Identification

A. Synthesis of Nitrite, Nitrate, and Nitrosamines from a Guanidino Nitrogen of L-Arginine

The nitrate that mammals excrete in excess of what they ingest (1) was thought to arise from intestinal flora until investigators at the Massachusetts Institute of Technology (MIT), tracking the origins of carcinogenic nitrosamines, demonstrated that even germ-free rats excreted more nitrate than they ingested (2). Interest in this observation was broadened by its extension to humans (3) along with the finding that the amounts increased during intercurrent infection (4). The latter observation sent the investigators back to rats: their injection with bacterial lipopolysaccharide (LPS), turpentine, or carrageenan led to marked increases in urinary nitrate (5).

Thus a link was established between immunostimulation and mammalian nitrate synthesis. In an affiliated laboratory at MIT, Stuehr and Marletta then carried out similar experiments in mice, injecting LPS or Bacille Calmette–Guérin (BCG). Nitrate levels rose markedly in blood and urine. Stuehr and Marletta went on to explant macrophages, cells long known to respond to such immunostimulants. Their demonstration that immunologically activated macrophages released copious nitrite and nitrate into the extracellular medium (6) left no doubt that mammalian cells, not just host-associated flora, could contribute to the nitrate in body fluids. Miwa *et al.* went on to demonstrate that macrophage-derived RNI could react with exogenous amines added to the tissue culture medium to generate micromolar quantities of nitrosamines (7).

Since 1987, the list of cells from mice, rats, guinea pigs, rabbits, dogs, and humans known to generate RNI under various circumstances has rapidly expanded to include endothelium, neurons, platelets, neutrophils, hepatocytes, adrenal cells, smooth muscle cells, fibroblasts, mesangial cells, and some tumor cells (8,9a). However, RNI production by human macrophages remains controversial, as discussed at the end of this chapter.

The MIT group went on to demonstrate that macrophages produce RNI from a guanidino nitrogen of L-arginine, yielding nitrite, nitrate, and L-citrulline. These precursor–product relationships were firmly established through gas chromatography–mass spectrometry (GC-MS) techniques using L-[*guanidino*-^{15}N]arginine (10).

Simultaneously, Hibbs and colleagues demonstrated that L-arginine was necessary and sufficient to sustain macrophage-mediated inhibition of tumor cell replication (11), and that the latter process was closely associated with L-arginine-dependent generation of nitrite by activated macrophages (12). Furthermore, L-arginine analogs bearing alkyl substitutions on the guanidino nitrogen(s) both inhibited the generation of nitrite and reversed the inhibition of tumor cell replication (11,12). These pharmacological studies provided complementary evidence that nitrite arose from the guanidino group of L-arginine. More important, the inhibitors introduced by Hibbs and colleagues (which were soon extended by others to include nitro- or amino-substituted analogs) have become the most widely used tools in NO research in biological systems, fueling a rapidly expanding appreciation of the widespread involvement of NO as a new autacoid system.

B. Nitric Oxide, or a Closely Related Species, as a Precursor of Nitrite and Nitrate

Although the foregoing studies from Hibbs' laboratory established that macrophage-mediated cytostasis was closely linked with nitrite production, nitrite itself was not cytostatic in the concentrations generated by macrophages in the medium in which it was found to accumulate (12). This apparent paradox prompted three groups of investigators to hypothesize that macrophages produce a more cytotoxic compound—NO or a species of similar reactivity, such as NO_2—as primary products of NO synthase (13–16). In this view, nitrite and nitrate are the accumulating products of the reaction of NO with oxygen and water.

Testing this hypothesis was not a simple task. The high chemical reactivity of NO makes its specific detection a methodological challenge. Its half-life is short (estimated at 6–30 sec in aerated, aqueous media); its reactions are nonenzymatic and hence of imited specificity. No definitive method has been employed in biological systems to distinguish NO from NO_2 or other similarly reactive oxides of nitrogen into which NO may quickly convert in oxygenated environments. Moreover, NO may nitrosate other species that can subsequently regenerate NO. In this chapter, for simplicity, the term "NO" is used to refer to all such species.

To demonstrate NO, Marletta and colleagues (13) and Hibbs *et al.* (14) adapted an approach used by Palmer *et al.* (17) to detect NO-like products from endothelial cells, namely, the generation of chemiluminescence on reaction of NO with ozone. In the study with endothelial cells (17), the samples were prepared by reflux in KI, which reduces nitrite to NO. Thus, this test did not distinguish NO from nitrite. However, in the studies with macrophages, KI was omitted (13) and the criterion of volatility was applied (14), thereby demonstrating that activated macrophages metabolize a guanidino N of L-arginine to a gas with the properties of NO.

Stuehr *et al.* in our laboratory used two other approaches (15). As Palmer *et al.* had shown with endothelial cells (17), Stuehr *et al.* demonstrated that activated macrophages used an L-arginine-dependent, N^{ω}-methyl-L-arginine-sensitive process to generate a labile compound that relaxed vascular smooth muscle (15). This is a property of authentic NO but not of nitrite or nitrate. Second, Stuehr *et al.* devised a spectrophotometric assay, the bleaching of the chromophore of clostridial ferredoxin. NO and NO_2 are active in this assay, but nitrite and nitrate are not (15). Activated macrophages bleached ferredoxin in a manner dependent on cell number, time, and the presence of L-arginine (15).

Collectively, these studies established that activated macrophages oxidize L-arginine to a gas with the chemical and biological reactivity of NO.

III. Biosynthetic Path for Formation of Nitric Oxide from L-Arginine

A. Cofactors and Cofactor-Cycling Accessory Enzymes

Before undertaking the purification of macrophage NO synthase, our laboratory decided to analyze in some detail the substrates and cofactors required by the enzyme for optimal activity. We reasoned that this information would prove invaluable for the assay of chromatographic fractions. In retrospect, the reasoning was sound, but the detour proved both more arduous and more interesting than anticipated: the chemical simplicity of NO contrasts with the complexity of the enzymatic five-electron oxidation by which macrophages generate it.

Postnuclear supernatants of activated primary macrophages or activated cells of the RAW 264.7 macrophage-like cell line were able to convert L-arginine to nitrite and nitrate, provided that NADPH was supplied (18). NADH, $NADP^+$, and NAD^+ would not suffice. Removal of a methylene group from the carbon backbone of L-arginine made it unsuitable as a substrate, as did removal of the α-amino or α-carboxyl or rotation to D-arginine. In contrast, addition of a methylene to the carbon backbone was tolerated (18).

There was a linear relation between amount of cytosol protein in the assay and amount of RNI detected. However, this relation broke down as the cytosol was further diluted (19). We hypothesized that a cofactor had been diluted out. Indeed, cytosol from nonactivated macrophages, itself incapable of generating RNI, could restore the specific activity of dilute cytosol from activated macrophages and could confer activity on specific chromatographic fractions of activated macrophage cytosol (we called these fractions inducible factor). The constitutive factors (i.e., those present in cytosol from nonactivated as well as activated macrophages) could be fractionated into species of greater than 30 kDa and less than 30 kDa. Neither fraction alone restored RNI-generating capacity to diluted or partially purifed cytosol from activated macrophages; only the combination of high and low mass fractions was effective (19).

We surmised that the higher mass constitutive factor was an enzyme. We were daunted by the prospect of having to purify this putative ancillary enzyme in order to move on to the purification of NO synthase itself. We reasoned that identification of the low mass constitutive factor might be simpler. If the low mass factor were a substrate for the high mass constitutive factor, we might be able to hypothesize the identity of the latter and then test our guess, without resorting to its purification.

These expectations were fulfilled, helped along substantially by a hunch growing out of earlier work (20) that tetrahydrobiopterin might be involved. First, Kwon *et al.* identified the low mass constitutive factor (21). The active principle was dialyzable, water soluble, and cationic at acidic to neutral pH, features consistent with a small amine, such as a pteridine. It eluted from a C_{18} reversed-phase column during high-performance liquid chromatography (HPLC) in a broad peak that contained a fluorophore with excitation and emission spectra identical to those of biopterin. Gas chromatography resolved a species with the mass spectrum of biopterin. Of 14 pteridines tested, only 7,8-dihydrobiopterin or 5,6,7,8-tetrahydrobiopterin could replace the low mass constitutive factor in synergism with the high mass constitutive factor and the inducible factor to generate RNI. The biopterin content of various cell lines corresponded to their content of the low mass factor, and lysate from a biopterin-deficient cell line contained no low mass factor until it was repleted with exogenous biopterin (21).

The redox state of biopterin proved critical. Fully oxidized biopterin was inactive. Partially reduced biopterin was active, but not in the presence of the dihydrofolate reductase inhibitors methotrexate or aminopterin. Fully reduced biopterin remained active even in the presence of methotrexate or aminopterin, but only if supplemented with dihydropteridine reductase, which is resistant to these inhibitors. Finally, the required concentrations of reduced biopterin were substoichiometric with the amount of product formed (21). These findings suggested the involvement of the biopterin redox cycle depicted in Fig. 1. The involvement of biopterin in macrophage NO synthesis was independently established by Tayeh and Marletta (22).

Dependence on tetrahydrobiopterin was undetectable in the first few minutes of the progress curve but became increasingly prominent the longer NO synthase was allowed to operate, reaching 75% from minute 60 to 90 (23) and nearly 100% thereafter. We speculated that this might reflect retention of some biopterin by the purified apoenzyme (21); this has subsequently been demonstrated for NO synthase from pig cerebellum (24).

Studies of cerebellar and endothelial NO synthase in which very short assays were used revealed no evidence for the participation of biopterin (e.g., Ref. 25). Later studies, however, have confirmed the participation of biopterin in the optimal action of NO synthase in brain (24,26) and fibroblasts (27).

The mechanism of action of biopterin in NO synthesis is not yet clear. In contrast to the situation with mouse macrophage NO synthase, NO synthase from rat cerebellum was said to depend on biopterin without redox cycling (26). It has not been established if biopterin merely maintains the enzyme in a catalytically competent form and/or donates electrons to the reaction.

Biopterin was previously identified as a cofactor for the hydroxylases acting on phenylalanine, tyrosine, and tryptophan in neurotransmitter synthesis. For years, it has seemed paradoxical that biopterin is much more widely distributed than the enzymes for which it was known to act as a cofactor. Since it is now apparent that NO synthases are widely

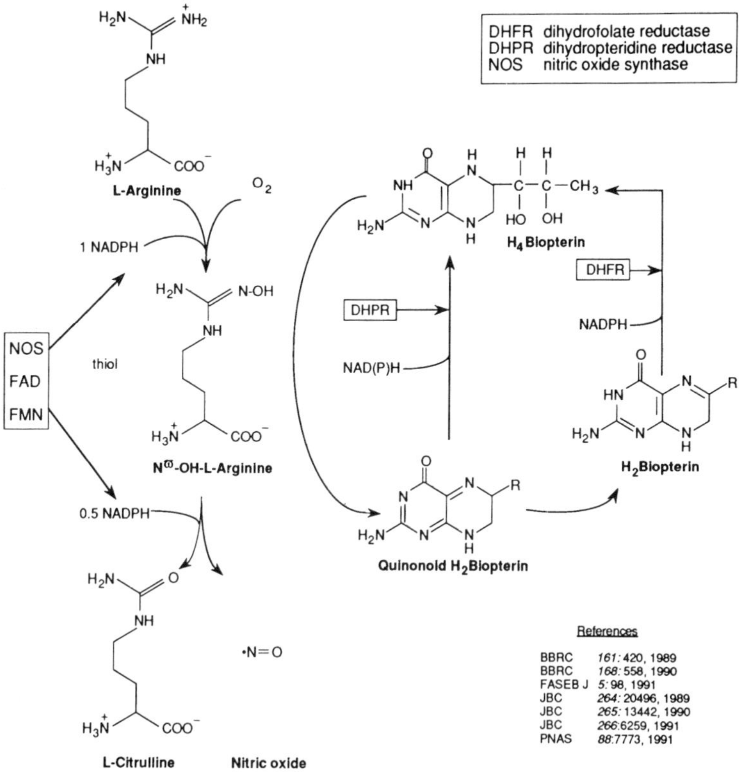

FIGURE 1

Biosynthesis of nitric oxide by inducible nitric oxide synthase.

distributed, it is likely that one of the major physiologic roles of biopterin is to facilitate the production of NO. Identification of tetrahydrobiopterin as a major component of the low mass constitutive factor led to identification of the major component(s) of high mass constitutive factor as the enzyme(s) needed to recycle partly oxidized biopterin to its fully reduced form, namely, dihydrofolate reductase and/or didhydopteridine reductase (21,28).

Finally, we showed that low and high mass constitutive factors were contributing additional components: FAD, reduced glutathione (GSH), and probably GSSG reductase, which recycles oxidized GSH (28). Dihydropteridine reductase could be omitted if large enough amounts of tetrahydrobiopterin were added, and GSSG reductase was dispensable when the reaction was supplemented with sufficient dithiothreitol. Thus, by adding L-arginine, NADPH, tetrahydrobiopterin, and dithiothreitol, we had an assay system in which the only uncharacterized macromolecular component was NO synthase itself.

B. Dioxygen as a Substrate

It seemed we were finally equipped to plunge into the purification of NO synthase. However, we were first seduced into undertaking additional studies of the enzyme reaction. The allure of this further detour consisted of the surprise of a new role for tetrahydrobiopterin, the novelty of NO synthesis in mammalian biochemistry, and the puzzle of a five-electron oxidation.

The literature contained two proposed reaction mechanisms for NO synthase. One involved an enzyme-catalyzed hydrolytic deimination of L-arginine to form L-citrulline and ammonia, with subsequent oxidation of the ammonia to form NO (12). The second mechanism involved formation of N^{ω}-hydroxy-L-arginine via a monooxygenase reaction, followed by abstraction of an electron and homolytic bond cleavage to yield NO and an amino acid carbodiimide. The latter would be hydrated to citrulline (13). In both schemes, the ureido oxygen of citrulline would come from water.

To test this, Kwon *et al.* used $H_2{}^{18}O$ and ${}^{18}O_2$, along with L-[*guanidino*-${}^{13}C$]arginine, and monitored citrulline formation by GC-MS. The results demonstrated that the ureido oxygen of the L-citrulline product of macrophage NO synthase derives from dioxygen, not from water (29). Thus, dioxygen is a substrate of NO synthase.

These results have recently been confirmed with endothelial NO synthase, then extended to show that the oxygen in NO also arises from dioxygen (30). However, it is not known if the same molecule of dioxygen donates the oxygens found both in citrulline and in NO. Thus, the stoichiometry of the reaction with respect to O_2 is unknown, and it is unclear if NO synthase is a dioxygenase as assumed (30) or, as seems more likely given our ability to isolate a hydroxylated intermediate (see below), a monoxygenase (24) that acts sequentially on the amino acid substrate and a resulting intermediate.

C. N^{ω}-Hydroxy-L-arginine as an Intermediate

The list of potential electron donors now included NADPH, FAD, tetrahydrobiopterin, and O_2. It was likely that a five-electron oxidation would occur in at least two steps. Identification of an intermediate might permit us to determine which of these compounds participated in the step(s) leading up to the formation of the intermediate, and which in a subsequent step(s).

As noted above, Marletta and colleagues had proposed that N^{ω}-hydroxy-L-arginine was an intermediate (13). To test this, Stuehr *et al.* (31) prepared authentic N^{ω}-hydroxy-L-arginine and found it competent as a substrate for NO synthase, with K_m and V_{max} values similar to those for L-arginine. The exogenous compound was also used to displace an endogenous product from NO synthase during oxidation of L-[^{14}C]arginine; this was identified by chromatographic techniques as N^{ω}-hydroxy-L-[^{14}C]arginine (31).

Having established that N^{ω}-hydroxy-L-arginine is an intermediate, Stuehr *et al.* (31) then tested which of the potential electron donors was required for the oxidation of this intermediate to citrulline. Surprisingly, no cofactor was dispensable. Moreover, with N^{ω}-hydroxy-L-arginine as substrate, molecular oxygen was still incorporated into the ureido group of citrulline. Finally, three inhibitors of NO synthase—two analogs of L-arginine and a flavoprotein inhibitor discussed below—blocked NO formation from the intermediate. In fact, the only detectable distinction between using L-arginine and N^{ω}-hydroxy-L-arginine as substrate was that the stoichiometry of NADPH utilization decreased, going from 1.5 mol NADPH oxidized per mole of NO formed from L-arginine to 0.5 mol NADPH oxidized per mole of NO formed from N^{ω}-hydroxy-L-arginine (31).

These results suggested that the same flavoprotein participates in an NADPH-dependent step to form N^{ω}-hydroxy-L-arginine and again in an NADPH-dependent step beyond this intermediate. Moreover, L-arginine binding, formation of the intermediate, and its subsequent oxidation to NO and L-citrulline may all take place within a single site.

IV. Purification of Nitric Oxide Synthase and Its Characterization as an FAD- and FMN-Containing Flavoprotein

A. Preliminary Evidence That Nitric Oxide Synthases Are Flavoproteins

As noted earlier, the activity of partially purified macrophage NO synthase was enhanced by adding FAD (28). To obtain additional evidence bearing on the possible participation of flavins, we tested the flavoprotein inhibitors diphenyleneiodonium, di-2-thienyliodonium, and iodonium-diphenyl (32). These proved to be extremely potent, irreversible inhibitors are not only of macrophage NO synthase (IC_{50} for diphenyleneiodonium, 50 n*M*) but also of endothelial NO synthase (IC_{50} 300 n*M*). NADPH or FAD could not reverse preestablished inhibition of NO synthase once the enzyme had been exposed to diphenyleneiodonium. However, when NADPH or FAD were added to the enzyme preparation simultaneously with diphenyleneiodonium, they blocked its inhibitory effect, even though diphenyleneiodonium did not react directly with NADPH or FAD. NADP and 2′,5′-ADP (structural fragments of NADPH) were effective blockers of inhibition by diphenyleneiodonium, but NADH was not. Similarly, FAD and its structural fragment FMN were both effective, but not the further structural fragments of FAD represented by riboflavin or adenosine 5′-diphosphoribose. This exquisite specificity, together with the lack of any direct interaction between diphenyleneiodonium and NADPH or FAD, suggested that diphenyleneiodonium competes with NADPH or FAD for binding site(s) on NO synthase (32).

B. Isolation of Inducible Nitric Oxide Synthase as a Dimer of 130-Kilodalton Constituents

For purification, we turned again to the macrophage-like cell line RAW 264.7 and induced NO synthase by exposing the cells to γ-interferon (IFN-γ) and bacterial lipopolysaccharide. The cells were lysed by freeze–thawing in the presence of protease inhibitors, and NO synthase was purified by sequential Mono Q anion exchange, 2′,5′-ADP Sepharose affinity, and TSK G3000 molecular sieve chromatography (23). The most important step was the affinity step that we had introduced earlier (19,21,28); subsequently, all reported purifications of various NO synthases have included this procedure. The active fraction from the final column eluted with an estimated mass of 250 kDa, but on sodium dodecyl sulfate–polyacrylamide gel electrophoresis (SDS-PAGE) yielded a closely spaced triplet at approximately 130 kDa. The protein peak eluting from the sizing column at 250 kDA shifted to about 121 kDa and lost enzyme activity when the elution buffer lacked L-arginine, FAD, and tetrahydrobiopterin. These results strongly suggested that the 130-kDa species associate(s) to form an enzymatically active dimer (23).

The 426-fold purification to homogeneity resulted in 8.7% recovery of activity. The specific activity of pure NO synthase was 1.3 μmol of nitrite plus nitrate/min/mg protein; its apparent K_m values for L-arginine and NADPH were 2.8 and 0.3 μ*M*, respectively. In contrast to results with the constitutive NO synthase(s) of brain and endothelium, the activity of macrophage NO synthase was minimally affected by EGTA, calmodulin inhibitors, or exogenous calmodulin (23).

C. Identification of FAD and FMN in Purified Nitric Oxide Synthase

On boiling, inducible NO synthase released fluorophores which were isolated by reversed-phase HPLC and identified by their retention times and fluorescence spectra as FAD and FMN. An average of 1.1 mol of FAD was recovered per 130-kDa monomer, along with an average of 0.55 mol of FMN (23). The latter most likely reflects partial loss of FMN during purification. Addition of both FAD and FMN was necessary for optimal activity of the purified enzyme (23). These results, which have been confirmed by Marletta and colleagues (33), establish that inducible NO synthase is indeed a flavoprotein. The negative tests for flavin in the purification reported by Yui *et al.* (34) probably resulted from insufficient amounts of enzyme.

Of special interest is the rarity of mammalian flavoproteins containing both FAD and FMN. Indeed, the only other example of which we are aware is cytochrome *P*-450 reductase. Constitutive NO synthase from rat cerebellum has been cloned by Bredt *et al.* (35). Its deduced amino acid sequence displayed extensive homology in its C-terminal region to cytochrome *P*-450 reductase, including putative flavin binding sites, leading Bredt *et al.* to speculate that constitutive brain NO synthase may also contain FAD and FMN (35); this has been confirmed by Mayer *et al.* (24).

D. Comparison of Inducible Mouse Macrophage Nitric Oxide Synthase with Constitutive Rat Cerebellar Enzyme

Purified mouse macrophage NO synthase was used to raise monospecific rabbit antibody. This Western-blotted the 130-kDa NO synthase in lysates of macrophages and EMT-6 mouse mammary adenocarcinoma cells, provided they had been exposed to IFN-γ and LPS (36,37). Bredt and Snyder have raised a rabbit antibody against the NO synthase from rat cerebellum. Their anticerebellar NO synthase antibody reportedly failed to react with macrophages (38). Likewise, our anti-macrophage NO synthase antibody filed to react with the recombinant rat brain enzyme (37).

We have cloned cDNAs encoding the inducible NO synthase from activated mouse macrophages (37). The same cDNA sequence has been reported by Lyon and Cunningham (37a). We confirmed 78% of the deduced amino acid sequence, using a combination of Edman degradation of tryptic peptides (36,37) and high performance liquid chromatography with electrospray ionization mass spectrometry of peptides generated by trypsin or protease Asp-N (37). The macrophage and cerebellular

NO synthases are only 51% homologous, and share only 16 of their 24 cysteines. These findings leave no doubt that the constitutive rat brain enzyme and the inducible mouse macrophage enzyme are products of different, albeit related, genes.

V. Immunologic Induction of Nitric Oxide Synthase

A. Stimuli for Induction

The most striking difference between macrophage NO synthase and the constitutive NO synthases of brain and endothelium is that the latter are transiently activated by any agonist that raises intracellular Ca^{2+}. Calcium ion promotes the binding of calmodulin to the enzyme; this presumably leads to a conformational change that permits NO synthase to begin catalysis. In contrast, the macrophage enzyme is indifferent to ambient Ca^{2+} in the physiological range and does not depend on exogenous calmodulin; rather, it is slowly and persistently activated by immunological stimuli (39).

Indeed, of the almost 100 known bioactive products released by macrophages (40), nitrite and nitrate are among those whose release is most profoundly affected by immunological activation. It was apparent from the early work of Stuehr and Marletta that RNI release was nearly undetectable in macrophages from untreated mice, but rose to levels several orders of magnitude above the limit of sensitivity of the assay on infection of the macrophage donors with BCG (6), or upon *in vitro* exposure of macrophages to IFN-γ or LPS. The combination of IFN-γ and LPS was synergistic (41).

A detailed comparison of 12 cytokines by Ding *et al.* (42) revealed that IFN-γ was the only one capable of inducing RNI release from mouse peritoneal macrophages when tested alone. However, tumor necrosis factors (TNF-α or TNF-β), themselves inactive, afforded marked synergy in enhancing the activity of IFN-γ. Also dramatically synergistic were combinations of IFN-α or IFN-β (themselves inactive) with LPS. The synergistic interaction of TNF-α with IFN-γ was independently noted by Drapier *et al.* (43). Green *et al.* (44) confirmed these observations and noted that ingestion of leishmania by IFN-γ-treated macrophages was a potent trigger for the release of TNF-α, which then acted in an autocrine manner to enhance RNI release by the same cell population.

Immunological induction of NO synthase also occurs in man, although, aside from vascular smooth muscle cells (45), the cell types involved have not been identified. Induction of human NO synthase *in vivo* was suggested by elevations in nitrate excretion by subjects who experienced apparently viral intercurrent illness (4), and it has been confirmed in studies in which cancer patients received experimental infusions of IL-2 (46,47).

B. Mechanism of Induction

There has been considerable debate on the mechanism of induction of NO synthase by immunological stimuli (48). Induction of transcription of the gene encoding NO synthase is not the only possibility. Control could also be expressed at the level of arginine transport, biopterin synthesis, posttranslational modification of preexistent NO synthase, or reduction in levels of an inhibitor or competing enzyme, such as arginase. Of all these alternative explanations, there is evidence only for the immunological enhancement of biopterin synthesis (49,50). However, Kwon *et al.* (21) identified tetrahydrobiopterin as a cofactor of NO synthase present in cytosol of nonactivated macrophages (hence a "constitutive factor"), strongly suggesting that inadequate levels of biopterin in nonactivated mouse peritoneal macrophages do not account for their failure to produce RNI. Instead, absence of NO synthase itself appears to be the explanation, in that the 130-kDa band corresponding to NO synthase monomer was undetectable when lysates from nonactivated macrophages were subjected to the same chromatographic procedures used to purify NO synthase (23).

Strong evidence that mouse macrophage NO synthase is immunologically inducible at the transcriptional level has been provided by recent experiments of Xie *et al.* (36,37). NO synthase enzyme activity was absent in nonactivated macrophages and was induced in IFN-γ- and LPS-treated macrophages, but not in the presence of actinomycin D. Both the induction of the mRNA and the protein, and the ability of actinomycin D to block their induction were further demonstrable by nuclear runoff assays, Northern blots, Western blots, and indirect immunofluorescence using monospecific rabbit antiserum against the 130-kDa NO synthase. In these experiments, actinomycin D was used briefly at low concentrations, and cell viability remained above 80%.

Thus it is clear that IFN-γ and LPS, separately and together, signal the transcription of the gene that encodes NO synthase. It remains to be determined by what mechanism the gene is induced.

C. Suppressive Cytokines

Long-standing interest in our laboratory in the phenomenon of macrophage deactivation (51) led us to search for cytokines that might suppress the ability of macrophages to release RNI. These proved to be at least as numerous as the cytokines known to induce RNI release. The suppressive factors we have identified to date are transforming growth factors (TGF-β1, TGF-β2, and TGF-β3), macrophage deactivation factor (MDF), and interleukin-10 (IL-10) (52,53).

In summary, macrophage RNI release is tightly controlled by the immune system through both inductive and suppressive signals, in a manner that closely correlates with the impact of the same signals on the cytotoxic capacity of the cell. It is hardly surprising that a molecule with the biochemical reactivity of NO is under strict control at the level of its production.

VI. Bioactivities and Molecular Targets of Macrophage-Derived Reactive Nitrogen Intermediates

A. Toxicity toward Mammalian Cells

The small amounts of NO produced briefly (over seconds to minutes) by endothelial cells and neurons in response to agonists cause transient modulations in the function of adjacent cells. These are attributable in large part to nitrosation of the heme group of soluble guanylyl cyclase, leading to enhanced production of cyclic GMP (54). Another enzyme whose function is enhanced by agonist-elicited NO production is mono(ADP-ribosyl)transferase (55), but in this case the impact on cell function is as yet unknown. Undoubtedly, there are additional important molecular targets critical to the cell-stimulatory actions of low-dose NO.

In contrast, macrophages release NO for up to 36 hr following immunological activation, in amounts that appear to be orders of magnitude larger than for comparable numbers of agonist-triggered endothelial cells or neurons (41). Uncertainty in the quantitative comparison arises because activity of the constitutive NO synthase in endothelial cells and neurons is usually measured by bioassay rather than chemical assay, and is not reported in molar terms. Macrophage-derived NO, as a rule, leads to inhibition of function, both in the macrophages that produce the NO (56,59), in microbial cells they have engulfed (reviewed in Ref. 60), and in mammalian cells with which they are coincubated (reviewed in Ref. 61).

In tumor cells, the best studied biochemical actions of macrophage-derived NO are inhibition of replication and respiration (11,12,14,16,57,

61–63), formation of iron–nitrosyl adducts (58,59), and loss of intracellular iron (64,65). The molecular targets believed to account for these effects include ribonucleoside reductase (63,66), *cis*-aconitase (61), and complex I and II of the mitochondrial electron transport chain (14,16,67).

The critical role of RNI generation in mouse macrophage antitumor activity *in vitro* was first established by Hibbs and associates (61). As noted earlier, these investigators demonstrated that macrophage-mediated cytotoxicity depended on L-arginine in the medium (11), was associated with nitrite production (12), and was inhibited by guanidino-N-substituted L-arginine analogs that block nitrite production (11,12). These findings have been widely confirmed (16,68,69), although it is clear both from earlier work (reviewed in Ref. 70) and from discordant results with arginine analogs (68) that other cytotoxic mechanisms are cooperative along with RNI production in some circumstances (69) or are of greater importance in others (70).

Our laboratory joined the study of antitumor effects of macrophage-derived RNI in order to address the paradox that macrophage-mediated cytotoxicity correlated with nitrite production but nitrite was not cytotoxic (12). As discussed earlier, we demonstrated that macrophages produce NO as a precursor of nitrite and nitrate (15), and went on to determine if NO could be implicated as the mediator of RNI-dependent, macrophage-mediated cytotoxicity.

First, we found that nitrite was profoundly cytostatic to L1210 mouse lymphoma cells, but only if the pH was lowered to 6.3 or below. Hydrogen ions alone were noninhibitory in the concentrations tested; instead, they interacted in true synergistic fashion with otherwise noninhibitory nitrite at the concentrations similar to those produced by activated macrophages. The combination of *nitrate* plus hydrogen ions was nontoxic under the same conditions (16). The most likely explanation for the specific synergy between hydrogen ions and nitrite was the protonation of nitrite to nitrous acid (pK_a 3.4). Nitrous acid is known to dismutate to NO and NO_2.

We next demonstrated that authentic NO gas was cytostatic and, moreover, that NO gas inhibited tumor cell respiration by blocking mitochondrial electron transport specifically at complex I and complex II (16). In this regard, NO gas reproduced the pattern of injury noted a decade earlier by Granger and Lehninger when they incubated activated macrophages with tumor cells (67).

Having shown that authentic NO mimicked effects of activated macrophages on tumor cells, we tried to test if NO actually accounted for these effects in macrophage–tumor cell cocultures. The experimental approach was not as facile as in the study of ROI, where one can sometimes resort to genetically deficient cells from patients with chronic granulomatous disease, and can add specific enzymes like superoxide dismutase and catalase to break down the cytotoxic mediators. In contrast, no genetic deficiency of NO production has been identified, and NO is probably too chemically reactive to be subject to catabolism by a specific enzyme. Thus, the methodological challenge was to select nonenzymatic NO scavengers with some specificity. Two were employed.

The first NO scavenger was superoxide anion itself, which reacts rapidly with NO (71). Superoxide was generated by the combination of $FeSO_4$ and ascorbate. Hydrogen peroxide, which is also generated in this reaction, was disposed of with catalase. This combination of reagents prevented macrophage-mediated tumor cell cytostasis in a dose-dependent fashion (16). At the time these experiments were carried out, the products of the reaction of superoxide with NO were not known. It has recently been proposed that NO and superoxide react to generate peroxynitrite radical, which is believed to break down to NO_2 and hydroxyl radical (72). If so, hydroxyl radical may react so quickly with components of the medium that it fails to reach intracellular targets in tumor cells. However, it is not clear why the proposed reaction of superoxide with NO would represent a detoxification, if it generates NO_2.

A challenge to the mechanism proposed to underlie these experiments (although not to the final interpretation) is the recent appreciation that NO may react nonenzymatically with the heme of catalase (72a). However, this does not appear to explain the NO-scavenging effect of $FeSO_4$/ascorbate/catalase in the experiments described, because we could reverse the effect of this cocktail by adding superoxide dismutase (16). Thus, superoxide anion almost certainly was the effective scavenger in this system, as originally believed.

The second intervention was the addition of myoglobin to the macrophage–tumor cell cocultures. Myoglobin reversed macrophage-mediated cytostasis almost completely, but only in the presence of ascorbate, which acts to keep myoglobin in the ferrous state. Ascorbate alone had no effect (15).

Tumor cells are not the only mammalian cell targets of macrophage-derived RNI. For one, RNI are autotoxic for the macrophages that produce them (56–59). Iron–nitrosyl complexes have been demonstrated within activated macrophages (58,59), whose own respiration is inhibited (57). Macrophage-derived RNI are also immunosuppressive toward lymphocytes (73–75). The biochemical basis of RNI-mediated inhibition of lymphocyte function has not been defined. Presumably this might involve either cyclic GMP elevation after exposure to low amounts of NO, or inactivation of heme-, iron–sulfur-, or sulfhydryl-dependent enzymes with exposures to higher levels of NO.

B. Mechanism of Nitric Oxide-Mediated Cytostasis

Finally, we tried to determine the mechanism of cytostasis by macrophage-derived NO. We speculated that ribonucleotide reductase might be a key target (16,63) because it is the rate-limiting enzyme in DNA synthesis and depends on thiols and nonheme iron in its reaction center. NO is known to react with thiols and nonheme iron.

First, we demonstrated that NO gas can inhibit ribonucleotide reductase from tumor cells (63). Next, we showed that NO synthase in lysates of activated macrophages also inhibited tumor cell ribonucleotide reductase, and did so in a manner dependent on L-arginine and inhibitable by *N*-methyl-L-arginine, *N*-nitro-L-arginine, or diphenyleneiodonium. Finally, we compared the effects of activated macrophages with the effects of the prototypic ribonucleotide reductase inhibitor hydroxyurea. Both inhibited tumor cell thymidine incorporation almost completely, and, in both cases, inhibition could be reversed to the same degree by exogenous deoxyribonucleosides, added to bypass the block created by inhibition of ribonucleotide reductase (63).

These results strongly supported the hypothesis that inhibition of ribonucleotide reductase by NO is a major contributor to the cytostatic effect of activated mouse macrophages under the conditions studied. The findings extended the observations of Lepoivre *et al.* (66), who used cytokines and LPS to induce NO synthesis within a tumor cell line and demonstrated an accompanying inhibition of ribonucleotide reductase.

Taking the analysis one step further, we noted a structural resemblance between hydroxyurea and the *N*-hydroxyguanidine moiety of N^{ω}-hydroxy-L-arginine, an intermediate in NO synthesis (31), and speculated that hydroxyurea might generate NO. Indeed, under oxidizing conditions, hydroxyurea produced nitrite. Nitrite formation was abolished by adding morpholine, which traps NO (the precursor of nitrite) to form nitrosomorpholine. Using GC-MS techniques, we identified nitrosomorpholine as a reaction product in the oxidation of hydroxyurea in the presence of morpholine. We conclude that hydroxyurea can generate NO when suitably oxidized (63). It is unknown whether such oxidation occurs in cells and, if so, whether it contributes to the mechanism of action of hydroxyurea.

C. Toxicity toward Microbes

Granger and colleagues pioneered in the demonstration of an L-arginine-dependent macrophage antimicrobial pathway; their target was extracellular cryptococci (76). This pathway was subsequently shown to contribute substantially to the ability of activated rodent macrophages to inhibit the growth of extracellular schistosomula (77) and intracellular leishmania (78), toxoplasmas (79), trypanosomes (80), and mycobacteria (81–83), including the agents of tuberculosis and leprosy.

These studies have relied heavily on the ability of *N*-methyl-L-arginine to reverse macrophage antimicrobial effects (60). It will be of interest to repeat such studies with macrophages rendered deficient in NO synthase through molecular biological techniques.

Little is known at the biochemical level about how macrophage-derived NO affects microbial metabolism. However, several potential targets are plausible, based on the known inhibitory effects of acid nitrite on bacteria, including ferredoxins, hydrogenases, and sulfhydryl-containing glycolytic enzymes (reviewed in Ref. 16). Indeed, early work on antimicrobial actions of acid nitrite stems from use of nitrite as a food preservative. Ribonucleotide reductase, identified as a target in tumor cells (63,66), may be an important target in microbes as well.

D. Regulation of Smooth Muscle Tone

Macrophage-derived NO need not always be cytotoxic. At lower fluxes, macrophage-derived NO will presumably activate guanylyl cyclase; neighboring cells will respond to cyclic GMP elevation in characteristic ways. Smooth muscle, for example, will relax. That macrophages can in fact generate vasorelaxant NO was directly demonstrated, using macrophages attached to Cytodex beads in a column through which a superfusate was directed onto preconstricted rings from rabbit aorta (15). Consideration of the strategic anatomic disposition of macrophages suggests that this phenomenon may be of considerable physiological importance. For example, macrophages are abundant in the renal juxtaglomerular apparatus and interstitium, gastrointestinal mucosa, uterine wall, bronchial epithelium, and pulmonary vasculature, interstitium, and alveoli. In all these sites, they may contribute to the regulation of smooth muscle tone, provided they have undergone immunological activation.

E. Inflammation

Roles have been proposed for RNI in neutrophil chemotaxis (84), the regulation of neutrophil adhesion to endothelium (85), and the elaboration of neutrophil-dependent tissue damage (86). The prevalence of macrophages in granulomas, atheromas, and wounds may position them to elicit regional hyperemia in inflammation, to inhibit the aggregation and adhesion of platelets, or to block the proliferation of lymphocytes. Much work is needed to test these speculations.

VII. The Puzzle of the Human Macrophage

Nitric oxide is currently touted as "the" mediator of macrophage antitumor and antimicrobial effects. This is the sort of exaggeration that often accompanies the enthusiasm engendered by genuinely new concepts in biomedical research. It is clear that NO is important in the *in vitro* cytotoxic reactions of mouse peritoneal macrophages against certain target cells, yet other mechanisms are also at work in these and other mononuclear phagocytes, especially when a wider range of targets is studied (70,87,88). In the human macrophage in particular, there has been only one report of immunologically inducible NO production, and that under very special circumstances (83). Other published efforts to detect human macrophage RNI production have been negative (89), as have many unreported efforts (e.g., N. S. Kwon and C. Nathan, unpublished observations, 1991). Thus, as reviewed above, inducible NO synthesis clearly exists in man, but perhaps not in the repertoire of the human macrophage, a cell with well-developed antitumor and antimicrobial capacities.

Hypotheses that attribute negative results with human macrophages to *in vitro* artifacts have been aired (48) and are being tested. The cloning of mouse macrophage NO synthase (37,37a) will hopefully lead us to the homologous human gene and give us tools to resolve this controversy.

Acknowledgments

We gratefully acknowledge the many people who contributed to the work summarized here. These include our present labmates, Hearn Cho and Aihao Ding; our former labmates, Nyoun-Soo Kwon and Dennis Stuehr; colleagues in other departments at Cornell, Owen Griffith, Stephen Gross, and Roberto Levi; and collaborators at Merck, Sharpe and Dohme Research Laboratories, Jimmy Calaycay, Philip Davies, Stephan Grant, and Richard Mumford. Much of the work reviewed here was supported by National Institutes of Health Grant CA43610 and by a grant from the Cancer Research Institute.

References

1. H. H. Mitchell, H. A. Schonle, and H. S. Grindly, *J. Biol. Chem.* **24,** 461–490 (1916).
2. L. C. Green, Tannenbaum, and R. Goldman, *Science* **212,** 56–58 (1981).
3. L. C. Green, K. R. de Luzuriaga, D. A. Wagner, W. Rand, N. Istfan, V. R. Young, and S. R. Tannenbaum, *Proc. Natl. Acad. Sci. U.S.A.* **78,** 7764–7768 (1981).
4. D. A. Wagner, V. R. Young, S. R. Tannenbaum, D. S. Schultz, and W. M. Deen, *in* "*N*-Nitroso Compounds: Occurrence, Biological Effects and Relevance to Human Cancer," (I. K. O'Neill, R. C. von Borstel, J. E. Long, C. T. Miller, and H. Bartsch, eds.), pp. 247–253. International Agency for Research on Cancer, Lyon, France, 1984.
5. D. A. Wagner, V. R. Young, and S. R. Tannenbaum, *Proc. Natl. Acad. Sci. U.S.A.* **80,** 4518–4521 (1983).
6. D. J. Stuehr and M. A Marletta, *Proc. Natl. Acad. Sci. U.S.A.* **82,** 7738–7742 (1985).
7. M. Miwa, D. J. Stuehr, M. A. Marletta, J. S. Wishnok, and S. R. Tannenbaum, *Carcinogenesis* **8,** 955–958 (1987).
8. D. J. Stuehr and O. W. Griffith, *Adv. Biochem. Relat. Areas Mol. Biol.* **65,** 287–346 (1992).
9. S. Moncada, R. M. J. Palmer, and E. A. Higgs, *Pharmacol. Rev.* **43,** 109–142 (1991).
9a. C. Nathan, *FASEB J.* In press, 1992.
10. R. Iyengar, D. J. Stuehr, and M. A. Marletta, *Proc. Natl. Acad. Sci. U.S.A.* **84,** 6369–6373 (1987).
11. J. B. Hibbs, Jr., Z. Vavrin, and R. R. Taintor, *J. Immunol.* **138,** 550–565 (1987).
12. J. B. Hibbs, Jr., R. R. Taintor, and Z. Vavrin, *Science* **235,** 473–476 (1987).
13. M. A. Marletta, P. S. Yoon, R. Iyengar, C. D. Leaf, and J. S. Wishnok, *Biochemistry* **21,** 8706–8711 (1988).
14. J. B. Hibbs, Jr., R. R. Taintor, Z. Vavrin, and E. M. Rachlin, *Biochem. Biophys. Res. Commun.* **157,** 87–94 (1988).
15. D. J. Stuehr, S. S. Gross, I. Sakuma, R. Levi, and C. F. Nathan, *J. Exp. Med.* **169,** 1011–1020 (1989).
16. D. J. Stuehr and C. F. Nathan, *J. Exp. Med.* **169,** 1543–1545 (1989).
17. R. M. J. Palmer, A. G. Ferrige, and S. Moncada, *Nature* (*London*) **327,** 524–526 (1987).
18. D. J. Stuehr, N. S. Kwon, S. S. Gross, B. A. Theil, R. Levi, and C. F. Nathan, *in* "Endothelium Derived Relaxing Factors" pp. 75–84 (G. Rubanyi and P. Vanhoutte, eds.), Karger, Basel.
19. D. J. Stuehr, N. S. Kwon, S. S. Gross, B. A. Thiel, R. Levi, and C. F. Nathan, *Biochem. Biophys. Res. Commun.* **161,** 420–426 (1989).
20. C. F. Nathan, *in* "Interferon" (I. Gresser and J. Vilcek, eds.), Vol. 7, pp. 125–143. Academic Press, New York, 1986.
21. N. S. Kwon, C. F. Nathan, and D. J. Stuehr, *J. Biol. Chem.* **264,** 20496–20501 (1989).
22. M. A. Tayeh and M. A. Marletta, *J. Biol. Chem.* **264,** 19654–19658 (1989).
23. D. J. Stuehr, H. J. Cho, N. S. Kwon, M. Weise, and C. F. Nathan, *Proc. Natl. Acad. Sci. U.S.A.* **88,** 7773–7777 (1991).
24. B. Mayer, M. John, B. Heinzel, E. R. Werner, H. Wachter, G. Schultz, and E. Bohme, *FEBS Lett.* **288,** 187–191 (1991).
25. D. S. Bredt and S. H. Snyder, *Proc. Natl. Acad. Sci. U.S.A.* **87,** 682–685 (1990).
26. J. Giovanelli, K. L. Campos, and S. Kauffman, *Proc. Natl. Acad. Sci. U.S.A.* **88,** 7091–7095 (1991).
27. G. Werner-Felmayer, E. R. Werner, D. Fuchs, A. Hausen, G. Rebinegger, and H. Wachter, *J. Exp. Med.* **172,** 1599–1607 (1990).

28. D. S. Stuehr, N. S. Kwon, H. J. Cho, and C. F. Nathan, *Biochem. Biophys. Res. Commun.* **168,** 558–565 (1990).
29. N. S. Kwon, C. F. Nathan, C. Gilker, O. Griffith, D. Matthews, and D. J. Stuehr, *J. Biol. Chem.* **265,** 13442–13445 (1990).
30. A. M. Leone, R. M. J. Palmer, R. G. Knowles, P. L. Francis, D. S. Ashton, and S. Moncada, *J. Biol. Chem.* **266,** 23790–23795 (1991).
31. D. Stuehr, N. S. Kwon, C. Nathan, O. Griffith, P. Feldman, and J. Wiseman, *J. Biol. Chem.* **266,** 6259–6263 (1991).
32. D. J. Stuehr, O. A. Fasehun, N. S. Kwon, S. S. Gross, J. A. Gonzalez, R. Levi, and C. F. Nathan, *FASEB J.* **5,** 98–103 (1991).
33. J. M. Hevel, K. A. White, and M. A. Marletta, *J. Biol. Chem.* **266,** 22789–22791 (1991).
34. Y. Yui, R. Hatori, K. Kosuga, H. Elizawa, K. Hiki, and C. Kawai, *J. Biol. Chem.* **266,** 12544–12547 (1991).
35. D. S. Bredt, P. M. Hwang, C. E. Glatt, C. Lowenstein, R. L. Reed, and S. H. Snyder *Nature (London)* **351,** 714–718 (1991).
36. Q.-w. Xie, H. Cho, J. Calaycay, R. Mumford, A. Ding, S. Grant, and C. Nathan, *in* "Biology of Nitric Oxide, Second International Meeting" (S. Moncada, M. A. Marletta, and J. B. Hibbs, Jr., eds.), Abstract, London, 1991.
37. Q.-w. Xie, H. J. Cho, J. Calaycay, R. A. Mumford, K. M. Swiderek, T. D. Lee, A. Ding, T. Troso, and C. Nathan, *Science* **256,** 255–228 (1992).
37a. C. R. Lyons, G. J. Orloff, and J. M. Cunningham, *J. Biol. Chem.* **267,** 6370–6374 (1992).
38. D. S. Bredt, P. M. Hwang, and S. H. Snyder, *Nature (London)* **347,** 768–772 (1990).
39. C. F. Nathan and D. J. Stuehr, *J. Natl. Cancer. Inst.* **82,** 726–728 (1990).
40. C. Nathan, *J. Clin. Invest.* **79,** 319–326 (1987).
41. D. J. Stuehr and M. A. Marletta, *J. Immunol.* **139,** 518–525 (1987).
42. A. H. Ding, C. F. Nathan, and D. J. Stuehr, *J. Immunol.* **141,** 2407–2412 (1988).
43. J.-C. Drapier, J. Wietzerbin, and J. B. Hibbs, Jr., *Eur. J. Immunol.* **18,** 1587–1592 (1988).
44. S. Green, R. M. Crawford, J. T. Hockmeyer, M. S. Meltzer, and C. A. Nacy, *J. Immunol.* **145,** 4290–4297 (1990).
45. R. Bussi, H. Kaufman, and A. Mulsch, *in* "Biology of Nitric Oxide, Second International Meeting" (S. Moncada, M. A. Marletta, and J. B. Hibbs, Jr., eds.), Abstract, IBC Technical Services Ltd., London, 1991.
46. J. B. Hibbs, Jr., C. Westenfelder, and W. Samlowski, *in* "Biology of Nitric Oxide, Second International Meeting" (S. Moncada, M. A. Marletta, and J. B. Hibbs, Jr., eds.), Abstract, IBC Technical Services Ltd., London, 1991.
47. T. R. Billar, J. B. Ochoa, B. Curti, A. B. Peitzman, R. L. Simmons, R. A. Hoffman, R. Rault, D. L. Longo, W. J. Urba, and A. C. Ochoa, *in* "Biology of Nitric Oxide, Second International Meeting" (S. Moncada, M. A. Marletta, and J. B. Hibbs, Jr., eds.), Abstract, IBC Technical Services Ltd., London, 1991.
48. C. Nathan, *Res. Immunol.* **142,** 553–602 (1991).
49. I. Ziegler, K. Schott, M. Lubbert, F. Herrmann, U. Schwulera, and A. Bacher, *J. Biol. Chem.* **265,** 17026–17030 (1990).
50. E. R. Werner, G. Werner-Fehlmayer, D. Fuchs, A. Hausen, G. Reibnegger, J. J. Yim, W. Pfleiderer, and H. Wachter, *J. Biol. Chem.* **265,** 3189 (1990).
51. C. Bogdan, Y. Vodovotz, and C. F. Nathan, *in* "Macrophages: Activation, Role and Cytokinetics" (R. van Furth, ed.) in press, Kluwer Academic Publishers, Dordrecht, The Netherlands (1992).
52. A. Ding, C. F. Nathan, J. Graycar, R. Derynck, D. J. Stuehr, and S. Srimal, *J. Immunol.* **145,** 940–944 (1990).

53. C. Bogdan, Y. Vodovotz, and C. Nathan, *J. Exp. Med.* **174,** 1549–1555 (1991).
54. L. J. Ignarro, *Biochem. Pharmacol.* **41,** 485–490 (1991).
55. B. Brune, and E. G. Lapetina, *J. Biol. Chem.* **264,** 8455–8458 (1989).
56. J. E. Albina, C. D. Mills, W. L. Henry, Jr. and M. A. Caldwell, *J. Immunol.* **143,** 3641–3646 (1989).
57. J.-C. Drapier and J. B. Hibbs, Jr., *J. Immunol.* **140,** 2829–2838 (1988).
58. J. R. Lancaster, Jr. and J. B. Hibbs, Jr., *Proc. Natl. Acad. Sci. U.S.A.* **87,** 1223–1227 (1990).
59. C. Pellat, Y. Henry, and J.-C. Drapier, *Biochem. Biophys. Res. Commun.* **166,** 119–125 (1990).
60. C. Nathan and J. B. Hibbs, Jr., *Curr. Opin. Immunol.* **3,** 65–70 (1991).
61. J. B. Hibbs, Jr., R. R. Taintor, Z. Vavrin, D. L. Granger, J.-C. Drapier, I. J. Amber, and J. R. Lancaster, Jr., *in* "Nitric Oxide from L-arginine: A Bioregulatory System" (S. Moncada and E. A. Higgs, eds.) pp. 189–223. Elsevier, Amsterdam, 1990.
62. D. L. Granger, R. R. Taintor, J. L. Cook, and J. B. Hibbs, Jr., *J. Clin. Invest.* **65,** 357–370 (1980).
63. N. S. Kwon, D. J. Stuehr, and C. F. Nathan, *J. Exp. Med.* **174,** 761–768 (1991).
64. J. B. Hibbs, Jr., R. R. Taintor, and Z. Vavrin, *Biochem. Biophys. Res. Commun.* **123,** 716–723 (1984).
65. D. W. Reif, and R. D. Simmons, *Arch. Biochem. Biophys.* **283,** 537–541 (1990).
66. M. Lepoivre, B. Chenais, A. Yapo, G. Lemaire, L. Thelander, and J.-P. Tenu, *J. Biol. Chem.* **265,** 14143 (1990).
67. D. L. Granger and A. L. Lenhinger, *J. Cell Biol.* **95,** 527–535 (1982).
68. R. Keller, M. Geiges, and R. Keist, *Cancer Res.* **50,** 1421–1425 (1991).
69. M. Higuchi, N. Higashi, H. Taki, T. Osawa, *J. Immunol.* **144,** 1425–1431 (1990).
70. C. Nathan, *Fed. Proc.* **41,** 2206–2211 (1982).
71. R. J. Grglewski, R. M. J. Palmer, and S. Moncada, *Nature (London)* **320,** 454–456 (1986).
72. J. S. Beckman, T. W. Beckman, J. Chen, P. A. Marshall, and B. A. Freeman, *Proc. Natl. Acad. Sci. U.S.A.* **87,** 1620–1624 (1990).
72a. J. Chan, Y. Xing, R. S. Magliozzo, and B. R. Bloom, *J. Exp. Med.* **175,** 1111–1122 (1992).
73. R. A. Hoffman, J. M. Langrehr, T. R. Billiar, R. D. Curran, and R. L. Simmons, *J. Immunol.* **145,** 2220–2226 (1990).
74. C. D. Mills, *J. Immunol.* **146,** 2719–2723 (1991).
75. J. E. Albina, J. A. Abate, and W. L. Henry, Jr., *J. Immunol.* **147,** 144–148 (1991).
76. D. L. Granger, J. B. Hibbs, Jr., J. R. Perfect, and D. T. Durack, *J. Clin. Invest.* **81,** 1129–1136 (1988).
77. S. L. James and J. Glaven, *J. Immunol.* **143,** 4208–4212 (1989).
78. S. J. Green, M. S. Meltzer, J. B. Hibbs, Jr. and C. A. Nacy, *J. Immunol.* **144,** 278–283 (1990).
79. L. B. Adams, J. B. Hibbs, Jr., R. R. Taintor, and J. L. Krahenbuhl, *J. Immunol.* **144,** 2725–2729 (1990).
80. P. Vincendeau and S. Daulouede, *J. Immunol.* **146,** 4338–4343 (1991).
81. L. B. Adams, S. G. Franzblau, V. Vavrin, J. B. Hibbs, Jr. and J. L. Krahenbuhl, *J. Immunol.* **147,** 1642–1646 (1991).
82. I. E. A. Flesch and S. H. E. Kaufmann, *Infect. Immun.* **59,** 3213–3218 (1991).
83. M. Denis, *J. Leukocyte Biol.* **49,** 380–387 (1991).
84. S. S. Kaplan, T. Billiar, R. D. Curran, U. E. Zdziarski, R. L. Simmons, and R. E. Basford, *Blood* **74,** 1885–1887 (1989).
85. P. Kubes, M. Suzuki, and D. N. Granger, *Proc. Natl. Acad. Sci. U.S.A.* **88,** 4651–4655 (1991).

86. M. S. Mulligan, J. M. Hevel, M. A. Marletta, and P. A. Ward, *Proc. Natl. Acad. Sci. U.S.A.* **88,** 6338–6342 (1991).
87. C. F. Nathan, *Trans. R. Soc. Trop. Med. Hyg.* **77,** 620–630 (1983).
88. J. Klostergard, M. E. Leroux, and M.-C. Hung, *J. Immunol.* **147,** 2802–2808 (1991).
89. M. L. Cameron, D. L. Granger, B. L. Weinberg, W. J. Kozumbo, and H. J. Koren *Am. Rev. Respir. Dis.* **142,** 1313–1319 (1990).

Index

ISBN 0-12-150404-2

90051

9 780121 504045